TEXTBOOK OF PROSTATE CANCER

Pathology, Diagnosis and Treatment

TEXTBOOK OF PROSTATE CANCER
Pathology, Diagnosis and Treatment

Edited by

AMIR V KAISARY, MA, ChM, FRCS
Consultant Urological Surgeon
Royal Free Hospital
London, UK

GERALD P MURPHY, MD, DSc
Director of Research
Pacific Northwest Cancer Foundation
Northwest Hospital
Seattle, Washington, USA

LOUIS DENIS, MD, FACS
Director
Oncology Centre Antwerp
Antwerp, Belgium

KEITH GRIFFITHS, PhD, DSc
Professor of Cancer Research
Tenovus Cancer Research Centre
Heath Park
Cardiff, UK

MARTIN DUNITZ

© Martin Dunitz Ltd 1999

First published in the United Kingdom in 1999 by
Martin Dunitz Ltd
The Livery House
7–9 Pratt Street
London NW1 0AE

A CIP catalogue record for this book is available from the British Library

ISBN 1–85317–422–X

Distributed in the United States by:
Blackwell Science Inc.
Commerce Place, 350 Main Street
Malden, MA 02148, USA
Tel: 1–800–215–1000

Distributed in Canada by:
Login Brothers Book Company
324 Salteaux Crescent
Winnipeg, Manitoba, R3J 3T2
Canada
Tel: 204–224–4068

Distributed in Brazil by:
Ernesto Reichmann Distribuidora de Livros, Ltda
Rua Coronel Marques 335, Tatuape 03440–000
São Paulo
Brazil

Composition by Wearset, Boldon, Tyne and Wear
Printed and bound in Great Britain by
Cambridge University Press

Contents

Foreword

There has been a revolution in the management of prostate cancer in the past decade. Ten years ago, most patients presented with disease that was too far advanced for local cure, and the benefit from radical treatment was far from certain. There was even doubt as to whether it was worth bothering with treatment in advanced disease: watch and wait was the byword, and many men died having had no effective therapy at all. Now all this has changed, thanks to an extraordinary burst of scientific and clinical research activity, much of it carried out in the face of widespread apathy or at worst active opposition from some of our most senior urological colleagues. But the pace of progress has been unstoppable, and now we are beginning to see the end product transmitted into real benefit for our patients.

The advent of PSA testing has truly changed the 'playing field' on which we look after this disease – a real paradigm shift. More and more men are appearing for treatment with disease that is imperceptible on examination, but with its pathological grade and its anatomical extent clearly defined. Of course this gives us the benefit of lead-time bias, but this is exactly what was needed, bearing in mind that over half of all men that we used to see presented with widely disseminated disease.

How do we know whether the disease is active, representing a threat to life, or an incidental discovery in an otherwise-healthy man who may be approaching the evening of his life? Assessment of malignant potential remains the biggest single challenge, but, with careful biological and histological studies, it seems likely that an accurate prediction of future behaviour will soon be possible. Modern imaging and accurately taken biopsies provide the necessary material upon which such assessments can be made.

Perhaps the most exciting prospect is the possibility of eliminating the disease. Careful genetic studies now enable us to define at-risk racial and family groups, in whom alterations in diet and lifestyle may delay or even prevent the emergence of overt disease. The androgen environment in the prostate can be altered by oral therapy, in effect changing the internal hormone milieu from a high-risk to a low-risk genetic category. Definition of racial or family groups with an increased likelihood of developing cancer, coupled with intensive screening in these individuals, may permit selective preventive measures to be introduced effectively.

Once early prostate cancer has been diagnosed, and the grade and stage accurately established, the most burning question remains 'How should the disease be eliminated?' There is a real dichotomy between those urologists who favour surgical removal of the prostate and its diseased portions, and our colleagues in radiotherapy and oncology who have developed increasingly sophisticated methods of delivering ionizing radiation. This is healthy rivalry that can only be resolved by carefully designed prospective clinical trials. The role of adjuvant treatment remains to be defined: preliminary hormone therapy reduces the incidence of positive resection margins, and appears to enhance the effects of radiotherapy, but will this be reflected in improved patient survival?

The effectiveness and the rapidity of onset of benefit of hormone therapy for advanced disease have long impressed urologists: How could a man riddled with metastases possibly derive benefit so fast? Improved understanding of the cell biology of prostate cancer has provided unparalleled insight into the dramatic effects of apoptosis. But what represents optimum treatment, which is the most cost-effective, and should therapy necessarily be given continuously or is there a place for intermittent treatment?

In this book, Amir Kaisary and his co-authors, representing a distinguished panel of internationally recognized experts, have assembled a team of contributors who have wide experience, and share between them a broad scientific background in the investigation and treatment of this disease. The field of prostate cancer has never been more alive, more bursting with questions waiting to be answered, with more problems asking to be addressed. All urologists interested in this field will eagerly seek out this book.

William F Hendry, MD, ChM, FRCS
Consultant Urologist
St Bartholomew's and Royal Marsden Hospitals
London, UK

Contributors

Jan Adolfsson, MD
Department of Urology
Huddinge Hospital
S-141 86 Huddinge
Sweden

Ronald Benoit, MD
Division of Urology
Allegheny University of the Health Sciences
Allegheny General Hospital
320 East North Avenue
Pittsburgh, PA 15222
USA

Laurent Boccon-Gibod, MD
Clinique Urologigue
L'Hôpital Bichat
46 Rue Henri Huchard
Paris 75788, Cedex 18
France

David G Bostwick, MD
Departments of Pathology and Urology
Mayo Clinic
200 First Street SW
Rochester, MN 55905
USA

Michael K Brawer, MD
Director, Northwest Prostate Institute
Northwest Hospital
Pacific Northwest Cancer Foundation
1560 North 115th Street
Seattle, WA 98133
USA

John Buscombe, FRCP
Department of Nuclear Medicine
Royal Free Hospital
Pond Street
London NW3 2QG
UK

Jeffrey K Cohen, MD
Division of Urology
Allegheny University of the Health Sciences
Allegheny General Hospital
320 East North Avenue
Pittsburgh, PA 15222
USA

Malcolm J Coptcoat, ChM, FRCS(Urol)
Honorary Consultant Urologist
King's College Hospital
Denmark Hill
London SE5 9RS
UK

E David Crawford, MD
University of Colorado
Health Sciences Center
4200 East Ninth Avenue
Denver, CO 80262
USA

Abhijit Darshane, MBBS, MS Gen Surgery, DNB (Urol)
Department of Urology
Burnley General Hospital
Burnley, Lancs BD10 2PQ
UK

Frans M J Debruyne, MD, PhD
Professor and Chaiman
University Hospital Nijmegen
Department of Urology
Geert Grooteplein 10
6500 HB Nijmegen
The Netherlands

Louis Denis, MD, FACS
Director
Oncology Centre Antwerp
Lange Gasthuisstraat 35-37
2000 Antwerp
Belgium

Peter Ekman, MD
Department of Urology
Karolinska Hospital
S-171 76 Stockholm
Sweden

Barry J A Furr, PhD, CBiol, FIBiol
Senior Vice President
Therapeutic Research Department
Zeneca Pharmaceuticals
Mereside
Alderley Park
Macclesfield, Cheshire SK10 4TG
UK

Keith Griffiths, PhD, DSc
Tenovus Cancer Research Centre
Tenovus Building
Heath Park
Cardiff CF4 4XX
UK

Henrik Grönberg, MD
Department of Oncology
Umeå University Hospital
S-901 85 Umeå
Sweden

Taz J Harmont, MD
Division of Urology
Department of Surgery
Washington University School of Medicine
4960 Children's Place
St Louis, MO 63110
USA

Kimberly B Hart, MD
Radiation Oncology Department
Wayne State University
School of Medicine
The Detroit Medical Center
3990 John R Detroit
Detroit, MI 48201
USA

Warren D W Heston, MD
George M O'Brien Urology Research
Center for Prostate Cancer
Memorial Sloan-Kettering Cancer Center
1275 York Avenue
New York, NY 10021
USA

Andrew J W Hilson, FRCP
Consultant in Nuclear Medicine
Royal Free Hospital
Pond Street
London NW3 2QG
UK

Alessandra Ianari, MD
San Raffaele Scientific Institute
Via Elio Chianesi 53
00144 Rome
Italy

Michael R Jarmulowicz, MBBS, MRCPath
Department of Histopathology
Royal Free Hospital
Pond Street
London NW3 2QG
UK

Amir V Kaisary, MA, ChM, FRCS
Consultant Urological Surgeon
Department of Urology
Royal Free Hospital
Pond Street
London NW3 2QG
UK

Saad Khoury, MD
7 Boulevard Flandrin
75116 Paris
France

Munekado Kojima, MD
Department of Urology
Kyoto Prefectural University of Medicine
Kawaramachi-Hirokoji
Kyoto 602-0841
Japan

Anna Kurowska, FRCP
Consultant in Palliative Medicine
Royal Free Hospital
Pond Street
London NW3 2QG
UK

Lori Merlotti
Division of Urology
Allegheny University of the Health Sciences
Allegheny General Hospital
320 East North Avenue
Pittsburgh, PA 15222
USA

Ralph Miller, MD
Division of Urology
Allegheny University of the Health Sciences
Allegheny General Hospital
320 East North Avenue
Pittsburgh, PA 15222
USA

Michael S Morton, PhD
Tenovus Cancer Research Centre
Tenovus Building
Heath Park
Cardiff CF4 4XX
UK

Gerald P Murphy, MD, DSc
Director of Research
Pacific Northwest Cancer Foundation
Northwest Hospital
120 Northgate Plaza
Seattle, WA 98125
USA

Don W W Newling, MBBChir, FRCS
Department of Urology
Academisch Ziekenhuis
Vrije Universiteit
De Boelelaan 1117
1081 HV Amsterdam
The Netherlands

Joseph E Oesterling, MD
Ann Arbor, MI 48105
USA

Arthur T Porter, MA, MD, FRCPC
Professor and Chairman
Radiation Oncology Department
Wayne State University
School of Medicine
The Detroit Medical Center
3990 John R Detroit
Detroit, MI 48201
USA

Timothy L Ratliff, PhD
Department of Urology
University of Iowa
Hospitals and Clinics
200 Hawkins Drive, 3234 RCP
Iowa City, IA 52242-1089
USA

Janak B Saada, MBBS, MRCP, FRCR
Department of Radiology
Norfolk & Norwich Hospital
Brunswick Road
Norwich
Norfolk NR1 3SR
UK

Sarbjinder S Sandhu, MBBS, FRCS(Eng)
Department of Urology
Royal Free Hospital
Pond Street
London NW3 2QG
UK

Justin Siegal, BS
School of Medicine
St Louis University
St Louis, MO 63110
USA

Baudouin Standaert, MD
Oncology Centre Antwerp
Lange Gasthuisstraat 35-37
2000 Antwerp
Belgium

Juan Stenner, MD
Coscomate 9
Col Toriello Guerra
Tlalpan
Mexico DF 14050
Mexico

Cora N Sternberg, MD
San Raffaele Scientific Institute
Via Elio Chianesi 53
00144 Rome
Italy

Adrian Tookman, MBBS, MRCP
Consultant in Palliative Medicine
Royal Free Hospital
Pond Street
London NW3 2QG
UK

Apoorva R Vashi, MD
Section of Urology
University of Michigan
1500 East Medical Center Drive
Ann Arbor, MI 48109-0330
USA

Hiroki Watanabe, MD
Third Department of Basic Medicine
Meiji University of Oriental Medicine
Hiyoshi-cho, Funai-gun
Kyoto 629-0392
Japan

Anthony F Watkinson, MBBS, FRCS, FRCR
Consultant Radiologist
Royal Free Hospital
Pond Street
London NW3 2QG
UK

Wim P J Witjes, MD, PhD
University Hospital Nijmegen
Department of Urology
Geert Grooteplein 10
6500 HB Nijmegen
The Netherlands

1

The natural history of prostate cancer

Peter Ekman, Jan Adolfsson, Henrik Grönberg

'The natural course of prostate cancer is highly variable and unpredictable' is a commonly used phrase when discussing various aspects of human prostate cancer. Generally regarded as a slow growing tumour, prostate cancer is one of the most common causes of cancer death in males in the Western World. As a consequence of an increasing number of elderly men in society, combined with a prolonged mean survival of men, partly due to a reduced incidence of cardiac and cerebrovascular deaths, the number of prostate cancer deaths is steadily increasing. The age-adjusted mortality remains relatively constant, however, so the major reason is that the total number of men at risk of dying from prostate cancer is increasing.[1]

Latent prostate cancer is extremely common. It has been estimated that approximately 50% of males aged 80 years have foci of prostatic carcinoma, of which only a fraction used to surface to clinical cancer.[2] However, following massive public information, prostate awareness campaigns, various screening protocols, etc., the number of newly detected prostate cancers has increased dramatically. In the USA, for instance, from 85 000 new cases detected in 1985, the number has increased to 317 000 new cases in 1996.[3,4] When comparing the mortality to incidence ratios for these years, 35 000/85 000 (41%) in 1985 versus 41 000/317 000 (13%) in 1996, a false impression of a successful improvement may be imagined.

Intense screening with prostate-specific antigen (PSA) will induce a lead-time bias, as numerous cancers will be detected, on average, perhaps 5 years earlier than previously.[5–7] Moreover, an increasing number of harmless cancers will be diagnosed. On the other hand, in areas having applied mass screening for several years, repeated screening reveals a substantially lower number of cases. Therefore, in areas like Washington State and Utah, with the most aggressive PSA-screening programmes, the incidence of prostate cancer has dropped almost to the numbers recorded before mass screening started.[8] This is probably explained by prevalent cases being detected at an early stage of the screening programme. Because screening detects an increasing number of patients with localized tumours, the absolute number of patients with metastatic disease at diagnosis has dropped substantially in areas with intense screening. Recently, the National Institutes of Health (NIH) presented mortality data from the Surveillance, Epidemology, and End Results Program (SEER) areas and, interestingly, a 12% decrease in age-adjusted mortality was recorded between 1990 and 1995 for white men under 70 years of age at diagnosis.[9] The interpretation of these data, which are preliminary and have not yet been scrutinized thoroughly, is difficult, as this drop in mortality comes too early to be caused by PSA screening. Hence, one explanation could be the expansion of aggressive local treatment during the 1980s. However, the same reduction in mortality was recorded in areas with a more conservative attitude to the treatment of localized prostate cancer, indicating that other explanations, such as changes in life-style during the 1970s, may be a more plausible explanation.

Prediction of the natural history of the cancer in an individual case would be of utmost importance in selecting patients who are most likely to benefit from major interventions. However, there are few reports in the literature on the true natural history of prostate cancer, without *any* antitumoural therapy. Moreover, various series are difficult to compare, partly due to highly variable selection criteria: 'Case selection is often the silent partner in the successful treatment of cancer.'[10] In previous years, the outcome for patients with prostate cancer was invariably poor.[11–13] As mentioned above, the recent development and introduction of new diagnostic tools, such as PSA, transrectal ultrasound (TRUS), public information, professional awareness, screening programmes, etc., have identified yet another large proportion of prostate cancers that would previously have been undetected. Therefore, the prostate cancer patients we see today have little in common with the patients of previous decades. Thus, as the data on the natural history of prostate cancer from the 1950s and 1960s can be compared only to a certain extent with that from the 1970s and 1980s, data from earlier decades must be judged cautiously if it is to be used to guide decision-making in the 1990s.

Most prostate cancers diagnosed today appear to be localized. Some controversial questions are yet to be answered; for example, what is the best treatment for men with localized prostate cancer, and can we reduce the mortality from prostate cancer by mass screening in combination with aggressive local treatment? The only way to answer these questions is by undertaking well-designed randomized trials comparing aggressive local treatment with deferred treatment in men with localized prostate cancer. Unfortunately, no results from such studies are available today. Two large studies are currently recruiting patients: the SPCG IV study (Scandinavian Prostate Cancer Group) in Sweden and Finland (more than 600 patients enrolled at 1996), and the PIVOT study (Prostate Intense Versus Observation Therapy) in the USA. Until the results become available, we have to rely upon data from earlier studies. In view of the statements above, however, it is likely that the results from, for example, the SPCG IV trial will be applicable only to a subgroup of future patients.

Before the era of endocrine therapy, the fate of patients with prostate cancer took what may be called 'the natural course'.[11–13] Even though some recent reports indicate a marginally better survival following early endocrine therapy, and in particular a reduced risk of serious complications,[14] until further proven, endocrine therapy should be regarded as purely palliative with little impact on patient survival. The main reason for the poor outcome in the early series was a selection of patients presenting late with locally advanced or metastatic disease.

In Scandinavia, an interesting comparison can be made between Sweden and Norway, where the incidence is high, and Denmark, where the incidence is comparatively low. This is due to little effort being made to detect asymptomatic prostate cancer in Denmark. The age-adjusted incidence, 5-year survival and age-adjusted mortality in these countries during the years 1983–1987 are listed in Table 1.1.[15,16] The similarities in overall mortality, despite the different incidence ratios, are noteworthy. Similar data have recently been reported from an analysis of the SEER data from various states in the USA.[17]

In many recent series, deferred treatment, or conservative treatment, 'surveillance only' or watchful waiting, has been employed for

Table 1.1 Age-adjusted incidence and mortality per 100 000 men and 5-year actual survival of prostate cancer patients in three different Scandinavian countries 1983–1987[15,16]

Country	Incidence	5-year relative survival rate (%)	Mortality rate* (%)
Sweden	81.6	61	18.2
Norway	71.8	52	19.3
Denmark	48.9	38	17.4

* Age-adjusted to the European standard population.

patients with clinically low-stage prostate cancer. 'Surveillance only', however, does not mean 'no therapy', but initial observation with antitumoural therapy given when, and if, the disease progresses symptomatically. Deferred treatment has customarily been androgen deprivation using various techniques, but sometimes more aggressive local therapy has been added. This treatment policy has been accepted, especially in the Scandinavian countries, and the rationale is that the disease usually has a protracted course with a high competing mortality due to a generally high age at presentation, and the quality of life of the patients being superior with a preserved hormonal milieu.[18]

INCIDENTAL, NON-PALPABLE, PROSTATE CANCER (T1)

Today the non-palpable prostate cancers are categorized as T1a and T1b, which are found after surgery for apparently benign prostatic hyperplasia, and T1c, a result of a positive prostatic biopsy, usually carried out due to an accidental finding of an elevated PSA value.[19] Long-term data are available for the first two categories only. In general, the prognosis for patients with these tumours is good, even when a conservative policy is applied. However, if

the patients are followed for long enough, a low but significant number of tumours will progress. Progression is clearly related to the tumour grade and volume of the disease.

T1a prostate cancer indicates tumours with low-volume or 'focal disease' (less than 5% cancer in the specimens) and T1b as high-volume or 'diffuse disease' (more than 5% tumour in the specimen). The categorization is based on the presumed volume of the tumour as judged from specimens obtained at transurethral resection of the prostate (TURP) or open adenoma enucleation for benign prostatic hyperplasia (BPH). The exact definition of the classes varies with different staging systems, and the uncertainty in the categorization is high since the sampling error in non-radical prostatectomies is impossible to assess.[20]

Series with long-term follow-up of patients with incidentally detected prostate cancer has reported an overall survival rate at 10 years ranging from 30% to 85%, a progression-free survival rate at 10 years ranging from 33% to 82% and, in one series, a disease-specific survival rate at 10 years of 93% (low-volume) and 77% (high-volume)[21–27] (Table 1.2, section I).

The outcomes in the three largest reported series on incidental prostate cancer[25,28,29] were largely comparable. Lowe and Listrom[25] reported on 232 patients, including both low- and high-volume disease, who were followed

Table 1.2 Overall survival, progression-free survival and disease-specific survival reported in the literature for deferred treatment of clinically localized prostate cancer

Reference	*n*	Stage (as reported)	Overall survival rate (%)			Progression-free survival rate (%)			Disease-specific survival rate (%)		
			5 years	10 years	15 years	5 years	10 years	15 years	5 years	10 years	15 years
I Incidental, non-palpable											
Heaney et al[21]	33	Incidental	80	54	50	–	–	–	–	–	–
Blute et al[22]	23	A	100	85	–	–	–	–	–	–	–
Moskovitz et al[23]	40	T0b	91	65	–	–	–	–	–	–	–
Goodman et al[24]	69	A	50	30	–	–	–	–	–	–	–
Lowe and Listrom[25]	236	A	–	–	–	84	68	48	–	–	–
Waaler et al[26]	13	T0f	–	–	–	100	–	–	100	–	–
	53	T0d	–	–	–	80	–	–	93	–	–
Johansson et al[27]	72	T01	72	39	–	89	82	–	95	93	–
	34	T0d	71	47	–	61	33	–	93	77	–
II Clinically confined, palpable											
Moskovitz et al[23]	44	T1–T2	61	34	–	–	–	–	–	–	–
George[34]	105	'Clinically localized'	–	–	–	–	–	–	80*	–	–
Graverson et al[35]	50	VACURG I–II	70	55	32	–	–	–	–	–	–
Warner and Whitmore[36]	68	B1–B3	–	–	43	–	–	54	–	–	–
Johansson et al[37]	223	T0d–T2	–	38	20	–	59	48	–	85	81
Johansson et al[27]	58	T0d–T2	78	58	–	60	50	–	94†	87†	–
Adolfsson et al[38]	122	T1–T2	–	51	–	–	–	–	99	84	–
Adolfsson and Carstensen[39]	61	T1–T2	–	85	–	–	–	–	98†	92†	–
Egawa et al[40]	52	A1–B	–	–	–	–	–	–	–	75	–
Stenzl and Studer[41]	34	T0–T2	67	34	–	–	–	–	89	87	–
Waaler and Stenwig[42]	28	T1–T3	–	–	–	–	–	–	70	–	–
Lundgren et al[43]	88	T0–T3	81	49	–	85‡	66‡	–	91	74	–
III Clinically unconfined											
Adolfsson[44]	50	T3	–	37§	–	–	–	–	–	70	–

* 90% in figure 4 in George.[34]
† Patients <70 years of age.
‡ Metastasis-free survival.
§ 9 years.

cancer. Cantrell et al[28] reported on 117 patients, also combining low- and high-volume disease, who were followed for 2–15 years. Fourteen patients (12%) progressed and five (4%) died from prostate cancer. Epstein et al[30] expanded the group of patients with low-volume disease in the aforementioned study[28] and reported on a total of 94 patients. Progression occurred in eight (9%) patients and six (6%) died from prostate cancer. However, in the 50 patients who survived more than 8 years and had not progressed before, the rates of progression and prostate cancer mortality were 16% and 12%, respectively (mean follow-up 10 years). Finally, Zhang et al[29] reported on 132 patients with low-volume disease with a mean follow-up of 8 years. Thirteen patients (10%) progressed, but none died from prostate cancer. A second TURP was performed in 52 patients. Of the 38 patients without tumour in the repeat TURP, 8% progressed, while of the 12 patients with tumour left in the repeat TURP specimens, 25% progressed. As expected, T1b patients with high-volume disease generally had a worse prognosis than those with low-volume disease. As mentioned above, the fate of patients with T1c tumours, which are usually detected due to an accidental finding of an elevated PSA, remains unknown. T1c cancers are often more advanced than expected from the digital rectal examination (DRE). In one series, capsular penetration was found in 35% of cases and seminal vesicle invasion in 10%, leaving just a little over half of cases where it was organ confined.[31] It is reasonable to believe that T1c cancers represent a more aggressive tumour type than T1a and T1b, and possibly even than T2a; however, long-term data are still awaited.

In summary, for patients with incidental prostate cancer the risk of progression and death from prostate cancer seems to be related to high grade[21,24–26,28,32] and high volume.[21,24,25,28,32,33] Nuclear roundness was found to be prognostic in one study,[32] and content of DNA (ploidy) in another.[33]

PALPABLE, CLINICALLY LOCALIZED PROSTATE CANCER (T2 AND T3)

There is a growing evidence to indicate that a conservative treatment strategy in patients with clinically localized, palpable prostate cancer results in a significant rate of local progression, a moderate rate of distant spread and a low rate of fatal disease during the first 10–15 years of follow-up after diagnosis. This experience is based on several series from various parts of the world[23,27,34–44] (Table 1.2, section II). The 10-year overall survival rate for patients with T2 tumours has been reported to range from 34% to 55%, and 10-year disease-specific survival rate ranges from 75% to 85% for patients with tumours clinically confined to the gland. One study reports a progression-free survival rate of 43% at the 10-year follow-up. The difference between overall and disease-specific survival rates indicates that many of the patients who die within up to 10 years of observation do so due to diseases other than prostate cancer. In two series, patients less than 70 years of age at diagnosis were analysed separately, and the disease-specific survival rate at 10 years was 88% and 92%, respectively.[27,39] Data on survival beyond 10 years after diagnosis are scarce. Recently, the 15-year follow-up of the Örebro series was published and the disease-specific survival rate at 15 years was continuously high: 81% for patients with T1–T2 tumours who were managed conservatively.[37] Also, during follow-up of up to 20 years, prostate cancer mortality did not increase substantially in the New York series.[36] In contrast, in the Stockholm series prostate cancer-related mortality continued to increase and disease-specific survival decreased, also beyond 10 years of follow-up (Figure 1.1) (J Adolfsson et al, unpublished data).

In one series, patients with prostate cancer clinically localized but palpably not organ confined (T3) were managed conservatively.[44] The overall survival rate at 9 years was 37% and disease-specific survival rate was 70%. As expected, in this series of more advanced cancers, a larger proportion of patients died from prostate cancer compared with the aforementioned series of

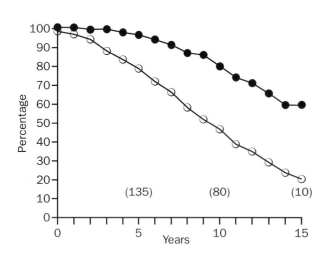

Figure 1.1 Disease-specific (●) and overall (○) survival rates of 172 patients with low-grade, T2–T3 prostate cancers, managed conservatively. Numbers in parentheses are numbers of patients at risk.

patients in whom tumours were clinically confined to the prostate gland.

During the 1990s, three separate reviews compiling data from the literature reporting on survival outcomes after various forms of treatment for clinically localized prostate cancer were published.[45–47] In two of the studies the compiled disease-specific survival rate at 10 years for patients with clinically confined tumours managed conservatively was 84% and 86%, respectively.[45,47] Two of the studies used different methods to calculate the incidence of distant progression and prostate cancer mortality in the available series on deferred therapy, but found similar values.[45,46]

Moreover, an international pooled analysis of original data from six different series employing deferred treatments in patients with clinically localized prostate cancer has been published.[48] Data from 828 patients were reanalysed. For patients with well or moderately differentiated tumours the disease-specific survival rate at 10 years was 87%; however, for patients with poorly differentiated tumours it was only 34%. In the same analysis the metastasis-free survival rate at 10 years was 81% for patients with well-differentiated tumours, 58% for patients with moderately differentiated

tumours and 26% for patients with poorly differentiated tumours. The series on deferred treatment have been subject to criticism because of a relatively high number of patients with well-differentiated tumours in the series, for including elderly patients with good prognosis and a high competing mortality, thereby reducing the risk of dying from prostate cancer, and for a relatively short-follow-up. At the time of patient enrolment (late 1970s to early 1980s), only approximately 25% of all newly diagnosed prostate cancers were well differentiated. However, of the organ-confined tumours, approximately 50% were well differentiated. As a consequence of today's increasing interest in early detection, an increasing number of newly detected prostate cancers will be well or moderately differentiated.

The general question of selection biases in series on deferred therapy for any management is difficult to address, since few authors give information on this aspect. One extreme is the Memorial Sloan–Kettering series,[36] which comprises 75 patients who were selected from presumably many hundreds or even thousands of patients over a long time period. The other extreme is the series studied by Johansson et al,[37] who used prospectively defined criteria when including patients from a defined population base over a limited period of time.

When comparing series on radical prostatectomy with series using external beam radiotherapy or deferred therapy, the latter groups seem to contain fewer patients with poorly differentiated tumours.[45] The tumours in the series on deferred treatment and radiotherapy are all based on results from biopsies (core or fine needle), whereas grading in radical prostatectomy series is performed on whole surgical specimens. It is well known that a substantial number of these will be upgraded as well as upstaged in comparison with the preoperative data,[49,50] thus, making comparisons virtually impossible, unless one compares data exclusively on the basis of the preoperative grading and staging. Furthermore, in most of these series radical surgery was discontinued when unexpected lymph node involvement was found (10–35%),[51,52] while lymph node involvement was unknown in deferred therapy series (Nx).

Some of the outcome data published for deferred treatment in patients with clinically localized prostate cancer are now available for up to 15 years of observation. The relatively low metastasis-free survival at 10 years for patients with moderately differentiated tumours, found in the aforementioned pooled analysis,[48] may indicate an increase in tumour-related mortality in this category beyond 10 years of observation. Even though the cancer-specific survival rate continues to drop, at 15 years the figure is still 60–80%[37] (J Adolfsson et al, unpublished data).

A recently published study from Gothenburg, Sweden has received great attention because the prostate cancer mortality rate was reported to be very high, about 50% in M0 disease patients offered deferred therapy.[53] An increasing risk of prostate-cancer-related deaths was also found with longer follow-up, for example, in men surviving beyond 15 years after diagnosis. These were said to have a 71% risk of dying from prostate cancer. If these data are correct, serious doubts must be raised questioning the ethics of advising deferred therapy for low-grade, low-stage prostate cancer

patients with a life expectancy of more than 10 years. These results indicate that the prostate cancer patient will eventually die from his disease, if he lives long enough. The results reported by Aus et al,[53] indicating a marked increase in cancer-specific mortality after 10 years of follow-up, are not compatible with some other studies on comparable populations, in which patients were offered deferred therapy.[36,37] Moreover, in a recent registry-based study from northern Sweden, 6514 prostate cancer patients, representing all grades and stages (including metastatic cases), diagnosed between 1971 and 1987, were reviewed.[49] A 55% overall prostate cancer mortality rate was recorded after a mean follow-up of 15 years (Figure 1.2).

A critical comparison of the studies by Aus et al,[53] Johansson et al[37] and that in northern Sweden is given in Table 1.3. Despite the fact that all these studies were based on presumably unselected population bases, with the intent to study the natural history of prostate cancer in patients diagnosed in the 1970s and 1980s, all offered non-curative treatment, there was a remarkable difference in cause-specific survival at 15 years of follow-up and in total prostate cancer mortality. However, at 15 years, only 28 patients were still at risk in the Gothenburg series, and hence the selection of patients is critical. The Gothenburg study used a retrospective selection, which has been criticized extensively by biostatisticians and others.[55] The selection of patients merely reflects the increase in relative survival over time, a phenomenon already known. The data do *not* prove an increase in prostate cancer mortality in patients surviving for more than 10 years, as claimed by the authors.

ADVANCED PROSTATE CANCER

The natural course of patients with metastatic prostate cancer is less controversial. Data in the literature almost invariably indicate a mean survival of 3–3.5 years. Patients with minimal metastatic load fare better, with an expected survival of 4–6 years. The survival is little influenced by mode of therapy given. At present,

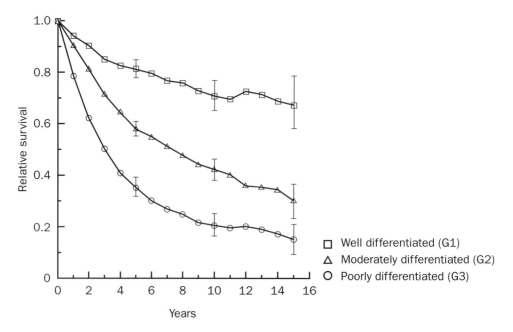

Figure 1.2 Relative survival rates in prostate cancer among all 6890 men diagnosed with the disease during the period 1971–1987 in northern Sweden up to 15 years after diagnosis, divided into tumour grades. (*Note:* all prostate cancer patients are included, not just those with localized cancer.)

the issue of whether early endocrine therapy may prolong anything but the time to progression is a matter of great controversy. As stated above, until otherwise proven, endocrine therapy should be regarded as purely palliative. Considering the side-effects of the therapy given, the quality of life of the patient should be in focus. For some years it was believed that in a specific subgroup of patients, namely those with minimal metastatic disease, survival could be significantly improved following total androgen blockade (luteinizing hormone-releasing hormone (LHRH) agonists plus a non-steroidal antiandrogen).[56,57] However, more

Table 1.3 A critical comparison of the percentage of prostate cancer deaths and 15-year cancer-specific survival rate in three different Swedish studies of the natural progression of prostate cancer

	Johansson et al[37]	Grönberg et al[54]	Aus et al[53]
No. of patients	643	6514	514
Percentage dead from prostate cancer	43	55	70*
Cancer-specific survival at 15 years	0.50	0.30	0.15
Cancer-specific survival at 15 years (M0)	0.81†	–	0.30‡

* Estimated from the data presented in the report.
† Including only localized tumours.
‡ Including only M0 tumours.

recent investigations have failed to confirm these data.[58] With regard to quality of life, intermittent androgen blockade is an attractive alternative, and has also (based on animal experiments) been claimed to delay the evolution of hormone-resistant cancer.[59] However, this regimen is still under investigation and evaluation. While in localized metastatic disease the tumour grade is an important prognostic parameter, in advanced disease with distant metastases the tumour grade seems to be less closely related to survival.

HORMONE-REFRACTORY CANCER

Patients escaping hormonal control invariably have an extremely poor prognosis. Mean survival is given as approximately 7–9 months, again regardless of the therapy given. The results reported in the literature are partly obscured by the introduction of PSA as a marker of tumour progression. PSA relapse usually precedes clinical relapse by up to 6 months, and this must be borne in mind when comparing results of various trials reported in the literature.

PROGNOSTIC MARKERS

Tumour grade and stage

In everyday practice, tumour grade and stage are probably the most important markers of final outcome for the patient (Figure 1.1). As stated above, patients with well-differentiated tumours with localized disease seem to have a survival very similar to that of a normal control population. In contrast, patients with poorly differentiated cancer invariably have a poor prognosis, with a 5-year cancer-specific survival rate of approximately 35%.[48]

In addition to the above, tumour stage is also of importance. Patients with tumours truly localized to the prostate gland seem to be doing pretty well in surveillance series. Patients with tumours penetrating the capsule have already acquired an aggressive tumour type and have a

less good prognosis. The 5-year disease-specific survival rate for patients with clinical T3 disease has been given as 85%, and 9-year survival rate as 70%.[44] For more detailed information the reader is referred to the discussion above.

DNA ploidy

The DNA content (ploidy) of prostate cancer cells has been proposed to be of prognostic value. There are, however, different techniques by which ploidy can be determined, and no consensus exists in the literature with regard to how the DNA content should be measured.[60] From the literature it is apparent that ploidy is well correlated both with tumour grade and with tumour stage, an increasing pattern of aneuploidy being closely linked to a lower grade and higher stage.[60] In a univariate analysis, ploidy was of prognostic importance for most categories of prostate cancer, but when combined with grade and stage in a multivariate setting the prognostic value of ploidy became less convincing.[60] Ploidy, in combination with grade and stage, is therefore probably not useful itself if one wants additional prognostic information for a general prostate cancer population, but may be useful in specific subgroups, for example in patients with an intermediate tumour stage.[60]

Serum markers

A number of serum markers have been introduced to estimate the biological activity of prostate cancer. In a multivariate analysis, Lewenhaupt et al[61] compared the efficacy of the markers neopterin, thymidine kinase, prostatic acid phosphatase (PAP), PSA, C-reactive protein and osteocalcin, and the non-specific markers CA-50 and tissue polypeptide antigen (TPA), and compared this with tumour grade and stage. Whereas all markers alone differed significantly between patients with a poor short-term prognosis and those with good prognosis, in a multivariate setting only neopterin, thymidine kinase, PSA and tumour grade were independent parameters useful for prognostic purposes. Thymidine kinase is a protein indicating the biological activity of the tumour, whereas neopterin reflects the immunological reaction of the patient. Somewhat surprisingly, the higher the neopterin value, the worse the prognosis. This is probably due to a reaction to tumour antigens: the higher the value, the more aggressive the tumour. Thymidine kinase reflects tumour proliferation and cell turnover: an elevated level signals a more aggressive tumour type.[62] In everyday practice, serum markers are of limited value in reflecting the prognosis in an individual case or in helping to design an appropriate therapeutic strategy.

The serum level of PSA has been studied extensively. However, this reflects the natural course poorly, except that low levels indicate a prognostically more favourable situation with a localized tumour, whereas a high value signals a generalized disease with short life expectancy. The best use of PSA monitoring in this setting is probably with regard to response to therapy. A PSA value dropping to undetectable levels indicates a very good response, be it following radical surgery, radiotherapy or endocrine therapy, with a long expected cancer-specific survival, whereas those not reaching this nadir are likely to relapse and have greatly shortened life expectancy.[63,64]

FACTORS INFLUENCING THE NATURAL COURSE OF PROSTATE CANCER

Age

If age is a prognostic factor, for instance if the disease is more malignant in younger men than in older men, the difference in mean age represents a confounding factor when comparing the outcomes of radical surgery and deferred treatment. To meet some of the criticisms about their use of non-representative patient material, with too many old men, Johansson et al[27] looked specifically at patients within their sample who were potential candidates for radical prostatectomy (T0–T2, G1–G2, <70 years old). The 5-year

disease-specific survival rate in this group was 95% and the 10-year survival rate was 88%, which is even better than the values for the whole series containing patients of all ages. The data in the literature almost invariably fail to demonstrate any difference in biological activity in younger prostate cancer patients and patients diagnosed at a later age.[48,65,66] However, this might not be true for hereditary prostate cancer. In a recent report on over 1000 patients with localized prostate cancer treated with radical prostatectomy, those who had a positive family history had a significantly lower relapse-free survival (29%) than did patients with no family history of this disease (52%). As familial cases have a younger age of onset, this might indicate that this phenotype produces a more aggressive disease.[65]

However, even if the relative survival is constant with age, the absolute impact of prostate cancer varies substantially, as indicated by a reduced life expectancy. On average, about 16 years are lost due to prostate cancer in patients aged 45–54 years at diagnosis, compared with only 2 years in men diagnosed between 75 and 84 years of age.[66] Needless to say, this is explained by the rapid increase in competing causes of death after the age of 65 years, and indicates that younger patients should be considered as candidates for a more aggressive treatment compared with older patients.

RISK FACTORS

Even though risk factors have, so far, mainly been discussed in relation to the risk of acquiring the disease, it is also most likely, albeit not proven, that life-style and environment may influence the natural course of prostate cancer. Hence, it is reasonable to mention a few risk factors.

Racial differences

In 1990, Carter et al[67] reported that prostate cancer was indeed as common in Japan as in the

USA. However, in Japan the prostate cancer usually remained latent and rarely progressed to clinical cancer. Apparently some hitherto unknown factor(s) might be protective against tumour progression, while other factors may promote it. Attempts have been made to explain the difference by referring to molecular genetic variations. It has been reported by Watanabe et al[68] and Konishi et al[69] that *p53* mutations are crucial for the evolution of clinical prostate cancer; this mutation is much more rare in Japanese men. Of interest also is the report by Takahashi et al[70] which demonstrates that androgen-receptor mutations were more common in latent prostate cancer than in clinically manifest cancer. The risk of acquiring clinical prostate cancer, and of promoting prostate cancer progression, is associated with the presence of short CAG repeats in the androgen receptor (AR). It has been shown that, as measured from serum samples, CAG repeats are short in Afro-Americans, intermediate in non-Hispanic whites, and longest in Chinese and Japanese men,[71] which is in close agreement with the incidence of clinical prostate cancer in these male populations.

The wide difference in the incidence of clinical prostate cancer between Westerners and Asians has been known for a long time and has usually been regarded as a genetic phenomenon. However, a more intriguing fact is that the incidence of clinical prostate cancer is increasing in Japanese men living in the USA, suggesting that environmental factors in general and dietary factors in particular play a determining role.[72] Differences in life-style between East Asian and the Western cultures have thus been much in focus.

Fat

Fat consumption is probably the most widely investigated parameter linked to the risk of developing clinical prostate cancer. Key,[73] reviewing the literature, found a mean relative risk (RR) of 1.25 in obese men in general. The RR associated with consumption of meat, milk and total fat became equal at 1.3. In particular,

it seems that consumers of animal fat carry the greatest risk, with an RR of 1.54, while consumption of vegetable fat does not seem to be linked to prostate cancer risk at all.[74,75] Grönberg et al[76] found a clear relationship between heavy eating in general and prostate cancer. As a consequence, the body mass index was found to be significantly related to prostate cancer. Red meat was also a significant risk factor. Experimental data support the importance of fat in prostate carcinogenesis. Dunning tumours in rats fed a fat-free diet grew significantly more slowly.[77,78]

Vitamin D

Ultraviolet (UV) radiation has also been linked to prostate cancer. Reported data have demonstrated an almost identical geographical variation in UV radiation and the incidence of prostate cancer, in an inverse relationship.[79,80] Presumably the explanation for this correlation is associated with a surplus of vitamin D induced by exposure to UV radiation.[81] Vitamin D_3 inhibits cell growth both in vitro and in vivo.[82,83] It has also been shown that vitamin D_3 causes rodent prostate cancer cells to differentiate to a less malignant phenotype, and that the expression of the *c-myc* oncogene is inhibited.[84,85]

Several studies involving the use of vitamin D for protection against tumour progression following radical prostatectomy are under way.

Molecular genetics

Patients subjected to radical prostatectomy whose tumours had retained a centromerically located potential tumour suppressor gene (TSG) locus on chromosome 8p, LPL, had only a 20% risk of tumour progression at 3 years as compared with 75% when LPL was lost.[86] The difference as measured from Kaplan–Meier curves was highly significant ($p < 0.01$). However, the same relationship was not seen at all for deletions on 16q. Deletions of parts of 16q are of great interest, because this chromosome carries the *E*-cadherin gene.[87] As described by Umbas et al,[88] loss of function of *E*-cadherin is likely to promote the spread of tumour metastases, since the *E*-cadherin protein is involved in cell–cell adhesion. Studies by Pan et al[89] demonstrated a loss of parts of 16q in 70% of the metastatic cancer patients, compared with 35% in patients with localized disease, and possibly these 35% were at risk of metastatic spread.

CONCLUSION

The natural course of prostate cancer is highly variable. No studies of the true natural course are reported in the literature. At present, not giving any therapy at all to a group of prostate cancer patients would be unethical. However, since hormone therapy seems to influence survival only marginally, the best information about the natural history can probably be extracted from series where deferred therapy is used in localized disease. In studies of this type prostate-cancer-specific mortality was low for low-grade tumours up to at least 10 years of observation.

Intense screening in many countries has markedly changed the panorama of newly diagnosed prostate cancers. This makes it very difficult to compare the natural history of prostate cancers today with those of previous decades. PSA screening has led to the identification of yet another group of prostate cancers, non-palpable T1c lesions, the fate of which we still know very little about.

In summary, at up to 15 years of observation patients with well-differentiated tumours seem to have a high disease-specific survival. Patients with poorly differentiated tumours or tumours clinically localized but not organ confined (T3) have a worse prognosis, indicating that deferred treatment may not be appropriate for this category of patients. The long-term follow-up of patients with moderately differentiated tumours has led to inconclusive results, as a fair number of these patients die after 10 years from diagnosis of prostate cancer. However, all the reported studies must be carefully scrutinized with respect to patient selection, definition of prostate cancer deaths, etc., before extrapolating the results of today's patients with prostate cancer. It can be stated, however, that advanced prostate cancer invariably has a poor prognosis, with severely reduced life expectancy.

Despite major research efforts involving the testing of numerous tissue and serum markers (including DNA ploidy), tumour grade and stage remain the most important indicators of the potential aggressiveness of the tumour in the individual case. Even though still not proven, it is likely that molecular genetic techniques will provide more reliable information about the potential course of an individual tumour. Epidemiological studies will reveal what life-style adjustments potential prostate cancer patients will need to make in order to delay the onset of the tumour for as long as possible and, once established, to reduce the rate of tumour growth as much as possible.

REFERENCES

1. Boyle P, Maisonneuve P, Napalkov P, Geographical and temporal patterns of incidence and mortality from prostate cancer. *Urology* 1995; **45**(suppl 3A): 47–55.
2. Sakr WA, Haas GP, Cassin BF, Pontes EJ, Crissman JD, The frequency of carcinoma and intraepithelial neoplasia of the prostate in young male patients. *J Urol* 1993; **150**: 379–85.
3. Parker SL, Tong T, Bolden S, Wingo PA, Cancer statistics, 1996. *CA* 1996; **46**: 5–27.
4. Mettlin CJ, Murphy GP, Ho R, Menck HR, The National Cancer Data Base report on longitudi-

nal observations on prostate cancer. *Cancer* 1996; **77**: 2162–6.

5. Pearson JD, Carter HB, Natural history of changes in prostate specific antigen in early stage prostate cancer. *J Urol* 1994; **152**: 1743–8.

6. Stenman UH, Hakama M, Knekt P, Teppo L, Leinonen J, Serum concentrations of prostate specific antigen and its complex with α-1-antichymotrypsin before diagnosis of prostate cancer. *Lancet* 1994; **344**: 1594–8.

7. Tibblin G, Welin L, Bergström R, Ronquist G, Norlen BJ, Adami HO, The value of prostate specific antigen in early diagnosis of prostate cancer. The study of men born in 1913. *J Urol* 1995; **154**: 1386–9.

8. Stephenson RA, Smart CR, Mineau GP, James BC, Janerich DT, Dibble RL, The fall in incidence of prostate carcinoma. On the downside of prostate specific antigen induced peak in incidence – data from the Utah Cancer Registry. *Cancer* 1996; **77**: 1342–8.

9. Shalala DE, Cancer death rate declined for the first time ever in the 1990s (press release). National Cancer Institute: Bethesda, MD, 14 November 1996.

10. Whitmore WF. Natural history of low-stage prostatic cancer and the impact of early detection. *Urol Clin N Am* 1990; **17**: 689–97.

11. Bumpus HC, Carcinoma of the prostate; a clinical study of 1000 cases. *Surg Gynecol Obstet* 1926; **43**: 150–5.

12. Nesbit RM, Plumb RT, Prostatic carcinoma: a follow-up on 795 patients treated prior to the endocrine era and a comparison of survival rates between these and patients treated by endocrine therapy. *Surgery* 1946; **20**: 263–73.

13. Hanash KA, Utz DC, Cook EN, Taylor WF, Titus JL, Carcinoma of the prostate: a 15-year follow-up. *J Urol* 1992; **107**: 450–3.

14. The Medical Research Council Prostate Cancer Working Party Investigators Group, Immediate versus deferred treatment for advanced prostatic cancer: initial results of the Medical Research Council trial. *Br J Urol* 1997; **79**: 235–46.

15. Engeland A, Haldorsen T, Tretli S et al, Prediction of cancer incidence in the Nordic countries up to the years 2000 and 2010. *APMIS* 1993; suppl 101: 1–124.

16. Engeland A, Haldorsen T, Tretli S et al, Prediction of cancer incidence in the Nordic countries up to the years 2000 and 2010. *APMIS* 1995; suppl 103: 1–163.

17. Lu-Yao GL, Greenberg ER, Changes in prostate cancer incidence and treatment in USA. *Lancet* 1994; **343**: 251–4.

18. Herr HW, Kornblith AB, Ofman U, A comparison of the quality of life of patients with metastatic prostate cancer who received or did not receive hormonal therapy. *Cancer* 1993; **71**: 1143–50.

19. Hermanek P, Sobin LH (eds), *TNM Classification of Malignant Tumors*, 4th edn, 2nd rev. Springer-Verlag: New York, 1992.

20. Paulson DF, Stage A prostatic adenocarcinoma. *World J Urol* 1989; **7**: 34–7.

21. Heaney JA, Chang HC, Daly JJ, Prout GR, Prognosis of clinically undiagnosed prostatic carcinoma and the influence of endocrine therapy. *J Urol* 1977; **118**: 283–7.

22. Blute ML, Zincke H, Farrow GM, Long-term followup of young patients with stage A adenocarcinoma of the prostate. *J Urol* 1986; **136**: 840–3.

23. Moskovitz B, Nitecki S, Richter Levin D, Cancer of the prostate: is there a need for aggressive treatment? *Urol Int* 1987; **42**: 49–52.

24. Goodman CM, Busuttil A, Chisholm GD, Age, and size and grade of tumour predict prognosis in incidentally diagnosed carcinoma of the prostate. *Br J Urol* 1988; **62**: 576–80.

25. Lowe BA, Listrom MB, Incidental carcinoma of the prostate: an analysis of the predictors of progression. *J Urol* 1988; **140**: 1340–4.

26. Waaler G, Ludvigsen TC, Stenwig AE, Prognosis of incidental prostatic cancer in Aust-Agder county, Norway. *Eur Urol* 1990; **18**: 179–83.

27. Johansson J-E, Adami H-O, Andersson S-O, Bergström R, Holmberg L, Krusemo UB, High 10-year survival rate in patients with early untreated prostatic cancer. *J Am Med Assoc* 1992; **267**: 2191–6.

28. Cantrell BB, DeClerk DP, Egglestone JC, Boitnott JK, Walsh PC, Pathological factors that influence prognosis in stage A prostatic cancer: the influence of extent versus grade. *J Urol* 1981; **125**: 516–20.

29. Zhang G, Wasserman NF, Sidi AA, Reinberg Y, Reddy PK, Long-term followup results after expectant management of stage A1 prostatic cancer. *J Urol* 1991; **146**: 99–103.

30. Epstein JI, Paull G, Eggleston JC, Walsh PC, Prognosis of untreated stage A1 prostatic carcinoma: a study of 94 cases with extended followup. *J Urol* 1986; **136**: 837–9.

31. Oesterling JE, Suman VJ, Zincke H, Bostwick DG, PSA-detected (clinical stage T1c or B0)

prostate cancer. Pathologically significant tumors. *Urol Clin N Am* 1993; **20:** 687–93.

32. Mohler JL, Partin AW, Epstein JI et al, Prediction of prognosis in untreated stage A2 prostatic carcinoma. *Cancer* 1992; **69:** 511–19.

33. McIntire TL, Murphy WM, Coon JS et al, The prognostic value of DNA ploidy combined with histologic substaging for incidental carcinoma of the prostate gland. *Am J Clin Pathol* 1988; **89:** 370–3.

34. George NJR, Natural history of localised prostatic cancer managed by conservative therapy alone. *Lancet* 1988; 5(8584): 494–7.

35. Graverson PH, Nielsson KT, Gasser TC, Corle DK, Madsen PO, Radical prostatectomy versus expectant treatment in stages I and II prostatic cancer. A fifteen-year follow-up. *Urology* 1990; **36:** 493–8.

36. Warner J, Whitmore WF Jr, Expectant management of clinically localized prostatic cancer. *J Urol* 1994; **152:** 1761–5.

37. Johansson JE, Holmberg L, Johansson S, Bergström R, Adami HO, Fifteen-year survival in prostate cancer. A prospective, population-based study in Sweden. *J Am Med Assoc* 1997; **277:** 467–71.

38. Adolfsson J, Carstensen J, Löwhagen T, Deferred treatment in clinically localized prostatic carcinoma. *Br J Urol* 1992; **69:** 183–7.

39. Adolfsson J, Carstensen J, Natural course of clinically localized prostate adenocarcinoma in men less than 70 years old. *J Urol* 1991; **146:** 96–8.

40. Egawa S, Go M, Kuwao S, Shoji K, Uchida T, Koshiba K, Long-term impact of conservative management on localized prostate cancer. *Urology* 1993; **42:** 520–7.

41. Stenzl A, Studer UE, Outcome of patients with untreated cancer of the prostate. *Eur Urol* 1993; **24:** 1–6.

42. Waaler G, Stenwig AE, Prognosis of localized prostatic cancer managed by 'watch and wait' policy. *Br J Urol* 1993; **72:** 214–19.

43. Lundgren R, Nordle Ö, Josefsson K, and the South Sweden Prostate Cancer Study Group, Immediate estrogen or estramustine phosphate therapy versus deferred endocrine treatment in non-metastatic prostate cancer. A randomized multicenter study with 15 years follow-up. *J Urol* 1995; **153:** 1580–6.

44. Adolfsson J, Deferred treatment of low grade stage T3 prostate cancer without distant metastases. *J Urol* 1993; **149:** 326–9.

45. Adolfsson J, Steineck G, Whitmore WF, Recent results of management of palpable clinically localized prostate cancer. *Cancer* 1993; **72:** 310–22.

46. Wasson JH, Cushman CC, Bruskewitz RC et al, A structured literature review of treatment for localized prostate cancer. *Arch Family Med* 1993; **2:** 487–93.

47. Middleton RG, Thompson IM, Austenfeld MS et al, Prostate Cancer Clinical Guidelines Panel summary report on the management of clinically localized prostate cancer. *J Urol* 1995; **154:** 2144–8.

48. Chodak G, Thiested R, Gerber G et al, Outcome following conservative management of patients with clinically localized prostate cancer. *N Engl J Med* 1994; **330:** 242–8.

49. Catalona WJ, Stein AJ, Fair WR, Grading errors in prostatic needle biopsies: relation to the accuracy of tumor grade in predicting pelvic lymph node metastases. *J Urol* 1982; **127:** 919–22.

50. Narayan P, Jajodia P, Stein R, Tanagho EA, A comparison of fine needle aspiration and core biopsy in diagnosis and preoperative grading of prostate cancer. *J Urol* 1989; **141:** 560–3.

51. Fowler JE, Barzell W, Hilaris BS, Whitmore WF Jr, Complications of ^{125}iodine implantation and pelvic lymphadenectomy in the treatment of prostatic cancer. *J Urol* 1979; **121:** 447–51.

52. Petros JA, Catalona WJ, Lower incidence of unsuspected lymph node metastases in 521 consecutive patients with clinically localized prostate cancer. *J Urol* 1992; **147:** 1574–5.

53. Aus G, Hugosson J, Norlén L, Long-term survival and mortality in prostate cancer treated with noncurative intent. *J Urol* 1995; **154:** 460–5.

54. Grönberg H, Damber L, Jonsson H, Damber JE, Prostate cancer mortality in Northern Sweden with special reference to tumor grade and patient age. *Urology* 1997; **49:** 374–8.

55. Abrahamsson P-A, Adami H-O, Taube A, Kim K, Zelen M, Kulldorf M, Re: Long-term survival and mortality in prostate cancer treated with noncurative intent. *J Urol* 1996; **155:** 296–7.

56. Crawford D, Eisenberger M, McLeod DG, Spaulding JT, Benson R, Dorr FA, A controlled trial of Leuprolide with and without Flutamide in prostatic carcinoma. *N Engl J Med* 1989; **321:** 419–24.

57. Denis LJ, Carnelro De Moura JL, Bono A et al, Goserelin acetate and flutamide versus bilateral orchiectomy: a phase III EORTC trial (30853). EORTC GU Group and EORTC Data Centre. *Urology* 1993; **42:** 119–30.

58. Crawford ED, Eisenberger MA, McLeod DG,

Wilding G, Blumenstein BA, Comparison of bilateral orchiectomy with or without Flutamide for the treatment of patients (pts) with stage D$_2$ adenocarcinoma of the prostate (CaP): results of NCI intergroup study 0105 (SWOG and ECOG). *J Urol* 1997; **157:** 336 (abstr 1311).

59. Goldenberg SL, Bruchovsky N, Gleave ME, Sullivan LD, Akakuro K, Intermittent androgen suppression in the treatment of prostate cancer: a preliminary report. *Urology* 1995; **45:** 839–45.

60. Adolfsson J, Prognostic value of deoxyribonucleic acid content in prostate cancer: a review of current results. *Int J Cancer* 1994; **58:** 211–16.

61. Lewenhaupt A, Ekman P, Eneroth P, Nilsson B, Tumour markers as prognostic aids in prostatic carcinoma. *Br J Urol* 1990; **66:** 182–7.

62. Larson A, Fritjofsson Å, Norlén BJ, Gronowitz JS, Ronquist G, Prostate specific acid phosphatase versus five other possible tumour markers: a comparative study in men with prostatic carcinoma. *Scand J Clin Lab Invest* 1985; **45**(suppl 179): 81–8.

63. Pound CR, Partin AW, Epstein JE, Walsh PC, Prostate-specific antigen following anatomical radical retropubic prostatectomy. Patterns of recurrence and cancer control. *Urol Clin N Am* 1997; **24:** 395–406.

64. Schellhammer PF, El-Mahdi AM, Kuban DA, Wright GL Jr, Prostate-specific antigen following radiation therapy. Prognosis by treatment level and post-treatment nadir. *Urol Clin N Am* 1997; **24:** 407–14.

65. Kupelain PA, Kupelain VA, Witte JS, Mecklis RM, Klein EA, Family history of prostate cancer in patients with localized prostate cancer: an independent predictor of treatment outcome. *J Clin Oncol* 1997; **15:** 1478–80.

66. Grönberg H, Damber JE, Jonsson H, Lenner P, Patient age as a prognostic factor in prostate cancer. *J Urol* 1994; **152:** 892–5.

67. Carter HB, Piantadosi S, Isaacs JT, Clinical evidence for and implications of the multistep development of prostate cancer. *J Urol* 1990; **143:** 742–6.

68. Watanabe M, Ushijima T, Kaiuchi H et al, p53 gene mutations in human prostate cancers in Japan: different mutations spectra between Japan and Western countries. *Jpn J Cancer Res* 1994; **85:** 904–10.

69. Konishi N, Hiasa Y, Hayashi I et al, p53 mutations occur in clinical, but not latent, human prostate carcinoma. *Jpn J Cancer Res* 1995; **86:** 57–63.

70. Takahashi H, Furusato M, Allsbrook WC Jr et al, Prevalence of androgen receptor gene mutations in latent prostatic carcinomas from Japanese men. *Cancer Res* 1995; **55:** 1621–4.

71. Irvine RA, Yu MC, Ross RK, Coetze GA, The CAG and GGC microsatellites of the androgen receptor gene are in linkage disequilibrium in men with prostate cancer. *Cancer Res* 1995; **55:** 1937–40.

72. Haenszel W, Kurihara M, Studies of Japanese migrants, I. Mortality from cancer and other diseases among Japanese in the United States. *J Natl Cancer Inst* 1968; **40:** 43–68.

73. Key T, Risk factors for prostate cancer. *Cancer Surveys* 1995; **23:** 63–77.

74. Kolonel LN, Nutrition and prostate cancer. *Cancer Causes Control* 1996; **7:** 83–94.

75. Morton MS, Griffiths K, Blacklock N, The preventive role of diet in prostatic disease. *Br J Urol* 1996; **77:** 481–93.

76. Grönberg H, Damber L, Damber JE, Total food consumption and body mass index in relation to prostate cancer risk: a case-control study in Sweden with prospectively collected exposure data. *J Urol* 1996; **155:** 969–74.

77. Clinton SK, Palmer SS, Spriggs CE et al, Growth and Dunning transplantable prostate adenocarcinomas in rats fed diets with various fat contents. *J Nutr* 1988; **118:** 908–12.

78. Pollard M, Luckert PH, Promotional effects of testosterone and dietary fat on prostate carcinogenesis in genetically susceptible rats. *Prostate* 1985; **6:** 1–5.

79. Schwartz GG, Hulka BS, Is vitamin D deficiency a risk factor for prostate cancer? *Anticancer Res* 1990; **10:** 1307–12.

80. Hanchette CL, Schwartz GG, Geographic patterns of prostate cancer mortality. *Cancer* 1992; **70:** 2861–9.

81. Preece MA, Tomlinson S, Ribot CA et al, Studies of vitamin D deficiency in man. *Q J Med, New Ser, XLIV* 1975; **176:** 575–89.

82. Eisman JA, Barkla DH, Tutton PJ, Suppression of in vivo growth of human solid tumor xenografts by 1α-25-dihydroxyvitamin D3. *Cancer Res* 1987; **47:** 21–5.

83. Abe M, Miyayra C, Sakagami H et al, Differentiation of mouse myeloid leukemia cells induced by 1α-25-dihydroxyvitamin D3. *Proc Natl Acad Sci USA* 1981; **78:** 4990–4.

84. Chida K, Hashiba H, Fukushima M, Suda T, Kuroki T, Inhibition of tumor promotion in mouse skin by 1α-25-dihydroxyvitamin D3. *Cancer Res* 1985; **45:** 5426–30.

85. Reitsma PH, Rothberg PG, Astrin SM et al, Regulation of myc gene expression in HL-60 leukaemia cells by a vitamin D metabolite. *Nature* 1983; **306:** 4992–4.

86. Matsuyama H, Yi P, Yoshihiro S et al, Deletion of chromosome 8p22 for the development of disease progression in prostate cancer. Submitted to *Cancer Research*.

87. Cher ML, Ito T, Weidner N, Carroll PR et al, Mapping of regions of physical deletion on chromosome 16q in prostate cancer cells by fluorescence in situ hybridization (FISH). *J Urol* 1995; **153:** 249–54.

88. Umbas R, Schalken JA, Aalders TW et al, Expression of the cellular adhesion molecule E-cadherin is reduced or absent in high-grade prostate cancer. *Cancer Res* 1992; **52:** 5104–9.

89. Pan Y, Matsuyama H, Naining W et al, Chromosome 16q deletion and E-cadherin expression in prostate cancer as related to tumor grade, stage and DNA ploidy. *Prostate* 1998; **36:** 31–8.

2

The role of pathology in biopsy, diagnosis and management of prostate cancer

Michael R Jarmulowicz

In previous years finger-guided transrectal or, more rarely, transperineal biopsies were performed on patients with symptoms of prostatism/outflow obstruction in whom a digital rectal examination was suggestive of malignancy or in whom metastatic disease was the presenting symptom and prostate cancer was suspected. The biopsy was to confirm the diagnosis of malignancy so that palliative hormonal therapy could be given. Following the success in identifying patients with small gland-confined carcinoma and the possibility of a curative radical prostatectomy, biopsies are now performed more frequently and are important in the preoperative diagnosis and staging of disease.

When faced with a patient with a possible carcinoma of the prostate, the surgeon not only needs to make the diagnosis of carcinoma, but also requires information to make the decision as to which is the most appropriate treatment to offer to the patient. The pathologist has a dual role when examining prostatic needle biopsies: making the diagnosis of carcinoma/ prostatic intraepithelial neoplasia (PIN), and providing information of the probable stage of the tumour in order to assist the surgeon in deciding on the best modality of treatment to be offered. The subsequent examination of a radical prostatectomy specimen will provide information on which possible additional therapy will be based. The histopathological assessment will also provide cancer staging, allowing comparison of surgical results and thus facilitating audit.

THE RISK OF DETECTING 'INSIGNIFICANT CANCER'

There is no widely accepted definition of 'insignificant cancer'. It was in 1954 that Franks first reported the high incidence of 'latent carcinoma' of the prostate when he found, in an autopsy series, that 30% of men had carcinoma of the prostate.[1] In 1993, a similar figure (40%) was found in a series of consecutive cysto-prostatectomy specimens removed for bladder cancer and in which prostatic carcinoma was not suspected. However, in the USA prostate cancer is clinically apparent in only 9% of men and kills only 3%.[2] Additional studies have demonstrated that the high incidence of histologically localized prostate cancer is observed throughout the world's male population. In contrast, the prevalence of clinically manifested prostatic cancer varies more than 15-fold between the high incidence in American men and the lower incidence in Japanese men, although their mean life spans are equal.[3] The problem is that the histological appearance of the 'latent' tumours is identical to that of fatal tumours, and so the difficulty has been in identifying those patients who will 'die *with* their cancer' and require no specific treatment, as opposed to those who, if left untreated, will 'die *of* their cancer'. In 1969, McNeal[4] proposed that there was a continuum of prostate cancer: as the cancer volume increased, so did its malignant potential. By 1986, he produced evidence which showed that prostate cancer metastasized only when the volume was larger than 4 cm^3 and when Gleason pattern 4 or 5 components were present.[5] Other studies reduced the significant volume to 3 cm^{3},[6,7] while others argued for 0.5 cm^3 and no Gleason pattern 4 tumour,[8] and some preferred a cut-off of 0.2 cm^3.[9] However, all these studies concentrated entirely on a 'still shot' of the tumour, and ignored the patient, his risk of death from other causes and the cancer dynamics. No-one would suggest that a tiny tumour in a 40 year old would remain clinically silent for the rest of his life; conversely, how many would treat an incidentally identified prostatic carcinoma in an elderly man with significant medical problems?

There are eight study series, using modern staging methods, in which patients were followed conservatively and so give an indication of untreated natural history.[10–17] The overall conclusion of these natural history studies is that disease progression, usually defined clinically, occurs in almost all patients who are left untreated. However, this equates only occasionally with metastatic disease and death due to prostate cancer, since the majority of patients will die of other causes. The most recent and largest study[17] with the longest follow-up is from a subgroup of 4000 patients treated for prostate cancer at the Memorial Sloan–Kettering Cancer Center. This group contained 75 patients who elected to have conservative therapy and received no treatment for at least a

year: 29 patients were classified as clinical stage B1 (palpable nodule less than 2 cm in diameter confined to one lobe), 37 patients were stage B2 (palpable nodule greater than 2 cm in diameter confined to one lobe), and 9 were stage B3 (nodule involving both prostatic lobes). The mortality details of this small group of patients are given in Table 2.1. The survival figures are within the normal mortality figures expected for the age group, which emphasizes the need for strict evaluation of the efficacy of aggressive treatments.

A new definition of 'insignificant prostate cancer', which takes the multiple factors into account, has been proposed by Duggan et al.[18] They define clinically insignificant prostatic cancers according to the cancer volume, grade, tumour-doubling time and the patient's predicted death using life-expectancy tables. Using the information that there is a 10% probability of a 5-cm^3 tumour having already metastasized, a 50% probability in a 13-cm^3 tumour and an 87% probability in a 20-cm^3 tumour, it is reasonable to predict that the majority of tumours would metastasize in the last doubling time from 10 to 20 cm^3. This logically leads to the definition that a clinically insignificant cancer is one which has a projected tumour volume at the expected time of death of less than 20 cm^3. The rate of tumour growth is probably proportional to the grade and, in order not to underestimate the relevance of small high-grade tumours, Duggan et al added the refinement that the Gleason score should be less than the tens digit of the patient's age (i.e. a 50-year-old man must have a Gleason score of less than 5, and a 70-year-old man must have one of less than 7). Using different tumour-doubling times they produced a series of graphs that defined the size of an 'insignificant cancer' in relation to age, Gleason score and rate of tumour growth. They then used these graphs to show, retrospectively, that patients received a radical prostatectomy for clinically insignificant disease in 0.3%, 3.9%, 7.4% and 14.5% of cases when using theoretical tumour-doubling times of 2, 3, 4 and 6 years, respectively. However these data cannot be used to select patients for radical surgery because cancer volume cannot

Table 2.1 Mortality of patients treated with expectant management of localized prostate cancer[17]

Follow-up period (years)	No. of patients	Prostate-cancer-related mortality (%)	Overall mortality (%)
1–5	75	0	7
5–10	61	18	25
10–15	31	22	35
15–20	14	0	29
≥20	2	0	50
Overall	75	24	48

be accurately predicted preoperatively and no definition has undergone sufficiently long-term follow-up to prove or disprove its validity. Furthermore, studies on what is insignificant cancer is compounded by the inevitable bias in any study group. In all studies the majority of patients have been recruited because of a palpable abnormality, a raised prostate-specific antigen (PSA) level or some abnormality on transrectal ultrasound examination.

BIOPSY

The optimum number of biopsies

The optimum number, sites and angle of biopsies necessary to detect and exclude cancers may become symptomatic or cause death are not known. The number of biopsies taken varies from sampling a suspicious lesion, be it palpable or apparent on transrectal ultrasound (TRUS), to systematic quadrant, sextant or even higher number of biopsies in patients with an elevated serum PSA. The general pattern is to use systematic sextant biopsies.[19]

Investigation of the degree of sampling necessary has been based on the relationship between tumour volume and metastases.

Sextant biopsies of clay models have indicated that cancer would be detected in 36%, 44% and all cases when tumour occupies 2.5%, 5% and 20% of the gland volume.[20] However, this model involves the assumption that the distribution of both the tumour and the biopsies would be random. The reality is that 80% of prostatic tumours arise in the posterior peripheral zone. A study of in vitro multiple core biopsies of radical prostatectomies, reproducing the usual transrectal route and subsequent mapping to the radical prostatectomy specimens, advocated a minimum of six systematic biopsies if tumour volume was to be projected reliably. A stronger correlation was obtained with ten biopsies, including four from the anterior aspect. Although in large studies there is a correlation between the amount of cancer in the sextant biopsies, and the volume of tumour in the prostate, in an individual patient these data may not be predictive.[21] One important reason for this discrepancy is that the tumour first expands in the transverse direction, across the posterior surface. The second extension occurs in a cephalad–caudal direction.[19] The standard TRUS biopsies therefore sample the tumour across its narrowest region, the dimension expected to have poor correlation to the overall volume. Cancer thickness measured in the anterior–posterior plane is not proportional to cancer volume until the tumour is greater than 4 cm³. A better sampling method would be to biopsy along the cephalad–caudal aspect of the gland, but this would involve a perineal biopsy which is both more time-consuming and uncomfortable for the patient, and would be clinically unacceptable as a routine procedure.

The risk of missing significant cancer on biopsy

When considering the problem of missing a significant cancer on biopsy, it is important to remember that patients have already been assessed by PSA level, digital rectal examination and TRUS. Despite some variation between studies, a systematic sampling of the prostate gland will reveal most peripheral-zone carcinomas. However, about 20% of prostate cancers arise in the transitional zone. This area would not be included in the routine biopsies. Many believe that the transition-zone carcinomas are a separate biological entity. They are more often of low grade, and the anatomical organization of the prostate gland, the compressed fibromuscular tissue between the central zone undergoing hyperplasia and the peripheral zone somehow limit the spread of transition-zone carcinomas into the neurovascular bundles and ejaculatory ducts – two major routes for extraglandular spread. Because of their location many, often large, transition-zone carcinomas are impalpable and show no ultrasound abnormality (clinical stage T1c). The consensus is that transition-zone sampling should not be recommended as a routine, but reserved for those patients who have a high PSA or rapidly rising PSA or a clinically suspected carcinoma, yet have had negative standard sextant biopsies.[19,22–24]

A SMALL FOCUS OF CANCER ON BIOPSY

It is difficult not to feel intuitively that focal cancer on biopsy (<3 mm in only one of six biopsy cores) is indicative of a small and possibly insignificant cancer in the prostate gland. This feeling was initially supported by a study by Terris et al,[25] which found that 41% of 17 patients who had a radical prostatectomy on the basis of a single focus of cancer in a single biopsy had an insignificant cancer (defined as <0.5 cm³ tumour volume). This is in complete contrast to the study by Weldon et al,[8] which showed that focal prostate cancer in a single biopsy correlated with an insignificant cancer in only 6% of cases. Other studies support this view, and also show that a proportion of 'focal cancer on biopsy' turn out to be significant cancers arising in the transition zone.[21,26,27]

If surgeons are considering offering conservative therapy for 'insignificant' tumours, then re-biopsy should be considered in order to establish whether the initial focal cancer on biopsy remains so on re-biopsy. The re-biopsy schedule should include the transition zone. The biopsy alone cannot be used to identify those with insignificant cancers, and better predictive values can be obtained using a combination of the biopsy findings together with serum PSA data.[9,19,28–30]

It is apparent from the numerous studies available that the two most important parameters which can be assessed preoperatively and are important in making treatment decisions are the Gleason score and the tumour volume. All modalities for measuring tumour volume preoperatively involve varying degrees of inaccuracy, but the pathologist can make a contribution to this assessment. Extensive tumour in several of the biopsies will equate with a significant tumour, while a small focus of cancer in a single biopsy cannot be interpreted as indicating a small tumour volume.

Gleason score

The histological grade of a carcinoma in a radical prostatectomy specimen is now well recognized as an important prognostic factor.[31–33] The important cut-off is in tumours that contain Gleason pattern 4 or 5 components, which usually equates with Gleason scores of 7 or above. In early series a 14-gauge biopsy needle was used, whereas common current practice is to use an 18-gauge needle because it gives rise to lower rates of infection and haemorrhage after biopsy. For the pathologist the problem is that the smaller needle provides less tissue on which to make an assessment.

Some would argue that, because there is variation in the Gleason patterns within any one tumour and because a needle biopsy only samples a small fraction of the tumour, giving a score on a nine-point scale (2–10) is theoretically unjustified. Furthermore, some find it difficult confidently to recognize the Gleason patterns when seen in a narrow-core biopsy. However, the surgeon needs to conclude from the preoperative assessment whether to recommend a radical prostatectomy to the patient, and each piece of data contributes to that assessment. The Gleason grading system is widely accepted and understood by workers in the field, and therefore there is pressure to report the tumour seen in the biopsy using the same system, with which the subsequent prostatectomy will be graded, albeit recognizing that discrepancies will arise.

Data from several sources show that, particularly in centres which see many prostate biopsies, there is an acceptable correlation between the grade on biopsy and subsequent radical prostatectomy.[34–38] All studies have found that, where discrepancies exist, there is an undergrading of well-differentiated tumours, which presumably reflects a sampling error, and good correlation of the moderately differentiated tumours and a lesser degree of overgrading in high-grade tumours. The author's experience is that the initial difficulty of grading biopsy specimens is that in a biopsy a good impression of the peripheral border of the tumour mass or of the overall architecture cannot be obtained, both of which are criteria in the Gleason system. To arrive at an accurate grade, it is important to concentrate on the appearance of the individual tumour glands and microarchitecture. The features have been well reviewed by Bostwick.[33]

Gleason pattern 1 is rarely recognized in biopsies, but has regular, round, closely packed glands. Although some Gleason 1 tumours have large prominent nucleoli, it is more common for them to have relatively small benign-appearing nuclei.

Gleason pattern 2 has simple round glands, which show only minimal variability in shape, but there is some definite separation of the glands by stroma. Both Gleason 1 and 2 tumours have abundant pale cytoplasm.

Gleason pattern 3 will have angulated glands with definite variation in their shapes. In addition, it is common to see some infiltration of malignant glands between benign elements. In Gleason 3 tumours the glands still form discrete units around which you can mentally draw a circle. Some difficulty may be experienced with cribriform pattern glands. To classify a cribriform pattern as Gleason 3, the nodule must be smoothly circumscribed and is nearly always accompanied by small infiltrating glands of pattern 3.

Gleason pattern 4 glands are no longer single and separate, but form ill-defined fused patterns with some chains and cords. In addition, glands with microacinar, papillary and cribriform patterns are seen.

In Gleason pattern 5 carcinoma it is difficult to identify the gland lumina and the tumour is composed of solid sheets, cords or single cells.

The biopsy report

The biopsy should offer more than the diagnosis or not of malignancy. There is valuable information that will not only help surgeons in their decision to proceed to radical prostatectomy, but also may help in the planning of surgery.

- *Site of the biopsies.* There is the temptation to put the three biopsies from each side into the same cassettes, which is a false economy. The presence of tumour in the apical biopsy is significant. The main purpose of a radical prostatectomy is to remove all tumour present. However, the surgeon is also keen to maintain continence if possible, and dissection will aim to preserve the external sphincter and nerves. The presence of tumour in the apical biopsy specimen will inform the surgeon that dissection of this area is likely to be difficult. If cost pressures favour processing all biopsies in the same cassette, then site information can be preserved by marking each biopsy with a different coloured ink.

- *Dimensions of biopsies.* The orientation with regard to the capsular end can be given by marking the capsular end on the biopsy with Indian ink (which sets instantly when placed into Bouin's fixative) as the biopsy is removed from the needle.
- *Presence of PIN.*
- *Length or proportion of the specimen invaded by carcinoma, and the number of cores involved in the tumour.* Extensive tumour in many cores indicates a large prostatic tumour, although the converse is not true on an individual basis.
- *Tumour grade.* Use the Gleason score by using both primary and secondary patterns. The crucial factor is the presence of Gleason pattern 4 or 5. In a series of 157 patients the presence of Gleason patterns 4 or 5, tumour in three or more biopsies or any core with more than 50% tumour involvement accurately predicted significant tumour in all cases.[9]
- *Presence of extracapsular spread.* Only occasionally will the biopsy identify the 'capsule' and tumour within periprostatic adipose tissue, but if present it will classify the tumour as already being outside the gland. This information is crucial for the surgeon in assessing the patient's suitability for a radical prostatectomy, or it may influence a decision to modify the operative procedure to include an increased amount of periprostatic tissue.[39]
- *Presence of perineural invasion.* Although only seen in 20% of malignant prostatic needle biopsies, perineural invasion should always be reported as its presence has a 96% specificity for predicting extracapsular spread.[40] If a radical prostatectomy is planned then this information may influence the decision about whether to sacrifice the neurovascular bundle. However, recent data suggest that this does not significantly alter the final outcome.[41]
- *Vascular invasion.*
- *Other pathology.* For example, atrophy and inflammation.

Fixatives

It has been suggested by some authors that specific fixatives that enhance nuclear detail should be used for prostate biopsies. However, the problem with using such fixatives is that they enhance the nuclear detail not only of the malignant glands but also of the benign glands. In using fixatives that enhance nuclear and nucleolar detail, the threshold for what constitutes prominent nucleoli becomes elevated. The author's preference is to use Bouin's fixative. In general, pathologists get used to their own material and artefacts and, therefore, the author does not believe that the choice of material has an impact on the accuracy of diagnosis. It is important to be comfortable and familiar with your laboratory techniques, and personal preference should prevail. Some have reported that Bouin's fixative decreases the sensitivity of high-molecular-weight cytokeratin immunohistochemistry to identify basal cells. The author finds no problem using the Dako LP34 antibody (against cytokeratins 6 and 18), provided that the specimen is fixed in Bouin's fixative for no more than 6 h.

Difficulties in diagnosing carcinoma at biopsy

The increase in prostatic biopsy referrals and requests from colleagues to audit such specimens indicates a level of diagnostic concern. The diagnosis of carcinoma involving the entire length of a needle biopsy rarely causes pathologists much difficulty, although occasionally Gleason 2 + 2 tumours cause problems. The main problems arise in what some have described as 'limited adenocarcinoma' on needle biopsy, where only a few malignant glands are present. This difficulty is compounded by the presence of numerous benign mimickers of adenocarcinoma of the prostate. Therefore, this section concentrates on the diagnosis and identification of 'limited' adenocarcinoma on biopsy.

Diagnosis

There is no single diagnostic feature of carcinoma, and diagnosis is achieved after assessing a number of features. To improve one's confidence in making this assessment, it is important to have a general feel for the architecture of the benign glands, concentrating both on their spatial arrangements and growth patterns as well as nuclear morphology. This will then allow a comparison to be made with the suspicious glands. This feel is best achieved by scanning at ×10 magnification. Scanning at high magnification will tend to emphasize the nuclear details, with the temptation that slight nuclear atypia will be taken out of context of the architectural pattern.

There are two common patterns that should alert the pathologist to the presence of carcinoma. The first is the presence of a focus of crowded glands, and the second is the presence of small glands situated between larger benign glands. In most cases neoplastic glands are smaller than adjacent benign glands, which also commonly show papillary infolding and branching. Comparison of overall nuclear size between the benign and malignant glands is an important feature.

Other helpful features are:

- *Crystalloids.* These are seen as slightly refractile, sharp-edged eosinophilic inclusions in the gland lumina, and are much more likely to be found in neoplastic than benign glands. When present they are more likely to be found in the lower-grade tumours.
- *Mitoses.* Mitotic figures are rare in hyperplasia, and their presence should increase the index of suspicion of malignancy.
- *Nucleoli.* Prominent nucleoli, although important in the diagnosis of carcinoma, should not be the sole criterion used to establish the diagnosis. Using nucleoli as

the dominant criterion will lead to the underdiagnosis in cases of well-differentiated tumour, but also to the possibility of overdiagnosis in cases of basal cell hyperplasia. The significance of prominent nucleoli must be taken in the context of the architectural pattern.

- *Luminal contents.* Depending on the haematoxylin used, blue-tinged mucinous secretions may be apparent in malignant glands, which is only rarely seen in benign glands. Although some have suggested that acid mucin stains can distinguish malignant from benign glands,[42] others have shown that acid mucin can be seen in adenosis and atrophic glands.[43]

Use of antibodies to high-molecular-weight cytokeratin

The normal prostate gland has an outer basal layer and an inner secretory cell layer. The basal cells are not myoepithelial as in other secretory glands.[44] The important diagnostic feature is that prostatic adenocarcinoma does not have any associated basal cells. The basal cells can be identified by antibodies to high-molecular-weight cytokeratin.[45–47] Many have shown the usefulness of this marker. In one large series this antibody established the diagnosis in 15% of cases, and changed the diagnosis from benign to malignant, or vice versa, in 3% of cases.[48]

Despite its great value, there are problems and cases can still remain equivocal. This is often due to the suspect glands no longer being present at deeper levels. In addition, examination of obviously benign glands will occasionally show some intermittent or absent staining of basal cells. This marker is most useful where there is a focus of atypical glands suspected for carcinoma, but the pathologist is unable to commit himself or herself to that diagnosis. The absence of basal cell staining in such a situation can often give the final impetus to make the diagnosis of cancer definitive. Conversely, its presence can be helpful when it identifies basal cells in mimickers of prostate cancer, such as atrophy and atypical adenomatous hyperplasia. In one study looking at this antibody in a non-academic setting, its use reduced the rate of diagnosis of 'atypical glands' from 8% to <1%.[49]

Differential diagnoses

Atrophy

Atrophy is the lesion that is most frequently misdiagnosed as carcinoma on needle biopsy. This is because glands are small and irregular, mimicking Gleason pattern 3 tumour. However, at low power atrophic glands have a very basophilic appearance due to their scant cytoplasm. Also at low power, particularly in marked atrophy, the glands give the impression of forming a patch of invasion, but proper assessment of the pattern will lead to the identification of a condensed lobule associated with sclerosis. The presence of chronic inflammation is helpful and points to a benign diagnosis. The danger is to evaluate atrophy at high magnification because atrophic nuclei are commonly enlarged and, particularly if associated with even mild chronic inflammation, nucleoli can be prominent. The two important features that prevent a misdiagnosis of carcinoma are the presence of atrophic cytoplasm and the presence of a double cell layer, which is sometimes obvious on the haematoxylin and eosin (H&E) stain. If there is any doubt, the basal cells of atrophic glands show uniform immunohistochemical staining for high-molecular-weight cytokeratin.

Atypical adenomatous hyperplasia

This condition is also known under a variety of other terms, such as adenosis, small gland hyperplasia, atypical adenosis and small acinar atypical hyperplasia. Although a consensus meeting agreed on the term 'atypical adenomatous hyperplasia',[50] other authors still prefer the term adenosis[51] because the former term implies a premalignant potential for which there is little, if any, supporting evidence.

After atrophy, atypical adenomatous hyperplasia (AAH) is another condition that is commonly confused and misdiagnosed as carcinoma, because it consists of a crowded focus of small glands that mimic low-grade adenocarcinoma. It is usually found in the transition zone and so is much more likely to be seen in curetting specimens performed for urinary obstruction. The diagnosis is based on a constellation of histological features, rather than on any single feature. At low power there is a lobular arrangement of small glands, which contrasts with the more haphazard and irregular arrangement of infiltrating malignant glands. However, despite the overall lobular pattern there may be some apparent infiltration by small glands into the surrounding stroma. Nucleoli are generally small, although occasional medium-sized nucleoli up to 1 μm in diameter are present.[52] The presence of huge nucleoli (>3 μm) is incompatible with a diagnosis of AAH, whereas they are occasionally seen even in low-grade carcinoma. An important observation to make is that the small suspect glands have cytoplasmic and nuclear features similar to the adjacent larger and obviously benign glands, and there is a gradual merging of the small glands into larger ones. Basal cells are focally present and are always seen in at least some small glands. If there are some small glands that are devoid of basal cells but otherwise appear identical to glands with basal cells, then this is an indication of AAH.[53,54] Corpora amylacea are commonly seen in AAH. The presence of crystalloids and blue staining mucin is unhelpful as these can be found both in AAH and in carcinoma. Atypical adenomatous hyperplasia should always be considered in the differential diagnosis of a low-grade prostatic adenocarcinoma.

Seminal vesicle epithelium

Occasionally the seminal vesicle or ejaculatory duct is included in a needle biopsy, and this can cause diagnostic problems to the unwary due to the presence of small glands and bizarre atypical nuclei. The normal seminal vesicle has a central large dilated lumen with numerous small glands clustered around the periphery. It is important to recognize this architectural pattern so as not to diagnose the small glands as carcinoma. The full architectural pattern is usually not seen in a thin-needle biopsy; commonly, there is part of a dilated gland surrounded by outpouchings of small glandular structures. In seminal vesicle epithelium the atypical nuclei are scattered and adjacent to normal nuclei. Prominent lipofuschin pigmentation is often seen. If diagnostic concern persists, immunohistochemistry is useful; seminal vesicle epithelium is negative for PSA and prostate-specific alkaline phosphatase.

Sclerosing adenosis

This is another uncommon condition that was first reported in 1983 as an adenomatoid prostatic tumour.[55] More recently, the term 'sclerosing adenosis' has been preferred because of the similar appearance of this condition to sclerosing adenosis of the breast.[56] As with atypical adenomatous hyperplasia, sclerosing adenosis is more commonly seen in transurethral resection specimens, but can occasionally be sampled in needle biopsies. Several features should prevent the misdiagnosis of adenocarcinoma. Sclerosing adenosis, if it were being considered as prostate cancer, would have a Gleason score of 8 or 9 because it comprises an admixture of glands, poorly formed glandular structures and single cells. However, this entity is seen as a focal lesion, which is virtually never seen in high-grade prostatic cancer. A distinctive feature of sclerosing adenosis, which is never seen in carcinoma, is the presence of a thick hyaline structure around at least some glands. The cytology of the cells is bland, and usually the diagnosis can be made on an H&E stain. However, if doubt persists then immunohistochemistry is diagnostic. Nearly all glandular structures will contain a basal layer staining with antibodies to high-molecular-weight cytokeratin. In addition, the basal cells react with actin and S100 protein, indicating that in this condition there is myoepithelial differentiation.

Clear-cell cribriform hyperplasia

Clear-cell cribriform hyperplasia is seen only rarely, and then typically occurs within the central region of the prostate and so is more likely to be seen in curetting specimens. It is composed of numerous cribriform glands separated from one another by a modest amount of stroma in a pattern typical of that of nodular hyperplasia. As its name suggests, the cytoplasm is strikingly clear. There is no nuclear atypia and there are either absent or small inconspicuous nucleoli. Usually the basal cells can be seen on H&E stain and will be clearly seen with high-molecular-weight cytokeratin. Although the presence of basal cells rules out carcinoma, the lack of cytological atypia is also important. If one was considering the diagnosis of carcinoma, then the Gleason pattern would be 3 or 4; these Gleason patterns always show nuclear atypia.

Verumontanum mucosal gland hyperplasia and nephrogenic adenoma

Both verumontanum mucosal gland hyperplasia and nephrogenic adenoma are rare lesions in the context of prostatic needle biopsies, but have been reported to have caused diagnostic problems and confusion with prostatic carcinoma. Both cause localized lesions beneath the urothelium and form closely packed glands. In the former condition there are basal cells,[57] and in the latter the epithelial cells are negative for PSA.[58]

Conclusion

It is important to stress that it is the constellation of features that should be used to make the diagnosis of carcinoma. There is no minimum number of atypical glands that is needed to make a diagnosis of malignancy. If all features are clearly present, then a single gland can be all that is necessary for a confident malignant diagnosis. Obviously there will always be a small percentage in which no definite diagnosis can be made. In these cases a report of 'suspicious but not diagnostic of carcinoma' should be made, and re-biopsy advised.

LYMPH NODE FROZEN SECTIONS

The literature on the accuracy of frozen sections to identify metastatic tumour is scanty. Studies quote false-negative rates of 7–28%,[59] but different methods of calculating the false-negative rate were used. When considering the false-negative rate, it is important to know the true incidence of metastases. One of the early studies found metastases in 70% of cases, whereas improved preoperative assessment has reduced the incidence to around 10%[60] or 12% (Dr Parkinson, personal communication); in these two studies the false-negative frozen section rates were 41% and 33%, respectively. In both these studies this high frozen section false-negative rate equated with 4% of patients undergoing radical prostatectomy with metastases present in lymph nodes. Pelvic lymph nodes are commonly very fatty, which makes frozen-section preparation difficult and time-consuming and produces suboptimal quality frozen sections. Review of false-negative results invariably shows them to be due to sampling error, where microscopic foci were not seen macroscopically and not sampled in the pieces submitted to frozen section. The concern, therefore, is that it is very likely that pathologists will have major problems identifying small metastases from frozen sections.[60]

RADICAL PROSTATECTOMY SPECIMENS

Methods of examination

What is the best method of examining a radical prostatectomy specimen? The information of prognostic value is Gleason score, tumour size/volume, extraglandular spread (some call this capsular penetration), involvement of seminal vesicles and the presence of tumour at the surgical margins. Although the ideal end-point for follow-up studies is survival or recurrent symptomatic disease, most studies use the surrogate end-point of disease progression, which is usually defined as a detectable PSA after surgery following undetected levels.

Many studies have repeatedly shown the significance of tumour size and McNeal et al[61] argued that capsular penetration was not a separate factor but directly related to the tumour size. Occasional positive surgical margins were found in small tumours, and in nearly all cases these were from the apex.

Although examination of prostate slices will usually reveal obvious areas of tumour, usually seen as granular yellow masses distinct from the spongy prostatic parenchyma, subsequent microscopy will nearly always reveal other areas of carcinoma not identified macroscopically. Similarly it is virtually impossible to identify possible areas of extraglandular or disease confidently at the surgical margins on naked-eye inspection and so macroscopic examination is of little value in selected blocks of 'nearest margin'. In practice, this would imply that embedding the entire prostate is required.

Some advocate 4-mm whole-mount preparations, while others state that alternate sections will provide the required prognostic information in 85% of cases.[62] Which sampling method is used will depend partly on the clinician's response to positive surgical margins or extraglandular spread. If the policy is to adopt a wait and see approach and only give further therapy when a recurrence is identified, usually by a rise in the PSA level, then it could be argued that a less thorough sampling would be adequate. However, if the surgeon plans to give adjunctive therapy on receipt of a positive surgical margin report, then it is imperative that full sampling of the resection specimen is necessary. However, for proper long-term follow-up and audit of results, a proper histological staging involving full sampling of the excised gland is necessary. With large-scale, long-term, follow-up data now being available from some centres, accurate prognostic staging will require full evaluation of the excision specimen.

Although the examination of whole-mount specimens is easier for the pathologist, the same information can also be obtained from embedding quadrants of the slices using standard sized cassettes and glass slides, although these generate many more slides.

Radical prostatectomy specimens vary widely in shape and size, and do not always conform to the stylized diagram of an inverted cone with the base at the bladder neck tapering to the apex adjacent to the external sphincter. Orientation of the specimen is necessary, and this is best achieved by identifying the seminal vesicles and recognizing that they are posterior and superior. By passing a sound through the urethra the anterior aspect is shorter than the posterior and commonly more rounded than the flatter posterior aspect.

The examination of prostatic specimens is well described in the Association of Clinical Pathologists' Broadsheet.[63] The prostate should be fixed in formol saline for a minimum of 24 h. The entire surface of the specimen is inked; different coloured inks can be used to identify laterality, although standard techniques can be used if strict care is taken to maintain orientation throughout the slicing and sectioning process. After slicing, further fixation is usually necessary. The author's preference is to leave the uncut specimen fixing for 72 h. This makes the whole gland very firm and easy to cut into uniform slices. In addition, there is little deformation of the slices on subsequent processing. The apical slice is the most difficult. Some advocate embedding the slice whole and reporting if tumour is present in the apical slice. The disadvantage is that this method limits the true identification of tumour at the surgical margin. If a slightly thicker slice is taken it can be cut further into parallel transverse slices, similar to a cervical cone biopsy, and in this way the true apical surgical margin is seen and the presence of tumour at the margin can be reported. The important features that should be included in the report are Gleason grade, tumour volume, spread outside the gland or at the surgical margins, and seminal vesicle involvement.

The Gleason grading system is the most widely used. The tumour is assigned two grades according to the predominant patterns present. The two scores are then summed to give the Gleason score, e.g. 2 + 3. The dominant pattern is given the first grade, with the second pattern which forms the lesser area being given the second grade. Where a number of different secondary grades are present, the highest grade should be recorded as the secondary pattern.

The measurement of tumour volume is approximate and will be partly affected by the degree of shrinkage in preparation of the specimen and preparation of the slides. It is possible to photocopy the original specimen slices, but an equally easy and more useful method is to use a flatbed scanner. The area of tumour can be mapped out and the surface area measured using either squared paper or, because the image is already in bit-map form, computer-aided techniques. Using the latter technique makes it easier to produce pictorial reports, which describe the state of tumour within the gland more clearly than written reports.

Interpretation of the outer limits of the gland is confused by the use of the word 'capsule', which is variable in structure and distribution and frequently absent. Identification of the capsule is made more difficult by the desmoplastic reaction commonly seen around tumours that invade periprostatic adipose tissue. Therefore, some are now adopting a terminology which avoids the use of the term 'capsule'. Regardless of whether one continues to use the term 'capsule' or not, three limits are defined, which correspond to three tumour classifications:

- *Gland confined.* The contour of the gland at low power is dictated by the muscle outline. Benign acini are virtually always within this limit and beyond it is adipose tissue. Rare exceptions do occur. It is important to remember that anteriorly towards the apex striated muscle fibres will be present. If the tumour is within this boundary it is classified as 'gland confined'.
- *Specimen confined but outside the gland/extracapsular spread.* This tissue external to the muscle outline consists of fibroadipose tissue within which run blood vessels and nerves. This zone, particularly posterolaterally, may be up to 1 cm wide. If tumour is present in this zone, it is classified as 'specimen confined but outside the gland' or 'capsular penetration'. In long-term follow-up studies there is a difference between those specimens that show just focal capsular penetration and those with more extensive or established capsular penetration.
- *Limit positive disease/positive surgical margins.* Essentially this is the inked resection margin. If tumour is present at this margin then it is classified as 'limit positive disease'. It is important to recognize that sometimes the surgical margin will be through the gland parenchyma and, therefore, limit positive

disease does not necessarily equate to tumour penetrating the 'capsule'.

Prognostic significance of features identified

Probably the largest long-term follow-up study is that by Epstein et al[64] involving 721 men. The larger cohort of patients and longer follow-up period have given statistical significance to variables that small studies did not have the power to identify. Patients with seminal vesicle invasion and/or lymph node metastases all show disease progression with time, and there is little further information of prognostic value to be obtained from analysis of the Gleason score and capsular spread.

The remainder of this discussion therefore applies to patients who have no lymph node spread or seminal vesicle involvement. The impact of the individual features taken in isolation is given in Table 2.2. Much better prognostic information is gained by stratifying patients

according to the Gleason score and then considering capsular spread and surgical margins. Although McNeal et al[61] had argued that capsular spread was not a separate entity but directly related to tumour volume, the larger and longer study has shown by multivariate analysis that capsular spread is of greater value than tumour volume.[65]

Gleason score

Those with Gleason scores of 2–4 do uniformly well and most would consider them cured by the radical prostatectomy, even in the rare cases that show capsular penetration or positive surgical margins. At the other extreme, those with Gleason scores of 8 and 9 do badly, but the reality is that the vast majority of these patients will have extensive capsular penetration and 50% will have positive surgical margins. Only about 10% of patients fall into the extreme ends of the Gleason spectrum and the vast majority will have Gleason scores of 5–7. It is in these patients that important prognostic information is gained from the other parameters.

Table 2.2 The impact of the individual features, considered in isolation, in the postoperative risk of progression in patients with negative seminal vesicles and negative lymph nodes[64]

Findings at radical prostatectomy	Progression-free risk at 5 years (%)	Progression-free risk at 10 years (%)
Organ confined	97.8	84.7
Focal capsular penetration	91.2	67.7
Established capsular penetration	77.8	58.4
Negative margins	94.6	79.4
Positive margins	74.0	54.9
Gleason score 2–4	100	95.6
Gleason score 5–6	96.9	81.9
Gleason score 7	76.9	51.5
Gleason score 8–9	59.1	34.9

Gleason score 5–6

Most studies exclude patients with Gleason 4 pattern tumour (i.e. Gleason 4 + 2) from the analysis as these behave in a more aggressive manner. If the disease is organ confined and the surgical margins are free then these patients are invariably cured with a disease-free outcome of 99% at 5 years and 92% at 10 years. An intermediate group is present where there is only focal penetration (regardless of the surgical margin) or established capsular penetration with negative margins. In these patients, 98% are still disease free at 5 years, but this falls to 77% by 10 years. Where there is extensive capsular spread and positive surgical margins the 5- and 10-year disease-free figures are 85% and 72%, respectively (Table 2.3).

Gleason score 7

A similar three-tier stratification can be used. The disease-free progression data are given in Table 2.4.

Surgical margins

Because of the significance of positive surgical margins, some pathologists feel that, because they are examining only a 4-µm section from a block 5 mm thick, they should emphasize when the tumour is very close to the surgical margin, with the implication that nearby there may be true surgical margin positivity. This problem has been examined in a cohort of 100 patients followed for 5 years, and it was demonstrated that tumour close to a margin added no extra information and these patients behaved as if they had clear surgical margins.[66] It can be seen from the follow-up data that surgical margins, although important, only significantly affect the prognosis in moderately differentiated tumours with established capsular spread.[65]

FUTURE PROGNOSTIC MARKERS

Because of the high prevalence of prostatic carcinoma in the elderly population, what is needed is a marker of virulence. An international workshop[67] on prostate cancer discussed the various issues, and areas that appeared most likely to be of value as clinical markers were the presence of: apoptosis, particularly its relationship with the bcl2 protein; metastases, which cause the important clinical problems; and microvascular invasion and neovascularization. Many cancers are now being recognized as having mutations with oncogenes or other areas, and it was agreed that androgen-receptor mutations should be given a high priority for funding, although data currently

Table 2.3 Postoperative risk of progression in Gleason score 5–6 tumours with negative seminal vesicles and negative lymph nodes[64]

Findings at radical prostatectomy (Gleason 5–6)	Progression-free risk at 5 years (%)	Progression-free risk at 10 years (%)
Organ confined, margin negative	98.7	92.4
Focal capsular penetration		
Established capsular penetration, margin negative	97.9	77.2
Established capsular penetration, margin positive	84.5	71.7

Table 2.4 Postoperative risk of progression in Gleason score 7 tumours with negative seminal vesicles and negative lymph nodes[64]

Findings at radical prostatectomy (Gleason 7)	Progression-free risk at 5 years (%)	Progression-free risk at 10 years (%)
Organ confined, margin negative	96.6	67.6
Focal capsular penetration		
Established capsular penetration, margin negative	82.8	47.9
Established capsular penetration, margin positive	50.0	41.6

available are insufficient for a definite conclusion. Tumours showing neuroendocrine differentiation appear to have a worse prognosis, and the presence of neuroendocrine markers either in serum or in tissue may be relevant. Although data are few, the production of soluble peptides may be of greater significance in determining tumour behaviour than tissue levels. The markers of most interest are chromagranin and serotonin.

Pathologists have traditionally analysed fixed, dead cells and tried to ascribe behaviour predictions to these observations. In order to evaluate metastatic potential fully it may be necessary to start analysing living cells. Mohler et al[68,69] have used computerized morphometrics to measure directly the in vitro motility of rat prostatic carcinoma cells using features such as membrane ruffling, pseudopodal extension and cellular translation to derive a visual motility grade. Using this grading system Mohler et al have been able to detect highly metastatic cells with a 94% sensitivity and 50% specificity. Although these experimental data apply only to animal material, they may have useful potential as they could be extrapolated to human investigations.

REFERENCES

1. Franks LM, Latent carcinoma of the prostate. *J Pathol* 1954; **68**: 603–16.
2. Seidman H, Mushinski MH, Gelb SK, Silverberg E, Probability of eventually developing or dying of cancer – United States, 1985. *CA* 1985; **35**: 36–56.
3. Denmeade SR, Isaacs JT, Prostate cancer: where are we and where are we going? *Br J Urol* 1997; **79**(suppl 1): 2–7.
4. McNeal JE, Origin and development of carcinoma of the prostate. *Cancer* 1969; **24**: 24–34.
5. McNeal JE, Kindrachuk RA, Freiha FS, Bostwick DG, Redwine EA, Stamey TA, Patterns of progression in prostate cancer. *Lancet* 1986: **i**: 60–3.
6. Stamey TA, McNeal JE, Freiha FS, Redwine EA, Morphometric and clinical studies on 68 consecutive radical prostatectomies. *J Urol* 1988; **139**: 1235–40.
7. Villers AA, McNeal JE, Redwine EA, Freiha FS, Stamey TA, Pathogenesis and biological significance of seminal vesicle invasion in prostatic adenocarcinoma. *J Urol* 1990; **143**: 1183–7.
8. Weldon VE, Tavel FR, Neuwirth H, Cohen R, Failure of focal prostate cancer on biopsy to predict focal prostate cancer: the importance of prevalence. *J Urol* 1995; **154**: 1074–7.
9. Epstein JI, Walsh PC, Carmichael M, Brendler

CB, Pathologic and clinical findings to predict tumour extent of non palpable (stage T1c) prostate cancer. *J Am Med Assoc* 1994; **271**: 368–74.

10. Cook GB, Watson FR, Twenty single nodules of prostate cancer not treated by total prostatectomy. *J Urol* 1968; **100**: 672–4.

11. Barnes R, Hirst A, Rosenquist R, Early carcinoma of the prostate: comparison of stages A and B. *J Urol* 1976; **115**: 404–5.

12. Moskovitz B, Nitecki S, Levin DR, Cancer of the prostate: Is there any need for aggressive treatment? *Urol Int* 1987; **42**: 49–52.

13. Marsden PO, Graverson PH, Gasser TC, Corle DK, Treatment of localised prostatic cancer. Radical prostatectomy versus placebo. A 15-year follow-up. *Scand J Urol Nephrol* 1988; **110**(suppl): 95–100.

14. George NJR, Natural history of localised prostatic cancer managed by conservative therapy alone. *Lancet* 1988; **i**: 494–7.

15. Johannsson JE, Adami HO, Andersson SO, Bergstrom R, Krusemo UB, Kraaz W, Natural history of localised prostatic cancer. A population-based study in 223 untreated patients. *Lancet* 1989; **i**: 799–803.

16. Adolfsson J, Carstensen J, Natural course of clinically localised prostate adenocarcinoma in men less than 70 years old. *J Urol* 1991; **146**: 96–8.

17. Whitmore WF, Warner JA, Thompson IM, Expectant management of localised prostatic cancer. *Cancer* 1991; **67**: 1091–6.

18. Dugan JA, Bostwick DG, Myers RP, Quian J, Bergstrain EJ, Oesterling JE, The definition and preoperative prediction of clinically insignificant prostate cancer. *J Am Med Assoc* 1996; **275**: 288–94.

19. Stamey T. Making the most out of six systematic sextant biopsies. *Urology* 1995; **45**: 2–12.

20. Stricker HJ, Ruddock LJ, Wan J, Belville WD, Detection of non-palpable prostate cancer. A mathematical and laboratory model. *Br J Urol* 1993; **142**: 43–6

21. Cupp MR, Bostwick DG, Myers RP, Oesterling JE, The volume of prostate cancer in the biopsy specimen cannot reliably predict the quantity of cancer in the radical prostatectomy specimen on an individual basis. *J Urol* 1995; **153**: 1543–8.

22. Lui PD, Terris MK, McNeal JE, Stamey TA, Indications for ultrasound guided transition zone biopsies in the detection of prostate cancer. *J Urol* 1995; **153**: 1000–3.

23. Fleshner NE, Fair WR, Indications for transition zone biopsy in the detection of prostatic carcinoma. *J Urol* 1997; **157**: 556–8.

24. Terris MK, Pham TQ, Issa MM, Kabalin JN, Routine transition zone and seminal vesicle biopsies in all patients undergoing transrectal ultrasound guided prostate biopsies are not indicated. *J Urol* 1997; **157**: 204–6.

25. Terris MK, McNeal JE, Stamey TA, Detection of clinically significant prostate cancer by transrectal ultrasound-guided systematic biopsies. *J Urol* 1992; **148**: 829–32.

26. Elgamal AA, van Poppel HP, Van de Voorde WM, Van Dorpe J, Oyen RH, Baert LV, Impalpable invisible stage T1c prostate cancer: characteristics and clinical relevance in 100 radical prostatectomy specimens – a different view. *J Urol* 1997; **157**: 244–50.

27. Dietrick DD, McNeal JE, Starmey TA, Core cancer length in ultrasound-guided systematic sextant biopsies: a preoperative evaluation of prostate cancer volume. *Urology* 1995; **45**: 987–92.

28. Goto Y, Ohori M, Arawaka A, Kattan MW, Wheeler TM, Scardino PT, Distinguishing clinically important from unimportant prostate cancers before treatment: value of systematic biopsies. *J Urol* 1996; **156**: 1059–63.

29. Terris MK, Haney DJ, Johnstone IM, McNeal JE, Stamey TA, Prediction of prostate cancer volume using prostate-specific antigen levels, transrectal ultrasound, and systematic sextant biopsies. *Urology* 1995; **45**: 75–80.

30. Esptein JI, *Prostate Biopsy Interpretation*, 2nd edn. Lippincott–Raven: Philadelphia, 1995.

31. Gleason DF, Mellinger GT, Prediction of prognosis for prostate carcinoma by combined histological grading and clinical staging. *J Urol* 1974; **111**: 58–64.

32. Murphy GP, Busch C, Abrahamson PA et al, Histopathology of localised prostate cancer. *Scand J Urol Nephrol* 1994; **162**(suppl): 7–42.

33. Bostwick DG, Grading prostate cancer. *Am J Clin Pathol* 1994; **102**(suppl I): S38–56.

34. Bostwick DG, Gleason grading of prostatic needle biopsies. Correlation with grade in 316 matched prostatectomies. *Am J Surg Pathol* 1994; **18**: 796–803.

35. Peller PA, Young DC, Marmaduke DP, Marsh WL, Badalament RA, Sextant prostate biopsies. A histopathological correlation with radical prostatectomy specimens. *Cancer* 1995; **75**: 530–8.

36. Cookson MS, Fleshner NE, Soloway SM, Fair WR, Correlation between Gleason score of needle biopsy and radical prostatectomy specimen: accuracy and clinical implications. *J Urol* 1997; **157**: 559–62.

37. Spires SE, Cibull ML, Wood DP, Miller S, Spires

SM, Banks ER, Gleason histologic grading in prostatic carcinoma. Correlation of 18-gauge core biopsy with prostatectomy. *Arch Pathol Lab Med* 1994; **118**: 705–8.

38. Lessells AM, Burnett RA, Howatson SR et al, Observer variability in the histopathological reposting of needle biopsy specimens of the prostate. *Human Pathol* 1997; **28**: 646–9.

39. Stephenson RA, Middleton RG, Abbott TM, Wide excision (non-nerve sparing) radical retropubic prostatectomy using an initial perirectal dissection. *J Urol* 1997; **157**: 251–5.

40. Bastacky SI, Walsh PC, Epstein JI, Relationship between perineural tumour invasion on needle biopsy and radical prostatectomy capsular penetration in clinical stage B adenocarcinoma of the prostate. *Am J Surg Pathol* 1993; **17**: 336–41.

41. Partin AW, Borland RN, Epstein JI, Brendler CB, Influence of wide excision of the neuromuscular bundle on prognosis in men with clinically localised prostate cancer with established capsular penetration. *J Urol* 1993; **150**: 142–8.

42. Pinder SE, McMahon RFT, Mucins in prostatic carcinoma. *Histopathology* 1992; **16**: 43–6.

43. Epstein JI, Fynheer J. Acidic mucin in the prostate: can it differentiate adenosis from adenocarcinoma? *Human Pathol* 1992; **23**: 1321–3.

44. Srigley JR, Dardick I, Warren R, Hartwick J, Klotz L, Basal epithelial cells of human prostate gland are not myoepithelial cells. *Am J Pathol* 1990; **136**: 957–66.

45. Brawer MK, Peehl DM, Stamey TA et al, Keratin immunoreactivity in the benign and neoplastic human prostate. *Cancer Res* 1985; **45**: 3663–7.

46. Shah IA, Schlageter M, Stinnett et al, Cytokeratin immunohistochemistry as a diagnostic tool for distinguishing malignant from benign epithelial lesions of the prostate. *Mod Pathol* 1991; **4**: 220–4.

47. Hedrick I, Epstein JI, Use of keratin 903 as an adjunct in the diagnosis of prostate carcinoma. *Am J Surg Pathol* 1989; **13**: 389–96.

48. Wojno KJ, Epstein JI, The utility of basal cell specific anti-cytokeratin antibody in the diagnosis of prostate cancer: a review of 228 cases. *Am J Surg Pathol* 1995; **19**: 251–60.

49. Kahane H, Sharp JW, Shuman GB, Dasilva G, Epstein JI, Utilisation of high molecular weight cytokeratin on prostate biopsies in an independent laboratory. *Urology* 1995; **45**: 981–6.

50. Bostwick DG, Algaba F, Amin MB et al, Consensus statement on terminology: recommendation to use atypical adenomatous hyperplasia in place of adenosis of the prostate. *Am J Surg Pathol* 1994; **18**: 1069–70.

51. Epstein JI, Adenosis vs. atypical adenomatous hyperplasia of the prostate. *Am J Surg Pathol* 1994; **18**: 1070–1.

52. Kramer CE, Epstein JI, Nucleoli in low-grade prostate adenocarcinoma and adenosis. *Human Pathol* 1993; **24**: 618–23.

53. Gaudin PB, Epstein JI, Adenosis of the prostate: histologic features in needle biopsy specimens. *Am J Surg Pathol* 1995; **19**: 737–47.

54. Gaudin PB, Epstein JI, Adenosis of the prostate: histologic features in transurethral resection specimens. *Am J Surg Pathol* 1994; **18**: 863–70.

55. Chen KTK. Adenomatoid prostatic tumour. *Urology* 1983; **21**: 88–9.

56. Sakamoto N, Tsuneyoshi M, Enjoji M, Sclerosing adenosis of the prostate: histopathological and immunohistochemical analysis. *Am J Surg Pathol* 1991; **15**: 660–7.

57. Gaudin PB, Epstein JI, Verumontanum mucosal gland hyperplasia in prostatic needle biopsy specimens. A mimic of low grade prostatic adenocarcinoma. *Am J Clin Pathol* 1995; **104**: 620–6.

58. Malpica A, Ro JY, Troncoso P, Ordonez NG, Amin AB, Ayala AG, Nephrogenic adenoma of the prostatic urethra involving the prostate gland: a clinicopathologic and immunohistochemical study of eight cases. *Human Pathol* 1994; **25**: 390–5.

59. Hersmansen DK, Whitmore WF, Frozen section lymph node analysis in pelvic lymphadenectomy for prostate cancer. *J Urol* 1988; **139**: 1073.

60. Davis GL, Sensitivity of frozen section examination of pelvic lymph nodes for metastatic prostate carcinoma. *Cancer* 1995; **76**: 661–8.

61. McNeal JE, Villers AA, Redwine EA, Freiha FS, Tamey TA, Capsular penetration in prostate cancer. *Am J Surg Pathol* 1990; **14**: 240–7.

62. Cohen MB, Soloway MS, Murphy WM, Sampling of radical prostatectomy specimens; how much is adequate? *Am J Clin Pathol* 1994; **101**: 250–2.

63. Harnden P, Parkinson MC, Macroscopic examination of prostatic specimens. *J Clin Pathol* 1995; **48**: 693–700.

64. Epstein JI, Partin AW, Sauvageot J, Walsh PC, Prediction of progression following radical prostatectomy. *Am J Surg Pathol* 1996; **20**: 286–92.

65. Ohori M, Wheeler TM, Kattan MW, Goto Y, Scardino PT, Prognostic significance of positive surgical margins in radical prostatectomy specimens. *J Urol* 1995; **154**: 1818–24.

66. Epstein JI, Sauvageot J, Do close but negative margins in radical prostatectomy specimens increase the risk of postoperative progression? *J Urol* 1997; **157**: 241–3.

67. von Eschenbach AC, Brawer MK, di Sant'Agnese PA et al, Exploration of new pathological factors in terms of potential for prognostic significance and future applications. *Cancer* 1996; **78**: 372–5.

68. Mohler JL, Partin AW, Isaacs WB, Coffey DS, Time lapse videomicroscopic identification of Dunning R-3327 adenocarcinoma and normal rat prostate cells. *J Urol* 1987; **137**: 544–7.

69. Mohler JL, Partin AW, Coffey DS, Prediction of metastatic potential by a new grading system of cell motility: validation in the Dunning R-3327 prostatic adenocarcinoma model. *J Urol* 1987; **137**: 168–70.

3

Prostatic intraepithelial neoplasia

David G Bostwick

CONTENTS • **Epidemiology** • **Prevalence and age** • **Serum PSA levels** • **Pathology** • **Evidence linking PIN and cancer** • **Molecular biology** • **Clinical significance** • **PIN as a risk factor for cancer** • **Elimination of PIN**

Prostatic intraepithelial neoplasia (PIN) has emerged as the most likely preinvasive stage of adenocarcinoma since its first formal description more than 10 years ago.[1-4] This microscopic finding refers to the precancerous (dysplastic) end of the morphologic continuum of cellular proliferations within prostatic ducts and acini, with cytologic changes mimicking cancer, including nuclear and nucleolar enlargement (Figure 3.1). It coexists with cancer in the majority of cases, but retains an intact or fragmented basal cell layer, unlike cancer, which lacks a basal cell layer.[3] Studies to date have not determined whether PIN remains stable, regresses, or progresses, although most investigators believe that, if left unchecked, it will progress. Early invasive carcinoma occurs at sites of glandular out-pouching and basal cell disruption. A model of prostatic carcinogenesis has been proposed based on the morphologic continuum of PIN and the multi-step theory of transformation.[2]

The term 'prostatic intraepithelial neoplasia' has been endorsed at multiple consensus meetings,[4-6] including a recent international conference sponsored by the American Cancer Society and the World Health Organization, which was held at the Mayo Clinic in November 1995.[7]

This chapter describes the epidemiology of PIN, its pathological features and clinical significance, and the evidence suggesting that it progresses to prostatic adenocarcinoma. Chemoprevention trials are ongoing that target patients with high-grade PIN in the hope that modulation of this morphologic finding will decrease or eliminate the risk of subsequent adenocarcinoma.

EPIDEMIOLOGY

Incidence of PIN in needle biopsies

High-grade PIN is a frequent finding in needle biopsies, being present in up to 16.5% of cases (Figure 3.2).[8,9] The incidence varies according to the patient population under consideration (screening population versus urology office population). The American Cancer Society's National Cancer Detection Project identified PIN and cancer in 5.2% and 15.8% men, respectively, from a series of 330 biopsies from men participating in an early detection project, although this is probably an underestimate because the findings were taken from

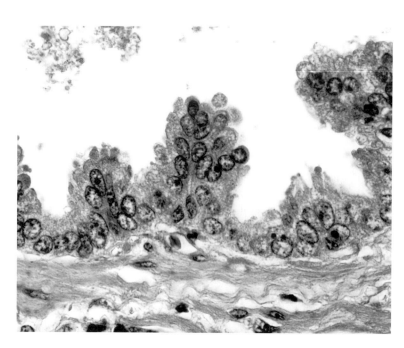

Figure 3.1 High-grade prostatic intraepithelial neoplasia.

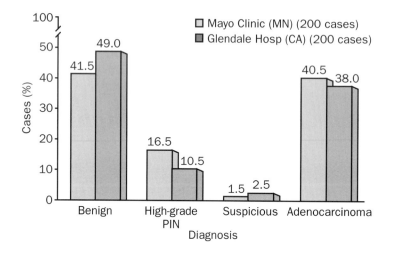

Figure 3.2 Pathologic findings in 200 consecutive prostate needle biopsies from an academic medical center (Mayo Clinic, Rochester, MN) and an equal number from a private practice laboratory (Glendale Memorial Hospital and Health Center, Glendale, CA). Note that high-grade prostatic intraepithelial neoplasia was identified in 10.5–16.5% of biopsies. (Data from Bostwick et al.[8])

pathology reports rather than a central slide review.[10] A urology practice study of 256 ultrasound-guided biopsies of hypoechoic lesions identified 27 cases of PIN (10.5%) and 103 cancers (40.2%); interestingly, those with PIN had a mean age of 65 years, whereas those with cancer were older, with a mean age of 70 years.[11] A recent European study of 148 consecutive biopsies identified high-grade PIN without cancer in 14% of specimens.[12]

Incidence of PIN in TURP specimens

The incidence of high-grade PIN in transurethral resections of the prostate (TURP) is 3.2–4.2% of cases, and is more often associated with prostatic cancer (10.2% of cases with cancer) than with nodular hyperplasia (benign prostatic hyperplasia, BPH) (2.8% of cases with BPH).[13,14] All cases of cancer with foci of PIN were well or moderately differentiated (Gleason score 3–5) and low grade (T1a or T1b).[13]

In radical prostatectomy specimens with cancer, high-grade PIN is present in the transition zone and peripheral zone simultaneously in 36% cases, and is found exclusively in the transition zone in 1% of cases.[15,16]

Association of BPH and high-grade PIN

High-grade PIN in transurethral resection specimens appears to be an important predictive factor for prostate cancer. Among 14 patients with PIN and BPH followed for up to 7 years (mean 5.9 years), three (21.4%) developed prostatic cancer.[13] The mean serum PSA concentration in these patients was higher (8.1 ng/ml) than in those who did not develop cancer (4.6 ng/ml). All subsequent cancers apparently arose in the peripheral zone and were detected by needle biopsy. These findings indicate that all additional tissue should be submitted for examination when high-grade PIN is found in TURP specimens. The high predictive value of PIN for development of subsequent prostatic cancer warrants reporting the presence of PIN in TURP specimens by the pathologist, as suggested by the Cancer Committee of the College of American Pathologists.[17] Serum prostate-specific antigen (PSA) concentration may further help in the identification of patients at risk for developing adenocarcinoma.

Association of BPH and prostate cancer

There are a number of similarities between BPH and cancer.[18] Both display a parallel increase in prevalence with patient age according to autopsy studies, although cancer lags by 15–20 years. Both require androgens for growth and development, and both may respond to androgen-deprivation treatment. Most cancers arise in prostates with concomitant BPH, and cancer is found incidentally in a significant number (10%) of TURP specimens. BPH may be related to prostate cancer arising in the transition zone, perhaps in association with certain forms of hyperplasia, but BPH is neither a premalignant lesion nor a precursor of carcinoma.

The optimal number of chips to submit for histologic evaluation from a TURP specimen remains controversial, with some authors preferring partial sampling and others advocating complete submission, even with large specimens which would require many cassettes. The Cancer Committee of the College of American Pathologists recommends a minimum of six cassettes for the first 30 g of tissue and one cassette for every 10 g thereafter.[17]

Clinical significance of cancer arising in BPH

The transition zone of the prostate, the region sampled by TURP, contains about 24% of all prostate cancers, including 75% of stage T1a and 79% of stage T1b cancers.[18] The high percentage of incidental cancers in the transition zone is probably due to selective sampling by TURP, and up to 30% stage T1 tumors could theoretically be removed completely by TURP. The majority of transition zone cancers arise in foci adjacent to BPH, with about one-third arising within BPH nodules; most are multifocal.

Transition-zone cancer is of lower malignant potential than cancer arising in the peripheral zone.[18–20] It is often of lower grade, and accounts for the majority of Gleason primary grade 1 and 2 cancers. Tumor volume tends to be smaller than that of tumors arising in the peripheral zone. Further, most transition-zone cancers display a distinctive columnar clear-cell pattern, which is infrequently observed in peripheral zone cancer; there is also a decreased likelihood of stromal fibrosis.

The confinement of transition-zone cancer to the anatomic site of origin may account in part for the favorable prognosis of clinical stage T1 cancer. The transition-zone boundary acts as a relative barrier to tumor extension, and malignant glands frequently fan out along this boundary before invasion into the peripheral and central zones. Transition-zone cancer preferentially clusters at the apex, similar to peripheral-zone cancer, but is less likely to show extraprostatic extension. Invasion into the anterior fibromuscular stroma can occur with small-volume tumors, but perforation is only seen with large tumors. Twenty-five percent of transition-zone cancers display extraprostatic extension of anterior fibromuscular stromal invasion, usually in the anterolateral and apical directions where the distance to the capsule is short. The risk of spread to the seminal vesicles and regional lymph nodes is significantly less than with peripheral-zone cancer.

The clinical significance of incidental carcinoma remains controversial. Recent studies indicate an increasing long-term risk for developing clinical carcinoma, progression, and death in patients with stage T1a tumors. In a series of 94 men with untreated stage T1a carcinomas identified by TURP, followed for more than 8 years, 16% developed progression, with a mean time to progression of 7 years.[21] Blute et al[22] found progression in 27% of 15 patients under 60 years of age with stage T1a carcinoma followed for 10 years or more. These studies indicate that patients with stage T1a prostate cancer are at risk for tumor progression.

The potential for significant clinical progression of stage T1b carcinoma is greater than that of stage T1a. Residual carcinoma has usually been found in subsequent prostatectomy specimens removed from patients with stage T1b carcinoma, with extraprostatic extension in up to 19% of cases. Most urologists aggressively treat stage T1b cancer, particularly when detected in younger patients. Long-term progression for untreated stage T1a cancer varies from 8% to 37%, with the risk of progression increasing with additional years of follow-up; survival at 10 years is 95%, similar to the age-specific survival, prompting the suggestion that treatment for this stage may be unnecessary.

Clinical understaging of incidental carcinoma can be a significant problem. The sensitivity of TURP in detecting stage T1 carcinoma is only 28%; in specimens for stage T1a carcinoma, 40–92% of patients will have residual carcinoma, and about 26% will be upstaged.[21] Even in those with substantial residual tumor, the location of the tumor in the peripheral and apical regions often makes it inaccessible to TURP.[21] The aggregate results challenge the utility of examining TURP specimens to stage prostatic carcinoma, due to the imprecision of this technique.

PREVALENCE AND AGE

The incidence and extent of PIN appear to increase with patient age.[11,23–26] Kovi et al[23] found that the prevalence of PIN in prostates with cancer increased with age, predating the onset of carcinoma by more than 5 years. Lee et al[11] found that the mean age of men with PIN (65 years) was significantly lower than the age of those with cancer (70 years). Qian et al[16] recently reported that the extent (volume) of high-grade PIN increased as patient age increased.

In a large study of forensic autopsy prostates, Sakr and colleagues[24–26] found that high-grade PIN was first identified in the third decade, and increased steadily with age. It was more prevalent and extensive in African–American men, being present in 18%, 31%, 69%, 78%, and 86% of these men in their fourth, fifth, sixth, seventh, and eighth decades, respectively; the corresponding figures for Caucasian men were 14%, 21%, 38%, 50%, and 63%, respectively. This differed from latent carcinoma, which increased steadily with age, but showed no significant difference between the two races. High-grade PIN in African–American men appeared to precede that of Caucasian men by about a decade. These racial differences have implications in epidemiology, screening, and chemoprevention of prostate cancer, and underscore the importance of race as a risk factor.

A large autopsy study of 180 Brazilian men revealed high-grade PIN in 84% of cases, with an equal prevalence in white and African–Brazilian males.[27]

SERUM PSA LEVELS

Conflicting findings have been reported regarding the relationship between PIN and serum PSA concentration. Brawer et al[28] studied 65 men undergoing TURP or open simple prostatectomy, and found that mean serum PSA concentration in patients with PIN alone (5.6 ng/ml) was intermediate between that of benign tissue (2.1 ng/ml) and carcinoma (35.1 ng/ml). They also found that a group of 87 patients who underwent needle biopsy of peripheral-zone hypoechoic lesions with a palpable prostatic abnormality with PIN alone had a mean serum PSA concentration that was intermediate (7.8 ng/ml), between that of benign glands (5.8 ng/ml) and carcinoma (18.3 ng/ml). Lee et al[11] evaluated 248 consecutive transrectal needle biopsy specimens, and found that the mean log(serum PSA) concentration in patients with high-grade PIN (1.85) was intermediate between that of patients with benign tissue (1.09) and those with carcinoma (2.79). These studies suggest that PIN contributes to serum PSA concentration.

Most recent studies suggest that there is no significant correlation between PIN and serum PSA concentration.[29–31] Ronnett et al[29] studied 65 patients with prostate cancer who underwent radical prostatectomy, and found that high-grade PIN volume did not correlate with serum PSA concentration or PSA density. Similarly, Alexander et al[30] studied a series of 194 radical prostatectomies, and found that PIN volume did not correlate with serum PSA concentration or PSA density after correcting for gland weight and cancer volume. They concluded that PIN does not contribute significantly to serum PSA concentration, and suggested that patients with high-grade PIN and elevated serum PSA concentration may benefit from early repeat biopsy; patients with high-grade PIN and normal serum PSA also need to be followed clinically, but the risk of subsequent cancer is lower. Marley et al[31] studied a total of 615 patients, and found that the ratio of free to total PSA distinguished PIN and carcinoma, but total PSA did not.

Immunohistochemical studies reveal that expression of PSA in PIN is less than that observed in benign epithelium and cancer.[32] PIN is an abnormality within pre-existing ducts and acini, and cytoplasmic secretory products such as PSA would be expected to wash into the lumina and travel downstream rather than escape into the stroma and blood vessels.

PATHOLOGY

PIN is divided into two grades (low grade and high grade) to replace the previous three-grade scale: prostatic intraepithelial neoplasia 1 is considered low grade, and neoplasia 2 and 3 are considered high grade. The term 'prostatic intraepithelial neoplasia' is usually used to indicate high-grade PIN. The high level of interobserver variability with low-grade PIN limits its clinical utility, and many pathologists do not report this finding.[33,34] Interobserver agreement for high-grade PIN is 'good to excellent'.

There are four architectural patterns of high-grade PIN: tufting, micropapillary, cribriform, and flat.[35] The tufting pattern is the most common, being present in 97% of radical prostatectomies with PIN and cancer, although most cases have multiple patterns. There is no prognostic difference between the architectural patterns of high-grade PIN, and their recognition appears to be only of diagnostic utility.

Crowding of the secretory cell layer is pronounced in PIN, in marked contrast with most benign acini. Along the luminal surface, the cells often display cytoplasmic apocrine-like blebs. The most striking cytologic findings are nuclear and nucleolar enlargement, these being diagnostic hallmarks of high-grade PIN. The nuclei are usually uniformly enlarged in the most severe foci, although some may be shrunken and hyperchromatic, probably representing degenerative changes; in less severe foci (formerly PIN grades 1 and 2) greater variability in nuclear size is observed, but some markedly enlarged forms are present. Nucleoli may be single or multiple, and are often eccentric or apposed to the chromatinic rim.

Early stromal invasion, the earliest morphologic indication of carcinoma, occurs at sites of glandular out-pouching and basal cell disruption in acini with high-grade PIN.[2,36] Such microinvasion is present in about 2% of high-power microscopic fields of PIN, and is seen with equal frequency with all architectural patterns.[35] A model of prostatic carcinogenesis has been proposed based on the morphologic continuum of PIN and the multistep theory of transformation.[2]

EVIDENCE LINKING PIN AND CANCER

Basal cell layer

Increasing grades of PIN are associated with progressive disruption of the basal cell layer.[2,37] Basal cell-specific monoclonal antibodies directed against high-molecular-weight keratin (e.g. clone 34 β-E12) immunohistochemically and selectively label the prostatic basal cell layer. Tumor cells consistently fail to be decorated with this antibody, whereas normal prostatic epithelial cells are invariably stained, with a continuous intact circumferential basal cell layer in most instances. Basal cell layer disruption is present in 56% of cases of high-grade PIN, and is more common in glands adjacent to invasive carcinoma than in distant glands. Also, the amount of disruption increases with increasing grade of PIN, there being a loss of more than one-third of the basal cell layer in 52% of foci of high-grade PIN. These findings have been confirmed by knowledge-guided histometry.[37]

The basal cell layer contains a subset of stem cells that acts as the proliferative compartment of the prostatic epithelium. In high-grade PIN, the apoptosis-suppressing bcl-2 oncoprotein extends from the basal cell layer into the secretory luminal cells, which, in turn, may increase the genetic instability of the dysplastic epithelium. PIN may arise from transformed stem cells in the basal cell layer, but this theory remains unconfirmed.

The basement membrane normally surrounding prostatic glands is intact in PIN and most cases of well-differentiated adenocarcinoma, indicating that this is not a prerequisite of early stromal invasion.[38,39] There is also increased expression of type IV collagenase in PIN and cancer compared with benign epithelium;[40] collagenase is a proteolytic enzyme that is thought to induce fragmentation of the stroma during invasion.

Microvessel density

Growth and metastasis of prostate cancer require new blood vessels for sustenance.[41] The number of microvessels in high-grade PIN is greater than that in benign or hyperplastic prostatic epithelium, but less than that in adenocarcinoma.[41,42] The microvessels in prostatic intraepithelial neoplasia are shorter than those in benign epithelium, with irregular contours and open lumina, an increased number of endothelial cells, and a greater distance from the basement membrane.

Cell proliferation and death (apoptosis)

Tumor growth represents a delicate balance between cell proliferation and cell death, which is dependent on a variety of influences, including patient age, nutritional status, hormonal status, and growth factor milieu. This balance is usually altered in malignant transformation, resulting in increased growth due to increased cell proliferation, decreased cell death, or a combination of these factors.

Prostate cancer has a relatively slow doubling time when compared with cancers from other organs, being estimated at between 6 months and 5 years, depending in part on tumor grade. Serial measurements of PSA indicate that prostate cancer has a constant log–linear growth rate, with mean doubling times of 2.4 years for localized cancer and 1.8 years for metastatic cancer.[43,44] Higher Gleason grades are associated with shorter doubling times. The mean growth fraction is 8.7–16.3%, according to immunohistochemical studies using antibodies directed against proliferating cell nuclear antigen (PCNA) and Ki-67, with the highest growth rates at the advancing edge.[45] By comparison, the growth fraction is 0.6% in atrophic prostatic glands, 3.2–4.0% in BPH, 6.0–9.5% in low-grade PIN, and 7.9–13.8% in high-grade PIN. The intermediate levels of doubling times in PIN when compared with BPH and cancer is considered evidence of the role of PIN as a putative premalignant lesion.

Mitotic figures are rare in the epithelium of the benign and neoplastic prostate, but there is a progressive increase from BPH through PIN to carcinoma.[46,47] Mitotic figures in BPH are present exclusively in the basal cell layer, with a mean value of 0.002%. In PIN, the number of mitotic figures was highest in the basal cell layer, with a progressive decrease through the cell layers to those at the luminal surface. For low-grade PIN, the mean value was 0.09% in the basal layer, 0.05% in the intermediate layer, and 0.02% in the superficial layer. For high-grade PIN, the mean value was 0.19% in the basal layer, 0.08% in the intermediate layer, and 0.05% in the superficial layer. In low-grade PIN, the percentages were slightly lower than those in high-grade PIN. The number of mitotic figures in the small acinar pattern of cancer was quite similar to that of low-grade PIN and close to that in the large acinar pattern of cancer, with mean values of 0.06% and 0.07%, respectively.

Apoptotic bodies are present throughout the normal prostatic epithelium and in gland lumina in all cases. They are usually seen in intercellular spaces and occasionally within the cytoplasm of epithelial cells, the latter being observed more often in PIN and carcinoma than in benign epithelium.[47] There is a progressive increase in the number of apoptotic bodies from BPH through PIN to adenocarcinoma, and the greatest frequency is invariably in the basal cell layer (or, in the case of carcinoma, in cells at the periphery of the malignant glands adjacent to the stroma); these trends are virtually identical to those seen with PCNA immunoreactivity.[45] The percentage of apoptotic bodies was greater in low-grade PIN, high-grade PIN, and adenocarcinoma than in BPH (0.68%, 0.75%, and 0.92–2.10% vs 0.26%, respectively).

There is no apparent association of mitotic figures and apoptotic bodies.

There was greater cytoplasmic expression of the apoptosis-suppressing oncoprotein bcl-2 in PIN (100% of epithelial cells) and cancer (62% of cells) than in benign and hyperplastic epithelium (basal cells only).[48] Expression of bcl-2 might play a role in the progression of PIN and/or low-grade cancer by interfering with apoptosis. Suppression of cell death by bcl-2 might result in accumulation of genetic abnormalities, perhaps increasing the clinical aggressiveness of cancer.

Phenotypic similarity

Virtually all studies of phenotypic biomarkers have indicated that high-grade PIN is more closely related to carcinoma than to benign epithelium (reviewed by Bostwick et al[49]). There is increased cytoplasmic expression of p160erbB3 and p185erbB2 in PIN and cancer compared with normal or hyperplastic epithelium,[50] similar to other biomarkers in the prostate, including epidermal growth factor, epidermal growth factor receptor,[51] and transforming growth factor-α. Increased cell proliferation is the most likely explanation for this phenotypic similarity of normal basal cells, PIN, and cancer, suggesting that the basal cells are the regenerative or stem cells of the prostate.[52]

Other biomarkers show progressive loss of expression with increasing grades of PIN and cancer, including markers of secretory differentiation such as PSA, secretory proteins, cytoskeletal proteins, glycoproteins, and neuroendocrine cells. Reduction of cytoplasmic differentiation markers during the preinvasive phase may be followed by abrupt re-expression at the site of microinvasion.[36,53] There is also a progressive decrease in the number of neuroendocrine cells in normal epithelium, high-grade PIN, and carcinoma.[54] These results indicate that there is progressive impairment of cell differentiation and regulatory control with advancing stages of prostatic carcinogenesis. Changes in cytoskeletal proteins in PIN may affect transport of cell products, accounting for the differences in secretory protein distribution.[55]

Morphometric similarity

Virtually all measures of nuclear abnormality by computer-based image analysis reveal the similarity of PIN and cancer, in contrast with normal and hyperplastic epithelium.[56–60] These changes include nuclear area, DNA content, chromatin content and distribution, nuclear perimeter, nuclear diameter, and nuclear roundness. Also, most measures of nucleolar abnormality reveal the similarity of PIN and cancer, in contrast with normal epithelium. Layfield and Goldstein[60] found that core and needle biopsies were more reliable than fine-needle aspiration biopsy in separating PIN from cancer, based on a morphometric study of 50 'atypical' cases. The cumulative data indicate that the morphologic continuum from PIN to cancer is characterized by progressive morphometric abnormalities of nuclei and nucleoli.

Ultrastructure

PIN and prostatic adenocarcinoma are morphologically heterogeneous, and this heterogeneity is reflected in the ultrastructural findings.[61,62] Cells with light and dark cytoplasm are present in varying proportions, probably reflecting the relative proportion of secretory vacuoles. The clear cells of PIN contain a large number of secretory vacuoles in the apical and basal portions, similar to the distinctive clear cells typically present in benign prostatic epithelium. Homogeneous dark cells are also often present in PIN, but these are much more common in prostate carcinoma. PIN and cancer both contain secretory vacuoles, a large number of mitochondria, lysosomes, microtubules, and free ribosomes.

PIN consists of a mixture of cells with clear and homogeneous dark cytoplasm and a decreased number of basal cells as compared with normal acini. Apocrine secretions are char-

acteristic of PIN. Prominent nucleoli are frequent, similar to cancer cells. Dilated nuclear envelopes and irregular stretched and multilobulated nuclei are infrequent in PIN and well to moderately differentiated cancer.[62]

The basement membrane in PIN is usually thin and intact, but shows occasional small foci of disruption, although not as much as that in adenocarcinoma; this loss of structural integrity in adenocarcinoma is apparently due to loss of type IV collagen,[38,63] but not heparan sulfate proteoglycan.[39] Basement membrane thinning and disruption occur only in sites with few or no basal cells, perhaps representing early stromal invasion. Such changes in the basement membrane may not be visible by light microscopy using immunohistochemical methods, probably due to differences in resolution from electron microscopy. Basement membrane disruption may result from defects in products of acquisition of membrane lysis activity, perhaps due to collagenase or matrix metalloproteinases such as pro-MMP-9.[64]

MOLECULAR BIOLOGY

The continuum that culminates in high-grade PIN and early invasive cancer is characterized by progressive basal cell layer disruption, abnormalities in markers of secretory differentiation, increasing nuclear and nucleolar alterations, increasing cell proliferation, variation in DNA content, and increasing genetic instability (reviewed by Bostwick et al[49]) (Figure 3.3). Some biomarkers show upregulation or gain in the progression from benign prostatic epithelium to high-grade PIN and cancer, whereas others are downregulated or lost. Existing data indicate that more biomarkers are upregulated, but the relative importance of each is unknown. There is a prominent clustering of changes in expression for many biomarkers between benign epithelium and high-grade PIN, indicating that this is an important threshold for carcinogenesis in the prostate; PIN shows marked genetic heterogeneity and impairment of cell differentiation and regulatory control. A smaller number of changes are

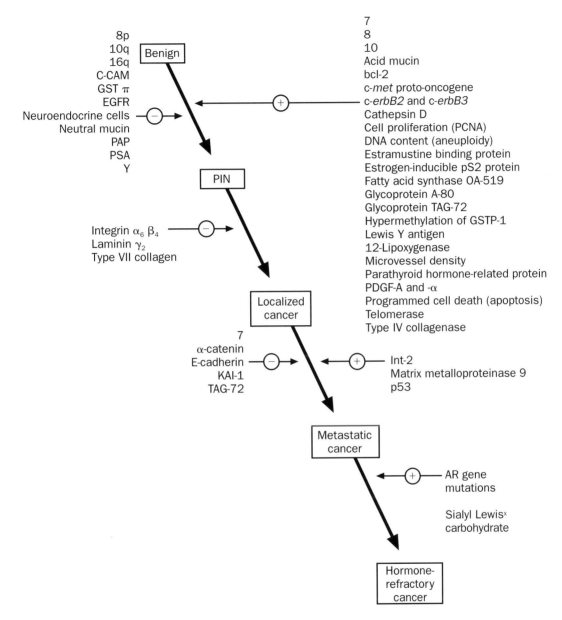

Figure 3.3 Genetic changes and other changes associated with progression of prostate cancer. Some biomarkers show upregulation or gain (+), whereas others are downregulated or lost (−). (Reprinted with permission from Bostwick et al.[49])

introduced in the progression from high-grade PIN to localized cancer, metastatic cancer, and hormone-refractory cancer. This scheme indicates the initial change in expression of a biomarker, but most of these changes become magnified in subsequent steps. The model is based chiefly on studies of human prostatic tissue, and excludes many biomarkers that have not been evaluated in PIN or different stages of cancer.

CLINICAL SIGNIFICANCE

The clinical importance of recognizing PIN is based on its strong association with prostatic carcinoma. Because PIN has a high predictive value as a marker for adenocarcinoma, its identification in biopsy specimens warrants further search for concurrent invasive carcinoma. This is particularly true for high-grade PIN; if this lesion is identified, close surveillance and follow-up biopsy appear to be indicated.

To examine the predictive value of high-grade PIN, Davidson et al[65] conducted a retrospective case-control study of 100 patients with needle biopsies with high-grade PIN and 112 biopsies without PIN matched for clinical stage, patient age, and serum PSA. Adenocarcinoma was identified in 35% of subsequent biopsies from cases with PIN, compared with 13% in the control group (Figure 3.4). The likelihood of finding cancer was greater in patients with PIN undergoing more than one follow-up biopsy (44%) than in those with only one biopsy (32%). High-grade PIN, patient age, and serum PSA level were jointly highly significant predictors of cancer, with PIN providing the highest risk ratio (14.93; 95% confidence intervals 5.6–39.8). No other candidate predictor was found to be significant, including patient race, digital rectal examination findings, transrectal ultrasound results, amount of PIN on biopsy, and architectural pattern of PIN.

Others have reported a high predictive value of PIN for cancer.[66–74] In one study of 37 patients with PIN identified on needle core biopsy, 14 (38%) had carcinoma identified on subsequent biopsy within 8 years.[69] Of 48 patients with a clinical suspicion of cancer and negative aspiration biopsies, follow-up aspiration revealed PIN in 15 (31%) and invasive carcinoma in 8 (17%). Another study of PIN diagnosed by fine-needle aspiration revealed that 13 or 32 patients with high-grade PIN developed cancer, compared with 3 or 23 with low-grade PIN; the patients were followed for 18 months with re-biopsy.[66] These data underscore the strong association of PIN and adenocarcinoma and indicate that diagnostic follow-up is needed. The optimal repeat biopsy strategy should include both sides of the prostate.[74]

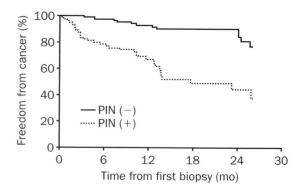

Figure 3.4 Freedom from cancer from time of first biopsy according to the presence or absence of high-grade PIN. (Reprinted with permission from Davidson et al.[65])

PIN AS A RISK FACTOR FOR CANCER

Increased frequency, severity, and extent of PIN with cancer

The frequency of PIN in prostates with cancer is significantly increased when compared with prostates without cancer.[1,15] McNeal and Bostwick[1] observed PIN in 82% of step-sectioned autopsy prostates with cancer, but in only 43% of benign prostates from patients of similar age. Qian et al[15] found that 86% of a series of 195 whole-mount radical prostatectomies with cancer contained high-grade PIN, usually within 2 mm of cancer. The severity of PIN in prostates with cancer was also increased when compared with prostates without cancer.[15] The extent of PIN was more extensive in lower stage tumors, presumably due to 'overgrowth' or obliteration of PIN by larger high-stage tumors.[75]

There have been conflicting reports concerning the relationship of volume of PIN and volume of cancer, probably due to differences in the method used for measurement or difficulty in identifying PIN in some fields with adenocarcinoma. The positive correlation between

PIN and cancer reported by Qian et al[15] was only significant for PIN within 2 mm of cancer; conversely, a negative correlation of PIN and cancer was found by others, and these results were attributed to overgrowth and replacement of PIN by cancer.[23,75,76]

The mean volume of PIN in prostates with cancer is 1.2–1.32 cm^3.[15] The volume of PIN increases with increasing pathologic stage, Gleason grade, positive surgical margins, and perineural invasion. These findings underscore the close spatial and biologic relationship of PIN and cancer, and may be secondary to the increase in PIN with increasing cancer volume.

Multifocality and location

PIN and cancer are usually multicentric. One study found that PIN was multicentric in 72% of radical prostatectomies with cancer, including 63% of those involving the non-transition zone and 7% of those involving the transition zone; 2% of cases had concomitant single foci in all zones.[35] These findings are in agreement with previous reports.[25,36]

The peripheral zone of the prostate, the area in which the majority of prostatic carcinomas occur (70%), is also the most common location for PIN.[16,23,35,36,75,76] Cancer and PIN are frequently multifocal in the peripheral zone, indicating a 'field' effect similar to the multifocality of urothelial carcinoma of the bladder. The majority of foci of high-grade PIN are exclusively in the peripheral zone (in one study, 63% of cases) or simultaneously in the transition and peripheral zones (36%); only rare cases (1%) are exclusively in the transition zone.[16]

The transition zone and periurethral area, the anatomic areas in which nodular hyperplasia occurs, account for about 20–25% of cases of prostate cancer, and harbor foci of PIN in 2–37% of cases.[16,23] The highest frequency of involvement of the transition zone (37%) is in radical prostatectomies with cancer; the lowest is in studies of transurethral resections or only small numbers of patients. These results have important implications for the origin of prostatic carcinoma in the transition zone; if PIN is the precursor for many cases of prostate cancer as has been proposed, this level of involvement of the transition zone by PIN is sufficiently high to account for the relative frequency (25%) of cancer at this site.

ELIMINATION OF PIN

There is a marked decrease in the prevalence and extent of high-grade PIN after androgen-deprivation therapy compared with untreated cases (Figure 3.5).[77–79] This decrease is accompanied by epithelial hyperplasia, cytoplasmic clearing, and prominent glandular atrophy, with decreased ratio of glands to stroma. These findings indicate that the dysplastic prostatic epithelium is hormone dependent. In the normal prostatic epithelium, luminal secretory cells are more sensitive to the absence of androgen than are basal cells, and these results show that the cells of high-grade PIN share this androgen sensitivity. The loss of some normal, hyperplastic, and dysplastic epithelial cells with androgen deprivation is probably due to acceleration of programmed single-cell death (apoptosis), with subsequent exfoliation into glandular lumina.[48,80]

Premalignant lesions such as high-grade PIN identify patients at high risk for developing invasive cancer, and these are ideal target populations for chemoprevention trials. The most efficient strategy for developing a chemoprevention program may be to perform two clinical trials concurrently, each based on the modulation of high-grade PIN but in different target populations. In patients with high-grade PIN associated with prostate cancer, a prospective, double-blind, placebo-controlled chemoactive pilot study designed to measure the response of a potential chemopreventive agent in the period (3–6 weeks) before radical prostatectomy could be performed easily. Androgen-deprivation therapy is commonly used in this population to downsize the prostate before radical prostatectomy. This study would determine the response of PIN to the agent in whole-mounted radical prostatectomy specimens.

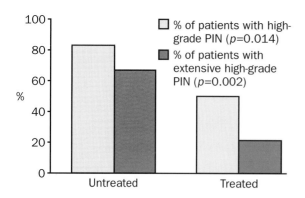

Figure 3.5 Histogram comparing the prevalence and extent of high-grade PIN following androgen deprivation in 24 treated and 24 untreated patients. Dark bars indicate prevalence; light bars indicate extent in high-power microscopic fields. (Reprinted with permission from Ferguson et al.[77])

A short-term, prospective, double-blind, placebo-controlled, phase II chemoprevention trial with cancer incidence as an end-point could be done simultaneously in patients with high-grade PIN without cancer. Chemo-prevention trials designed to reverse high-grade PIN may be confounded by the presence of underlying but undetected prostate cancer. This difficult problem is addressed by requiring a second biopsy with negative findings for cancer before entry into the study (preferably sextant biopsies with special attention to areas of abnormality on ultrasonogram or digital rectal examination) and by including enough subjects in the study and control groups to equalize the risk of coexistent cancer between the two groups.[81–83] PIN is routinely monitored by repeat biopsy in contemporary urologic practice. Periodic re-evaluation would be necessary, including physical examination, re-biopsy, and surrogate intermediate end-point biomarkers. If subsequent biopsy reveals prostate cancer, these patients need active treatment. Those

with PIN or no malignancy need continued observation.

This approach, utilizing concurrently performed chemopreventive and chemoactive trials, would provide valuable complementary information. Findings would be immediately applicable to long-term treatment for patients with high-grade PIN. These study methods are consistent with current urologic practice and would allow other promising chemopreventive agents to be evaluated in a comparable design. The information gained could provide the basis for additional clinical trials directed at the prevention and elimination of the prostate cancer in other high-risk target populations and in the general population.

Blockade of 5α-reductase with finasteride appears to have less effect than other forms of androgen-deprivation therapy. The incidence of PIN was unchanged after 1 year of finasteride, and there was a significant increase in the number of patients with subsequent cancer on biopsy after this treatment.[84]

SUMMARY

High-grade PIN is the most likely precursor of prostatic adenocarcinoma, according to virtually all available evidence. It has a high predictive value as a marker for adenocarcinoma, and its identification in biopsy specimens of the prostate warrants further search for concurrent invasive carcinoma. Most studies suggest that PIN will, if left untreated, progress to early carcinoma. Androgen-deprivation therapy decreases its prevalence and extent, suggesting a role for this therapy in chemoprevention. Prostatic intraepithelial neoplasia does not appear to elevate serum PSA concentration.

PIN is associated with progressive abnormalities of phenotype and genotype that are intermediate between those of normal prostatic epithelium and cancer, indicating impairment of cell differentiation and regulatory control with advancing stages of prostatic carcinogenesis.

REFERENCES

1. McNeal JE, Bostwick DG, Intraductal dysplasia: a premalignant lesion of the prostate. *Human Pathol* 1986; **17:** 64–71.
2. Bostwick DG, Brawer MK, Prostatic intra-epithelial neoplasia and early invasion in prostate cancer. *Cancer* 1987; **59:** 788–94.
3. Bostwick DG, High grade prostatic intraepithelial neoplasia: the most likely precursor of prostate cancer. *Cancer* 1995; **75:** 1823–36.
4. Graham SD Jr, Bostwick DG, Hoisaeter A et al, Report of the Committee on Staging and Pathology. *Cancer* 1992; **70**(suppl): 359–61.
5. Drago JR, Mostofi FK, Lee F, Introductory Remarks and Workshop Summary. *Urology* 1989; **34**(suppl): 2–3.
6. Algaba F, Epstein JI, Fabus G, Helpap B, Nagle RB, Polito M, Working standards in prostatic intraepithelial neoplasia and atypical adenomatous hyperplasia. *Pathol Res Pract* 1995; **91:** 836–7.
7. Montironi R, Bostwick DG, Bonkhoff H et al, Origins of prostate cancer. *Cancer* 1996; **78:** 362–5.
8. Bostwick DG, Qian J, Frankel K, The incidence of high grade prostatic intraepithelial neoplasia in needle biopsies. *J Urol* 1995; **154:** 1791–4.
9. Wills ML, Hamper UM, Partin AW, Epstein JI, Incidence of high-grade prostatic intraepithelial neoplasia in sextant needle biopsy specimens. *Urology* 1997; **49:** 367–73.
10. Mettlin C, Lee F, Drago J, Murphy GP, and the Investigators of the American Cancer Society National Prostate Cancer Detection Project, The American Cancer Society National Prostate Cancer Detection Project. Findings on the detection of early prostate cancer in 2425 men. *Cancer* 1991; **67:** 2949–58.
11. Lee F, Torp-Pedersen ST, Carroll JT, Siders DB, Christensen-Day C, Mitchell AE, Use of transrectal ultrasound and prostate-specific antigen in diagnosis of prostatic intraepithelial neoplasia. *Urology* 1989; **24**(suppl): 4–8.
12. Perachino M, di Ciolo L, Barbetti V et al, Results of rebiopsy for suspected prostate cancer in symptomatic men with elevated PSA levels. *Eur Urol* 1997; **32:** 155–9.
13. Pacelli A, Bostwick DG, The clinical significance of high-grade prostatic intraepithelial neoplasia in transurethral resection specimens. *Urology* 1997; **50:** 355–9.
14. Gaudin PB, Sesterhenn IA, Wojno KJ et al, Incidence and clinical significance of high-grade prostatic intraepithelial neoplasia in TURP specimens. *Urology* 1997; **49:** 558–63.
15. Qian J, Bostwick DG, The extent and zonal location of prostatic intraepithelial neoplasia and atypical adenomatous hyperplasia: relationship with carcinoma in radical prostatectomy specimens. *Pathol Res Pract* 1995; **191:** 860–7.
16. Qian J, Wollan P, Bostwick DG, The extent and multicentricity of high grade prostatic intraepithelial neoplasia in clinically localized prostatic adenocarcinoma. *Human Pathol* 1997; **28:** 143–8.
17. Henson DE, Hutter RV, Farrow G, Practice protocol for the examination of specimens removed from patients with carcinoma of the prostate gland. *Arch Pathol Lab Med* 1994; **118:** 779–83.
18. Bostwick DG, Cooner WH, Denis L, Jones GW, Scardino PT, Murphy GP, The association of benign prostatic hyperplasia and cancer of the prostate. *Cancer* 1992; **70**(suppl): 291–301.
19. McNeal JE, Redwine EA, Freiha FS, Stamey TA, Zonal distribution of prostatic adenocarcinoma: correlation with histologic pattern and direction of spread. *Am J Surg Pathol* 1988; **12:** 897–906.
20. Greene DR, Wheeler TM, Egawa S, Dunn JK, Scardino PT, A comparison of the morphological features of cancer arising in the transition zone and in the peripheral zone of the prostate. *J Urol* 1991; **146:** 1069–76.
21. Epstein JI, Oesterling JE, Walsh PC, The volume and anatomical location of residual tumor in radical prostatectomy specimens removed for stage A1 prostate cancer. *J Urol* 1988; **139:** 975–9.
22. Blute ML, Zincke H, Farrow GM, Long-term follow-up of young patients with stage A adenocarcinoma of the prostate. *J Urol* 1986; **136:** 840–3.
23. Kovi J, Mostofi FK, Heshmat MY, Enterline JP, Large acinar atypical hyperplasia and carcinoma of the prostate. *Cancer* 1988; **61:** 555–61.
24. Sakr WA, Haas GP, Cassin BJ, Pontes JE, Crissman JD, Frequency of carcinoma and intraepithelial neoplasia of the prostate in young male patients. *J Urol* 1993; **150:** 379–85.
25. Sakr WA, Haas GP, Grignon DJ et al, High grade prostatic intraepithelial neoplasia (HG prostatic intraepithelial neoplasia) and prostatic adenocarcinoma between the ages of 20–69. An autopsy study of 249 cases. *In Vivo* 1994; **8:** 439–44.
26. Sakr WA, Grignon DJ, Haas GP et al, Epidemiology of high grade prostatic intraepithelial neoplasia. *Pathol Res Pract* 1995; **191:** 838–41.

27. Billis A, Age and race distribution of high-grade prostatic intraepithelial neoplasia. An autopsy study in Brazil (South America). *J Urol Pathol* 1996; **5:** 1–7.

28. Brawer MK, Lange PH, Prostate-specific antigen and premalignant change: implications for early detection. *CA* 1989; **39:** 361–75.

29. Ronnett BM, Carmichael MJ, Carter HB et al, Does high grade prostatic intraepithelial neoplasia result in elevated serum prostate specific antigen levels? *J Urol* 1993; **150:** 386–9.

30. Alexander EE, Qian J, Wollan PC, Myers RP, Bostwick DG, Prostatic intraepithelial neoplasia does not appear to raise serum prostate specific antigen. *Urology* 1996; **47:** 693–8.

31. Marley GM, Miller MC, Smith J, O'Dowd GJ, Veltri RW, Free/total prostate specific antigen serum ratios distinguish high-grade prostatic intraepithelial neoplasia from prostate cancer. *J Urol* 1997; **157**(4 suppl): 61(abstr).

32. McNeal JE, Alroy J, Leave I et al, Immuno-histochemical evidence for impaired cell differentiation in the premalignant phase of prostate carcinogenesis. *Am J Clin Pathol* 1988; **90:** 23–32.

33. Epstein JI, Grignon DJ, Humphrey PA et al, Interobserver reproducibility in the diagnosis of prostatic intraepithelial neoplasia. *Am J Surg Pathol* 1995; **19:** 873–86.

34. Allam CK, Bostwick DG, Hayes JA et al, Interobserver variability in the diagnosis of high-grade prostatic intraepithelial neoplasia and adeno-carcinoma. *Mod Pathol* 1996; **9:** 742–51.

35. Bostwick DG, Amin MB, Dundore P, Marsh W, Schultz DS, Architectural patterns of high grade prostatic intraepithelial neoplasia. *Human Pathol* 1993; **24:** 298–310.

36. McNeal JE, Villers A, Redwine EA, Freiha FS, Stamey TA, Microcarcinoma in the prostate: its association with duct–acinar dysplasia. *Human Pathol* 1991; **22:** 644–52.

37. Thompson D, Bartels PH, Bartels HG, Montironi R, Knowledge-guided histometry of the basal cell layer in prostatic intraepithelial neoplasia. *Anal Quant Cytol Histol* 1996; **18:** 177–84.

38. Schultz DS, Amin MB, Zarbo RJ, Basement membrane type IV collagen immunohistochemical staining in prostatic neoplasia. *Appl Immunohistochem* 1993; **1:** 123–6.

39. Bostwick DG, Leske DA, Qian J, Sinha AA, Prostatic intraepithelial neoplasia and well differentiated adenocarcinoma maintain an intact basement membrane. *Pathol Res Pract* 1995; **191:** 850–5.

40. Boag AH, Young ID, Increased expression of the 72-kd type IV collagenase in prostatic adenocarcinoma. Demonstration by immunohistochemistry and in situ hybridization. *Am J Pathol* 1994; **144:** 585–91.

41. Bigler SA, Deering RE, Brawer MK, Comparison of microscopic vascularity in benign and malignant prostate tissue. *Human Pathol* 1993; **24:** 220–6.

42. Montironi R, Magi Galluzzi C, Diamanti L et al, Prostatic intraepithelial neoplasia. Qualitative and quantitative analyses of the blood capillary architecture on thin tissue sections. *Pathol Res Pract* 1993; **189:** 542–8.

43. Hanks GE, D'Amico A, Epstein BE, Schultheiss TE, Prostatic-specific antigen doubling times in patients with prostate cancer: a potentially useful reflection of tumor doubling time. *Int J Rad Oncol Biol Phys* 1993; **27:** 125–7.

44. Schmid HP, McNeal JE, Stamey TA, Observations on the doubling time of prostate cancer. The use of serial prostate-specific antigen in patients with untreated disease as a measure of increasing cancer volume. *Cancer* 1993; **71:** 2031–40.

45. Montironi R, Magi Galluzzi C, Diamanti L et al, Prostatic intraepithelial neoplasia. Expression and location of proliferating cell nuclear antigen (PCNA) in epithelial, endothelial and stromal nuclei. *Virchow Arch [A] Pathol Anat* 1993; **422:** 185–92.

46. Gainnulis I, Montironi R, Galluzzi CM et al, Frequency and location of mitoses in prostatic intraepithelial neoplasia (PIN). *Anticancer Res* 1993; **13:** 2447–52.

47. Montironi R, Magi Galluzzi C, Scarpelli M, Giannulis I, Diamanti L, Occurrence of cell death (apoptosis) in prostatic intra-epithelial neoplasia. *Virchows Arch [A] Pathol Anat* 1993; **423:** 351–7.

48. Colombel M, Symmans F, Gil S et al, Detection of the apoptosis-suppressing oncoprotein bcl-2 in hormone-refractory human prostate cancers. *Am J Pathol* 1993; **143:** 390–400.

49. Bostwick DG, Pacelli A, Lopez-Beltran A, Molecular biology of prostatic intraepithelial neoplasia. *Prostate* 1996; **29:** 117–34.

50. Myers RB, Srivastava S, Oelschlager DK et al, Expression of p160erbB-3 and p185erbB-2 in prostatic intraepithelial neoplasia and prostatic adenocarcinoma. *J Natl Cancer Inst* 1994; **86:** 1140–4.

51. Maygarden SJ, Strom S, Ware JL, Localization of epidermal growth factor receptor by immunohis-

tochemical methods in human prostatic carcinoma, prostatic intraepithelial neoplasia, and benign hyperplasia. *Arch Pathol Lab Med* 1992; **116:** 269–73.

52. Bostwick DG, Devaraj L, Basal cell proliferations and tumors of the prostate. In: *Pathology of the Prostate* (Foster C, Bostwick DG, eds). WB Saunders: Philadelphia, PA, 1998: 157–71.

53. McNeal JE, Villers A, Redwine EA, Freiha FS, Stamey TA, Microcarcinoma in the prostate: its association with duct-acinar dysplasia. *Human Pathol* 1991; **22:** 644–52.

54. Bostwick DG, Dousa M, Crawford B et al, Neuroendocrine differentiation in prostatic intraepithelial neoplasia and adenocarcinoma. *Am J Surg Pathol* 1994; **18:** 1240–6.

55. Yang Y, Hao J, Liu X, Dalkin B, Nagle RB, Differential expression of cytokeratin mRNA and protein in normal prostate, prostatic intraepithelial neoplasia, and invasive carcinoma. *Am J Pathol* 1997; **150:** 693–704.

56. Helpap B, Observations on the number, size and location of nucleoli in hyperplastic and neoplastic prostatic disease. *Histopathology* 1988; **13:** 203–11.

57. Montironi R, Scarpelli M, Sisti S et al, Quantitative analysis of prostatic intra-epithelial neoplasia on tissue sections. *Anal Quant Cytol Histol* 1990; **12:** 366–72.

58. Deschenes J, Weidner N, Nucleolar organizer regions (NOR) in hyperplastic and neoplastic prostate disease. *Am J Surg Pathol* 1990; **14:** 1148–55.

59. Petein M, Michel P, Van Velthoven R et al, Morphonuclear relationship between prostatic intraepithelial neoplasia and cancers as assessed by digital cell image analysis. *Am J Clin Pathol* 1991; **96:** 628–34.

60. Layfield LJ, Goldstein NS, Morphometric analysis of borderline atypia in prostatic aspiration biopsy specimen. *Anal Quant Cytol Histol* 1991; **13:** 288–92.

61. DeVries CR, McNeal JE, Bensch K, The prostatic epithelial cell in dysplasia: an ultrastructural perspective. *Prostate* 1992; **21:** 209–21.

62. Bostwick DG, Pacelli A, Lopez-Beltran A, Ultrastructure of prostatic intraepithelial neoplasia. *Prostate* 1997; **33:** 32–7.

63. Fuchs ME, Brawer BK, Rennels MA, Nagle RB, The relationship of basement membrane to histologic grade of human prostatic carcinoma. *Mod Pathol* 1989; **2:** 105–11.

64. Hamdy FC, Fadlon EJ, Cottam D et al, Matrix metalloproteinase 9 expression in primary human prostatic adenocarcinoma and benign prostatic hyperplasia. *Br J Cancer* 1994; **69:** 177–82.

65. Davidson D, Bostwick DG, Qian J et al, Prostatic intraepithelial neoplasia is a risk factor for adenocarcinoma: predictive accuracy in needle biopsies. *J Urol* 1995; **154:** 1295–9.

66. Markham CW, Prostatic intraepithelial neoplasia: detection and correlation with invasive cancer in fine-needle biopsy. *Urology* 1989; **24**(suppl): 57–61.

67. Brawer MK, Bigler SA, Sohlberg OE, Nagle RB, Lange PH, Significance of prostatic intraepithelial neoplasia on prostate needle biopsy. *Urology* 1991; **38:** 103–7.

68. Weinstein MH, Epstein JI, Significance of high grade prostatic intraepithelial neoplasia on needle biopsy. *Human Pathol* 1993; **24:** 624–9.

69. Berner A, Danielsen HE, Pettersen EO, Fossa SD, Reith A, Nesland JM, DNA distribution in the prostate. Normal gland, benign and premalignant lesions, and subsequent adenocarcinomas. *Anal Quant Cytol Histol* 1993; **15:** 247–52.

70. Aboseif S, Shinohara K, Weidner N, Narayan P, Carroll PR, The significance of prostatic intraepithelial neoplasia. *Br J Urol* 1995; **76:** 355–9.

71. Keetch DW, Humphrey P, Stahl D, Smith DS, Catalona WJ, Morphometric analysis and clinical follow-up of isolated prostatic intraepithelial neoplasia in needle biopsy of the prostate. *J Urol* 1995; **154:** 347–51.

72. Raviv G, Zlotta AR, Janssen Th, Descamps F, Verhest A, Schulman CC, Does prostate-specific antigen and prostate-specific antigen density enhance the detection of prostate cancer in patients initially diagnosed to have prostatic intraepithelial neoplasia? *Cancer* 1996; **77:** 2103–8.

73. Raviv G, Janssen Th, Zlotta AR, Descamps F, Verhest A, Schulman CC, Prostatic intraepithelial neoplasia: influence of clinical and pathological data on the detection of prostate cancer. *J Urol* 1996; **156:** 1050–5.

74. Shepherd D, Keetch DW, Humphrey PA, Smith DS, Stahl D, Repeat biopsy strategy in men with isolated prostatic intraepithelial neoplasia on prostate needle biopsy. *J Urol* 1996; **156:** 460–3.

75. Qian J, Huang S, Immunohistochemical and quantitative morphological studies of duct-acinar dysplasia in the prostate. *Chin J Pathol* 1992; **21:** 198–202.

76. De La Torre, Haggman M, Brandstedt S et al, Prostatic intraepithelial neoplasia and invasive

carcinoma in total prostatectomy specimens: distribution, volume and DNA ploidy. *Br J Urol* 1993; **72:** 207–13.

77. Ferguson J, Zincke H, Ellison E, Bergstrahl E, Bostwick DG, Decrease of prostatic intraepithelial neoplasia (prostatic intraepithelial neoplasia) following androgen deprivation therapy in patients with stage T3 carcinoma treated by radical prostatectomy. *Urology* 1994; **44:** 91–5.

78. Montironi R, Magi-Galluzzi C, Muzzonigro G, Prete E, Polito M, Fabris G, Effects of combination endocrine treatment on normal prostate, prostatic intraepithelial neoplasia, and prostatic adenocarcinoma. *J Clin Pathol* 1994; **47:** 906–13.

79. Vaillancourt L, Tetu B, Fradet Y et al, Effect of neoadjuvant endocrine therapy (combined androgen blockade) on normal prostate and prostate carcinoma. A randomized study. *Am J Surg Pathol* 1996; **20:** 86–93.

80. Van der Kwast TH, Ruizeveld de Winter JA, Trapman J, Androgen receptor expression in human prostate cancer. *J Urol Pathol* 1995; **3:** 200–22.

81. Bostwick DG, Target populations and strategies for chemoprevention trials of prostate cancer. *J Cell Biochem* 1994; **19**(suppl): 191–6.

82. Bostwick DG, Burke HB, Wheeler TM et al, The most promising surrogate endpoint biomarkers for screening candidate chemopreventive compounds for prostatic adenocarcinoma in short-term phase II clinical trials. *J Cell Biochem* 1994; **19**(suppl): 283–9.

83. Aquilina JW, Lipsky JJ, Bostwick DG, Androgen deprivation as a strategy for prostate cancer chemoprevention. *J Natl Cancer Inst* 1997; **89:** 689–96.

84. Slem CE, Cote RJ, Skinner EC et al, The effect of finasteride on prostate gland peripheral zone histology and proliferation rates in men at high risk for prostate cancer. *J Urol* 1997; **157:** 228.

4

Aspects of the cell biology of prostate cancer

Keith Griffiths, Michael S Morton

CONTENTS • **The sites of origin of cancer within the prostate gland** • **Some growth regulatory processes in the prostate** • **Androgens and the prostate gland** • **The biology of androgen action: androgens and the genome** • **Growth factor signalling pathways** • **The stromal–epithelial interaction** • **Regional variation of epithelial and stromal function** • **Progression of prostate cancer** • **Dietary components and the pathogenesis of prostate cancer**

Carcinoma of the prostate gland is now recognized as one of the principal medical problems confronting the male population of the world, with evidence[1–3] indicating that in many countries of the world, the disease is the second most prevalent form of cancer in men. In the male population of the USA, cancer of the prostate is the second most commonly diagnosed cancer after skin cancer, and the second most common cause of death from cancer after that of the lung. The age-adjusted mortality rates per 100 000 can differ widely in the various regions of the USA,[4] with a low rate of 18.9 for white males in the state of Arkansas, contrasting with a rate of 55.5 for black men in other states, the latter probably being one of the highest mortality rates in the world.

The incidence of prostate cancer is rising,[5] a trend seen particularly in data from the USA (Figure 4.1); around the world overall, the annual rate of increase is 2–3%.[3] It has been reported that the lifetime risk of a North American male developing clinically relevant disease is close to 10%.[3,6] Furthermore, it has also been estimated[7] that if the prevalence of prostate cancer is defined such that the figures include patients alive up to 5 years after diag-

nosis, then 1 014 000 patients are alive, around the world, with prostatic cancer that requires medical care, i.e. approximately 16% of all the 5-year prevalent male cancer cases. Of these cases, it is reported[7] that 896 000 will have originated in the developed countries and 118 000 in the developing regions of the world.[8]

The public health importance of carcinoma of the prostate, as we approach a new millennium, has been well identified and emphasized by Boyle.[3] He indicates that with an increasing life expectancy[9] leading to more cases of prostate cancer being diagnosed, together with the absence of any marked improvement in treatment and with prevention by changing lifestyle only just now being discussed,[10] the consequence will be an increase in mortality from cancer of the prostate world-wide.

It is extremely important continually to reiterate the need to understand better the natural history, not only of prostate cancer, but also of benign prostatic hyperplasia (BPH) and the biological and molecular processes that are associated with the pathogenesis of these diseases. More attention must be directed to the influence of environmental factors on these biological processes, and to the role of the diet and

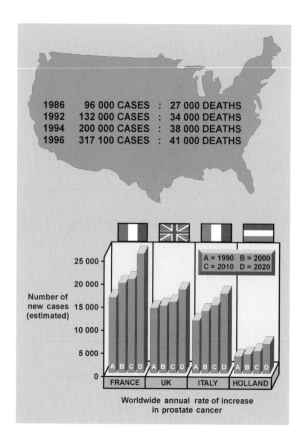

1986	96 000 CASES	:	27 000 DEATHS
1992	132 000 CASES	:	34 000 DEATHS
1994	200 000 CASES	:	38 000 DEATHS
1996	317 100 CASES	:	41 000 DEATHS

Figure 4.1 Some data to illustrate the rate of increase in prostate cancer incidence and mortality in certain countries. Data from the USA clearly show this increase and those from Boyle[4,7] provide the predicted new cases through to the year 2020 in European Community countries.

dietary constituents on the molecular endocrinology associated with prostatic dysfunction.[10] A fundamental issue, only now being addressed, is the influence of race and geographical variation on the world-wide incidence of carcinoma of the prostate.[4,7] In comparison to the USA and the countries of northern Europe, the disease is rarely seen in the Asian people of, for example, China, Japan, Thailand and India, and a reported 200-fold difference in the incidence worldwide[7] emphasizes

the need to understand the inherent biology that must be implicated[10] in this racial and geographical variation. The mortality rate from cancer of the prostate gland increases (Figure 4.2) to at least half of that of the indigenous North American males for those Japanese and Chinese migrants who settle in the USA.[11,12]

THE SITES OF ORIGIN OF CANCER WITHIN THE PROSTATE GLAND

It was the careful, precise dissection of the human prostate that allowed McNeal, some 25 years ago,[13–15] to elaborate on his concept of the zonal anatomy of the gland (Figure 4.3), which today forms the basis on which newer insights regarding the natural history of prostatic disease can be developed. At that time it was believed[13] that the peripheral zone of the gland was the site of origin of the major proportion of cancers, with the transition zone being the region in which BPH developed.

In the 1970s, there was controversy[16,17] as to whether cancer and BPH were independent diseases with separate distinct aetiologies, although the general consensus was that they did constitute independent disorders. However, recognizing particular biological and endocrinological features common to both, together with a more rigorous reassessment of the epidemiology and pathology of prostatic disease, there now appears to be good evidence[18–20] of a potential relationship between transition zone cancer and the early, nonclinical phase in the development of BPH.

A recent report[18] has indicated that, whereas approximately 70% of cancers do develop in the peripheral zone, it is now recognized that up to 25% originate in the centrally located transition zone – these cancers are termed *incidental*, when found in tissue removed at transurethral resection of the prostate (TURP) for the treatment of bladder outflow obstruction.

These T1 transition-zone cancers were once considered of low, insignificant malignant potential. A more recent detailed morphological analysis[21] has revealed a range of volume

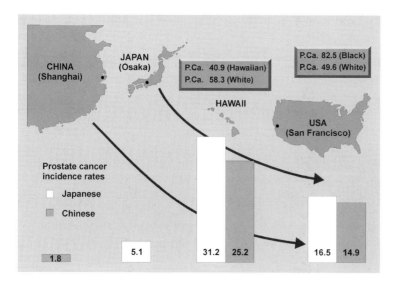

Figure 4.2 Different incidence rates for prostate cancer (P.Ca.) in Chinese and Japanese migrating populations relative to the rates for certain indigenous peoples.

and grade similar to T2 cancers, offering little support for the belief that the T1 cancers are intrinsically different from the T2 cancers of the peripheral zone that are identified by digital rectal examination (DRE). The essential difference would appear to be related simply to their relative rates of growth.[22] Progressive disease is recognized in 33% of stage T1b cancer patients within 4 years,[23] a higher frequency than that shown by the stage T2a cancer,[24] as recognized by DRE.

Controversy surrounds the clinical significance of the putative lesions of 'premalignancy', referred to as atypical adenomatous hyperplasia (AAH) and prostatic intraepithelial neoplasia (PIN). Tissue resected at prostatectomy for BPH contains the AAH lesions, which are similar to low-grade acinar carcinoma.[25] PIN is recognized in the peripheral zone. The prevalence and grade of both types of lesion are greater in prostates containing cancer than in those without,[26,27] and it would seem reasonable

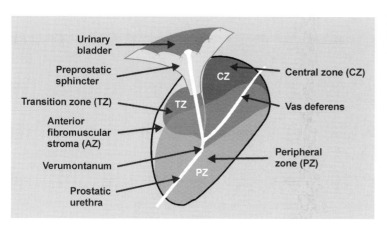

Figure 4.3 Anatomical zones of the human prostate gland. (As depicted by McNeal.[13–15])

that both AAH and PIN should be recognized as premalignant lesions.[28,29]

It is interesting to consider the potential relationship between BPH and AAH and to question whether BPH is causally related to transition zone cancer.[18] Both diseases show an increasing incidence with age, have related natural histories and are androgen dependent, in that they respond to androgen withdrawal therapy. Moreover, cancer is found incidentally in up to 10% of TURP specimens, with an incidence that relates to ageing, and neither BPH nor cancer of the prostate develop in males castrated early in life. There is growing evidence[18–20] that microscopic BPH, rather than the clinical symptomatic enlarged gland, may well be an early phase in the pathogenesis of transition-zone cancer, but there is still controversy as to whether AAH is a premalignant lesion implicated in these processes.

Although it would generally be agreed that our knowledge of the natural history of prostatic disease is poor,[7] it is important to establish a basis for discussion, and Figure 4.4 simply illustrates a pattern which many could well support. Furthermore, it offers a concept against which the rapidly accumulating knowledge of prostatic molecular biology can be assessed.

The concept of 'latent carcinoma' is also illustrated, this essentially being small microscopic foci of well-differentiated cancer cells, which are not latent, but would now be recognized as very slowly growing lesions. These foci of cancer cells were reported to be present in approximately 30% of prostates of men over 50 years of age[30] and, moreover, in men of all races from Eastern and Western countries.[31] More detailed studies[32–34] have indicated that smaller 'latent' cancers were present in 12–16% of men from the East and West, but the prevalence of the larger foci increased with age, and the geographical variation resembled that observed for more advanced prostate cancer incidence.

It is clear that, although prostate cancer becomes clinically manifest in the later period of life, beyond 50 years of age, its origins will have been present many years earlier. It is important that we understand better the molecular events that are concerned in the initiation of AAH and PIN, their development to focal well-differentiated cancer and the ultimate progression of the slow-growing 'latent' cancer to the malignant phenotype.

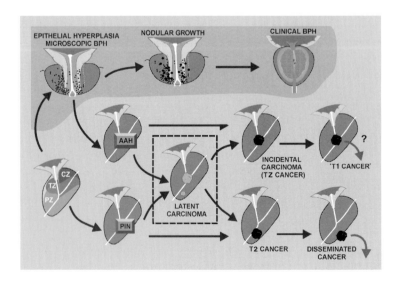

Figure 4.4 Simplistic representation of the possible pathways implicated in the natural history of prostate disease.

SOME GROWTH REGULATORY PROCESSES IN THE PROSTATE

The androgen-dependent nature of cancer of the prostate was established by the biological studies of Charles Huggins more than 50 years ago.[35,36] His investigations provided the scientific basis for the treatment of metastatic disease by androgen ablative therapy. The clinical behaviour of prostatic cancer reflects androgen responsiveness, and first-line endocrine therapy, such as surgical or medical castration, offers effective short-term palliative treatment.

Classically, therefore, it is accepted that prostatic growth is regulated by androgens, and there is little doubt that an adequate level of circulating testosterone is necessary to sustain the growth, development, differentiation and function of the prostate gland.[37,38] Bilateral orchidectomy results in apoptosis, or programmed cell death, and involution of the gland.[39,40] Subsequent administration of exogenous testosterone causes regrowth, but only to the normal adult size.[37] Moreover, exogenous testosterone will similarly promote prostatic growth in the immature male rat, but again only to the normal adult size.

The response of the gland to exogenous testosterone does not therefore produce prostate overgrowth,[19,20] and the normal size is maintained through a balance between cell proliferation and cell death, in the presence of adequate levels of plasma androgen.[41]

Tissue growth, whether normal or malignant, is dependent on the balance between the rate of cell proliferation and that of programmed cell death. Normal prostatic homeostasis, whereby there is no increase in size with time, is regulated by a complex relationship between growth stimulatory and growth inhibitory factors, of both systemic and local origin.[19,20]

The androgenic hormones are undoubtedly important mitogenic factors within the prostate, a necessary prerequisite for cellular proliferation, but evidence is accumulating to suggest that they do not stimulate directly the proliferation of isolated epithelial cells in culture, but rather the cells respond to a range of peptide growth factors such as:

- epidermal growth factor (EGF),
- keratinocyte growth factor (KGF), and
- insulin-like growth factors I and II (IGF-I and IGF-II).

Systemic agents, the *extrinsic factors*, such as the steroid hormones testosterone, oestradiol and cortisol, are transported to the target organ in the plasma. Within the microenvironment of the prostate, the extrinsic factors influence the production and action of the *intrinsic factors*, i.e. the peptide growth regulatory factors (Figure 4.5). These then act through *paracrine* effects on adjacent, different types of cells, by an *autocrine* action on the same type of cell from which the growth factor is produced, or through an intracellular *intracrine* effect, acting within the cell of origin.

Although the rate of cellular proliferation of the prostate cancer will therefore be greater than the rate of cell death, during the early phases of growth the cancer cells will inherently respond to the same growth regulatory factors. Clearly the dysfunctional growth regulatory processes of the cancer do reflect some degree of abnormal responsiveness to these growth factors, a process that ultimately leads to the development of autonomous clones of malignant cells.

It was the conviction of Charles Huggins in 1967[42] that the slow, but consistent, rate of growth of prostate cancer was determined by the balance between the biological effects of intraprostatic factors and other growth-restraining components of the 'soil' in which a tumour resided and grew, a concept consistent with current attitudes relating to the pathogenesis of prostatic cancer.[43,44] It would seem that homeostasis within the complex intracellular structure of the prostate gland is maintained by a balance between the actions of growth-stimulatory factors and those of growth-restraining components such as transforming growth factor-β (TGF-β), the former promoted by androgens, whereas androgens exercise an antagonistic effect on programmed cell death.[39] Androgens orchestrate the interactions between

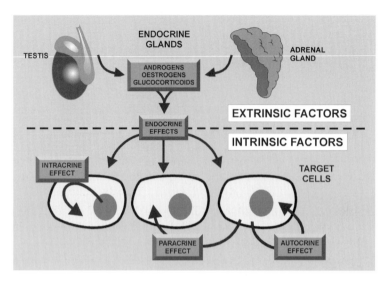

Figure 4.5 Secreted hormones are transported to the prostate. These extrinsic factors regulate the activity of the intrinsic factors, such as the growth regulatory factors, which are produced by prostate cells; in turn, these intrinsic factors then influence the gland through paracrine effects on adjacent cells, by an autocrine effect on the cell from which the factor is produced, or in an intracrine manner within the cell of origin.

the growth regulatory factors (Figure 4.6), probably with the oestrogens and glucocorticoids also eliciting some influence and with the protein products encoded by the growth-suppressor genes also having a major role in the regulation of prostate growth.

ANDROGENS AND THE PROSTATE GLAND

Although the prostate grows and functions within a complex multihormonal environment, responding to a range of growth-regulatory factors, the functional activity of the human gland is primarily dependent on the provision of an adequate level of testosterone in the plasma. Of the 6–7 mg testosterone that is synthesized daily and appears in the plasma, approximately 90–95% is produced by Leydig cells of the testis[45,46] under the control of luteinizing hormone (LH) by way of the hypothalamic–pituitary axis (Figure 4.7). The remainder originates in the adrenal gland, either by direct synthesis, or from the peripheral metabolism in

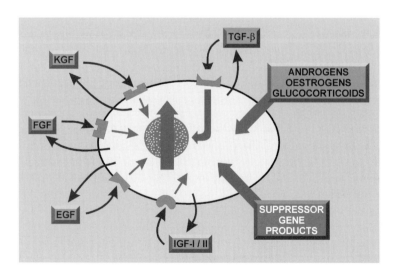

Figure 4.6 A simple concept to illustrate that certain growth-regulatory factors stimulate growth of prostate cells and that TGF-β restrains epithelial cell proliferation. The balance between the effects of such growth-regulatory factors under the modulating influence of 5α-dihydrotestosterone (DHT) sustains homeostasis. DHT promotes epithelial cell proliferation and exercises an antagonistic effect on the influence of TGF-β on apoptosis. The protein products of the growth-suppressor genes restrain growth. FGF, fibroblast growth factor.

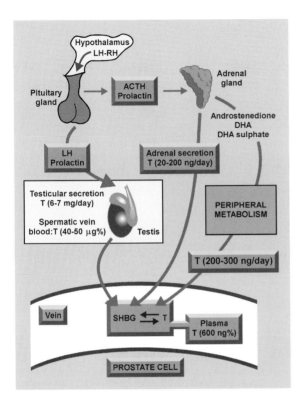

Figure 4.7 Testosterone (T) production in the human male.

muscle and adipose tissue, of the adrenal androgens, dehydroepiandrosterone (DHA) sulphate, DHA and androstenedione, which are C_{19} steroids synthesized and secreted by the human adrenal gland.

LH synthesis and secretion by the pituitary gland is regulated by LH-releasing hormone (LHRH), a decapeptide released by the hypothalamus in a pulsatile manner, thereby promoting a corresponding pulsatile secretion of LH.[47] Both androgens and oestrogens are concerned in the regulation of LH secretion through negative-feedback control processes.

In the human male, about 30% of the oestrogens in plasma also originate in the testis,[48,49] but with the larger proportion being generated[50] from the peripheral aromatization of androstenedione and testosterone (Figure 4.8).

The principal androgen in plasma is testosterone but, more specifically, the free, non-protein-bound form that is generally accepted to be the biologically active moiety that diffuses into a target tissue. The concentration of free testosterone provides a reasonable index of the androgenic status of the male.[51-54] As illustrated in Figure 4.9, only 2% of the total plasma concentration of testosterone and oestradiol is free, the remainder being specifically bound to sex-hormone-binding globulin (SHBG), or less specifically and avidly to albumin. SHBG is synthesized by the liver, with oestrogens, insulin and the thyroid hormones appearing to exercise some control over the process.

Testosterone is therefore taken up by the prostate, where it is converted by the 5α-reductase enzyme system to 5α-dihydrotestosterone (DHT), the principal androgenic hormone within the gland, although it acts directly as an androgenic hormone in other tissues of the body.

Testosterone in plasma is, however, further metabolized by other tissues:[55,56] it is catabolized (Figure 4.10) by the liver to the inactive metabolites, the 17-oxosteroids androsterone and aetiocholanolone, and also to DHT and 5α-androstane-3α,17β-diol, generally referred to as 3α-androstanediol. These metabolites are converted to their sulphate or glucuronide conjugates before excretion in the urine.

Testosterone is also metabolized to DHT in the seminal vesicles, the sebaceous glands, skin and by certain regions of the brain. Of the DHT produced each day, approximately 300 μg, less than 50% is synthesized and secreted by the testis.[57]

THE BIOLOGY OF ANDROGEN ACTION: ANDROGENS AND THE GENOME

The free testosterone is therefore transferred into the target prostate cells by a process of passive diffusion,[58] although there is still much to be understood about this process, with reports[59] that the testosterone–SHBG complex can specifically associate with cell membrane receptors to

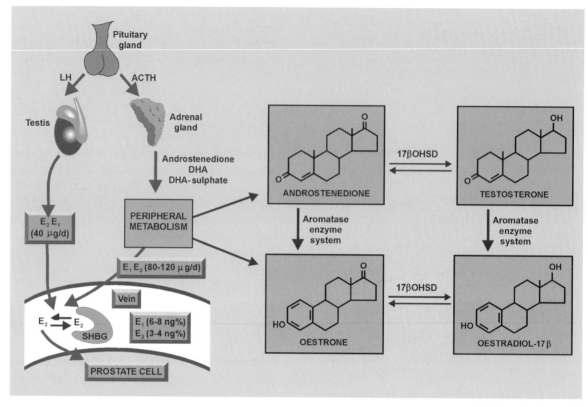

Figure 4.8 Production of oestrogens in the human male. E_1, oestrone; E_2, oestradiol-17β; 17βOHSD, 17β-hydroxysteroid dehydrogenase; SHBG, sex-hormone-binding globulin.

activate second-messenger production and signal transduction.

Within the prostate cells, the testosterone is converted by the 5α-reductase localized on the nuclear membrane to DHT, the biologically active, intracellular androgenic hormone.[60,61] DHT preferentially binds to the androgen receptor protein (AR) of the prostate (Figure 4.11) with a three- to fivefold greater affinity than testosterone. The DHT–AR complexes then specifically associate with particular nucleotide-recognition sequences on the genome, referred to as hormone response elements (HREs), which are sited adjacent to androgen responsive genes.

In the prostate, therefore, it is the DHT–AR complex that modulates gene expression.[19,20] The formation of the DHT–AR complex and its specific association with the HREs is central to the activation and efficacy of the normal growth-regulatory processes of the prostate gland and during the early androgen-dependent phases in the natural history of prostatic cancer.[20,62–66]

The association of DHT to the AR results in a conformational change that unmasks the DNA-binding domain of the receptor protein revealing the 'zinc fingers'[67,68] that specifically facilitate the high-affinity association of the DHT–AR with the HRE. HREs are generally located upstream (Figure 4.12) from the transcription start sites of androgen-responsive genes.[69,70] The association of the DHT–AR to these specific enhancer sequences of the HRE in the promoter region of such genes enables the complex to function as a ligand-dependent transcription factor, thereby modulating gene expression.

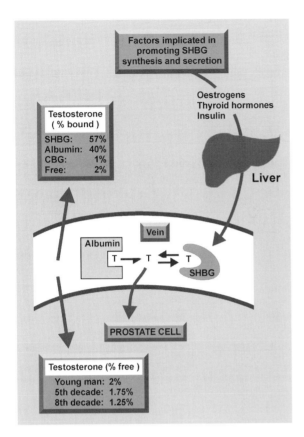

Figure 4.9 The concentration of free, non-protein-bound steroid hormone in plasma that is considered to be the biologically active moiety that enters the target cell. CBG, corticosteroid-binding globulin; SHBG, sex-hormone-binding globulin.

expression, influencing either the rate of gene transcription or transcription initiation. The DHT–AR thereby acts as a *trans*-acting modulator to influence gene expression and, as such, acts within the promoter region in concert with other transcription factors, e.g. the Fos and Jun proteins that are encoded by the c-*fos* and c-*jun* proto-oncogenes. Such proteins are concerned in growth-regulatory processes and are depicted in Figure 4.11 in juxtaposition to the DHT–AR on the genome.

It is envisaged[64] that the efficacy by which androgens influence gene transcription and growth regulation resides in their capacity to affect the spatial orientation of DNA strands in order to facilitate easier access of the transcription factors to their own specific nucleotide sequences or recognition sites on the genome. The transcription factors are expressed by proto-oncogenes through the activation of growth factor signalling pathways.

Therefore DHT has a major role in growth-regulatory processes within the prostate and the gland fails to grow if DHT is absent. Neither BPH nor prostatic cancer develops in men castrated early in life. Investigations also indicate[77] that the prostate gland remains vestigial in men in the Dominican Republic with an inherited 5α-reductase deficiency that causes male pseudohermaphroditism. Although reasonable musculature and adequate genitalia develop, and the subjects manifest libido and erections, presumably the biological effects of testosterone, the prostate fails to grow in the absence of DHT.

The binding of DHT to the AR is related to the release of the associated heat shock protein 90 (hsp90),[71–75] and conformational changes that lead to DHT–AR complex dimerization[76] on the genome involving dimerization domains on the AR, a prerequisite that gives stability to the process of gene transcription. The particular symmetry of specific sequences of nucleotide bases within the HRE facilitates the interaction between the zinc fingers of the AR and the major grooves of the DNA (Figure 4.13).

The association between the DHT–AR and the HRE can thereby promote or suppress gene

GROWTH FACTOR SIGNALLING PATHWAYS

Steroid hormones are therefore seen to modulate the production and biological action of the growth regulatory factors (see Figure 4.5). It must also be understood that there exists a quite complex interrelationship between the steroid-hormone signalling pathways and those activated by the growth-regulatory factors.[19,20]

Many of the known peptide growth-regulatory factors and their corresponding cell-membrane-associated receptors have been identified

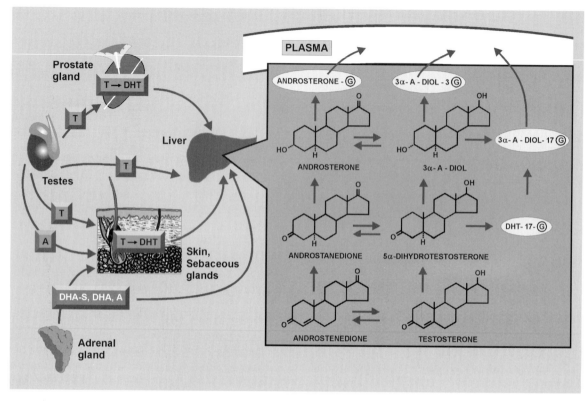

Figure 4.10 Metabolism of androgens.

in prostatic tissue.[77,78] The binding of the growth factor to the external domain of the receptor with its associated tyrosine-specific protein kinase triggers a cascade of intracellular signalling events (Figure 4.14) that result in the activation of proto-oncogenes which encode various proteins such as the Fos, Jun and Myc proteins.[79–82] These proteins are intimately involved in growth regulatory processes. The proto-oncogenes also encode for growth-regulatory peptides and their complementary receptors, and for the various components of the signal transduction pathways (Figure 4.14).

Imbalance between the finely tuned growth stimulatory and inhibitory mechanisms could result in cellular hyperplasia, with genetic instability and subversion of the complex regulatory processes. Dysfunction of the proto-oncogenes through point mutations, deletions or amplification, or gene impairment that alters the structure or expression gives rise to oncogenes that would then be implicated in the pathogenesis of cancer.

The cross-talk between the signalling pathways, those activated by peptide growth factors and through the biological action of DHT is fundamental to normal glandular homeostasis and growth control, with the DHT–AR facilitating easier access of the transcription factors to the DNA (Figure 4.15). In the normal gland, DHT–AR is therefore involved in growth factor function.

THE STROMAL–EPITHELIAL INTERACTION

The prostate gland is composed of secretory acini lined by epithelial cells, essentially a com-

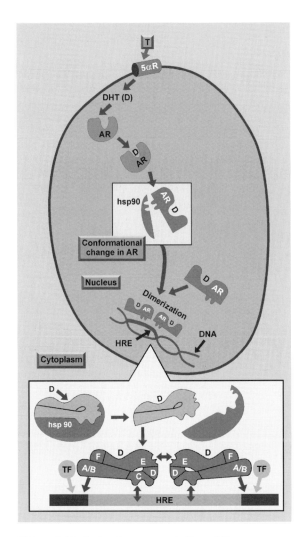

Figure 4.11 A simple representation of the intracellular processes relating to the binding of DHT (D) to the androgen receptor (AR) and to the dimerization of the DHT–AR complex when binding to the hormone response elements (HRE), the nucleotide recognition sequences on the genome. TF, the transcription factors are illustrated binding to the DNA adjacent to the DHT–AR complexes; 5αR, 5α-reductase.

plex branching system of ducts that drain into the prostatic urethra (see Figure 4.13). The epithelium-lined ducts are embedded in a matrix of stromal components[83] and it is now

recognized[84–87] that the stroma has a role in the regulation of epithelial cell proliferation.[20]

This interrelationship is illustrated in Figure 4.16, which indicates that DHT-mediated effects on the stromal compartment promote the production of growth stimulatory factors, probably KGF or EGF,[20] that exercise a paracrine influence on epithelial cell growth and differentiation. Glandular homeostasis is maintained through a balance between this stimulatory effect on cell proliferation and the growth-restraining influence of factors such as TGF-β, which promotes cell death. Recent studies[88,89] suggest that the smooth muscle cells of the stromal compartment produce the TGF-β. The quantitative interaction between the rates of cell proliferation and of programmed cell death will govern overall tissue growth. A steady-state homeostasis exists in the normal adult prostate, but, in hyperplasia or cancer, the rate of proliferation overrides the rate at which cells die.

A synergistic effect of both DHT and oestradiol would appear to exercise some autocrine control over stromal cell growth and function, through the production and action of fibroblast growth factor 2 (FGF-2), or bFGF.[20,90]

There is mounting evidence[91–95] that KGF, a member of the FGF family and referred to as FGF-7, is the androgen-induced paracrine mediator that promotes epithelial proliferation. KGF elicits a mitogenic effect on epithelial cells in culture, but not stromal cells and this effect on epithelial cell proliferation is inhibited by TGF-β. KGF is produced by fibroblasts, where its expression is regulated by androgens. Moreover, epithelial cells produce a cell membrane receptor which specifically recognizes KGF.[93] The epithelial cells express a splice variant of the FGF receptor-2 (FGF-R-2) (*bek*) gene, which encodes an FGF-R referred to as FGF-R2-exonIIIb. In contrast, stromal growth appears to be controlled by FGF-2 (bFGF) through the FGF-R1 (see Figure 4.16).

It has been suggested[20] that, after the rapid phase of prostatic growth between adolescence and the early twenties, when the gland attains its maximum adult size, homeostasis would normally be established, with TGF-β then promoting growth restraint. From the studies of

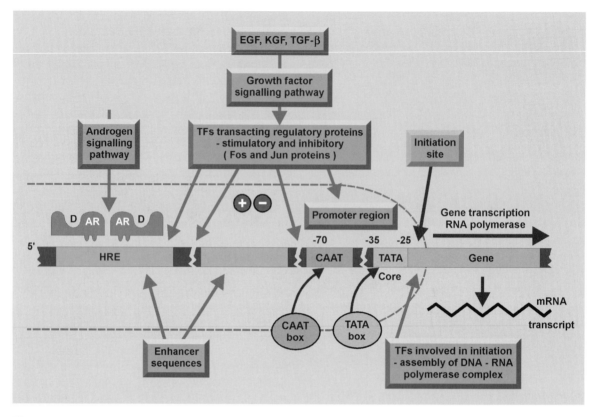

Figure 4.12 A simple illustration of the influence of various factors on the promoter region of an androgen-responsive gene. Represented are the DHT–AR homodimers and the possible stimulatory or inhibitory influence of growth-regulatory factors that could influence gene transcription. TFs, transcription factors.

Coffey and colleagues,[96,97] it would seem that homeostasis is not always established, and that growth factor imbalance, excessive epithelial cell proliferation or an inability of TGF-β to restrain growth results in microscopic BPH, epithelial hyperplasia leading to nodular hyperplasia in the transition zone. This increases in prevalence with increasing age. It could be envisaged that microscopic BPH could constitute a dysfunctional premalignant lesion (see Figure 4.4). Any relationship to AAH is unclear, but it seems reasonable that AAH in the transition zone, like PIN in the peripheral zone, represents an early stage in the escape of epithelial cells from growth control.

The molecular events related to the expression of the FGF-R proteins with structural variation and differing ligand specificity for members of the FGF family could well be implicated in the loss of growth control, particularly during the initiation and early progression of prostatic cancer. This would involve the differential splicing of FGF-R mRNA transcripts. Such a concept suggests that in this multi-step process, epithelial hyperplasia, resulting from an imbalance of growth factor regulatory mechanisms, leads to premalignancy as the epithelial cells lose the growth-restraining influence of, first, the stromal factors represented by KGF and TGF-β and, second, the regulatory control

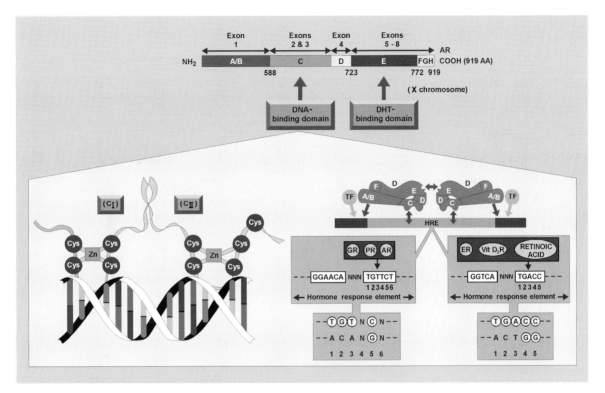

Figure 4.13 Diagrammatic representation of the AR protein and of the AR–DHT complex association with the HRE, the 'zinc fingers' of the DNA-binding domain of the AR interacting with the major grooves of the DNA, a process in which specific nucleotides of the androgen response element (ARE) are implicated. The illustration shows the interaction of other members of the receptor family with the HRE.

from the molecular cross-talk associated with DHT–AR and Fos–Jun dimers at the level of the genome (see Figure 4.15).

Paracrine intercellular signalling between stroma and epithelium is therefore fundamental to growth regulation in the prostate. It is interesting that the well-differentiated, androgen-responsive Dunning R-3327 PAP tumour, with its associated stromal elements, also expresses the FGF-R2-exonIIIb receptor that specifically 'sees' KGF. The undifferentiated, androgen-unresponsive, malignant Dunning tumour expresses the splice variant FGF-R2-exonIIIc receptor, together with FGF-R1, normally located in the stromal cells, both of which respond to FGF-2 (Figure 4.17), but not KGF. Such molecular events could be regarded as stages in the severing of the intimate interaction between stromal and epithelial compartments with the associated loss of the growth-restraining influence of the stroma.

REGIONAL VARIATION OF EPITHELIAL AND STROMAL FUNCTION

The physiological importance of the epithelial–stromal interaction in the regulation of growth is clearly important. Recent studies[98–100] re-emphasize the importance and

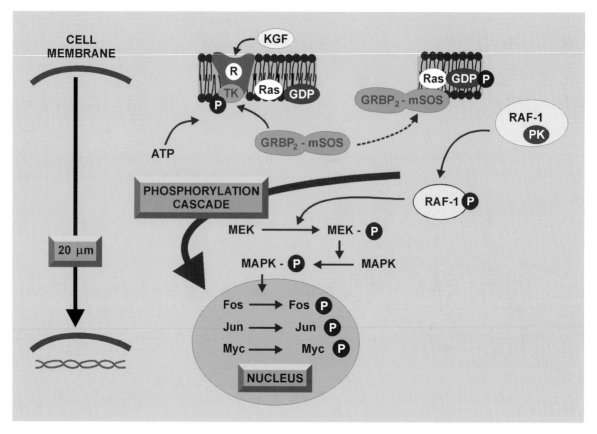

Figure 4.14 Diagrammatic representation of the influence of various growth-stimulatory factors on the activity of growth-related proto-oncogenes. The influence of the growth factors on signal transduction pathways within the cell is effected through the cell-membrane-localized specific receptors. The complex range of interactions implicated in the molecular events associated with the transduction of signals from the cell membrane to the nucleus is illustrated.

complexity of the interrelationship, in that evidence now indicates a regional variation in the functional activity of the epithelial cells in regions of the rat ductal system. In segments relative to the urethra, active epithelial cell proliferation was located in the distal region, programmed cell in the segment proximal to the urethra and secretory activity in the major component, the middle intermediate region. The concept (Figure 4.18) implies a migration of epithelial cells along the duct and a regional variability in response to androgen, KGF and TGF-β. If a similar relationship prevails in the human gland, the distant active proliferative activity could explain the high prevalence of PIN and cancer in the peripheral zone.

A corresponding heterogeneity of the stromal elements has also been reported,[101,102] with multiple layers of smooth muscle in the proximal region and a single layer of cells adjacent to the basement membrane in the distal segment. Evidence indicates that the smooth muscle cells are the origin of TGF-β, which promotes programmed cell death[88,103,104] in low concentrations of androgen. Prostatic fibroblasts were found to be evenly distributed along the duct.

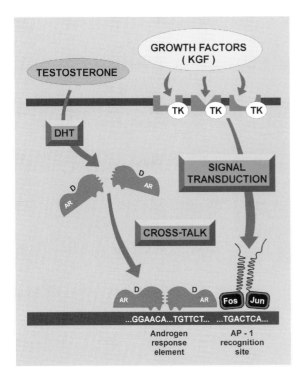

Figure 4.15 The concept of cross-talk and the regulation of gene transcription by the particular arrangement of regulatory sequences of nucleotides. The DHT is shown influencing the genome through the AR. Signal transduction pathways are also activated by various growth factors such as KGF, and thereby activate proto-oncogenes like c-*fos* and c-*jun*. The Fos/Jun heterodimer binds to AP-1 recognition sites. The relative positioning of these regulatory sequences can result in competition or cooperation. An inhibitory growth factor can introduce a regulatory agent that may prevent the association of a transcription factor to DNA. The nucleotides of the ARE that are implicated in the recognition of the AR are highlighted.

The precise physiological roles of androgens and oestrogens within the stromal compartment remain to be elucidated, but it is clear that TGF-β exercises a pivotal role in the growth-regulatory processes. The mechanisms by which the androgen-mediated production of KGF, or other growth-stimulating factors, interact with the growth-restraining influence of TGF-β feature prominently in maintaining growth control. The negative regulatory influence of DHT on the expression of TGF-β would also seem to be of importance.

PROGRESSION OF PROSTATE CANCER

The studies of Lee and coworkers[105–107] have shown that, as with the more aggressive Dunning tumour, the proliferation of the well-differentiated, androgen-responsive human LNCaP cancer cells is also promoted by FGF-2 in the presence of low DHT levels. This stimulatory effect is inhibited by TGF-β, under an androgen-dependent influence. Although the LNCaP cells cannot be seen as a precise model system that relates to early hormone-dependent cancer, since the cells express a mutant AR with a point mutation in the steroid-binding domain[108] that allows the activation of the receptor by oestradiol, progesterone and antiandrogens as well as DHT, it does, however, represent an androgen-sensitive model system independent of stromal growth-regulatory influence.

It is well accepted[109] that cancer progresses through a series of progressive changes that occur over a long period of time, from early epithelial hyperplasia, through premalignancy to the aggressive malignant phenotype. In the early phases of prostatic carcinogenesis, the cells retain some degree of androgen dependence and respond to androgen ablative therapy. The inexorable disease progression with the associated genetic mutations ultimately produces clones of autonomous cells with autocrine growth-promoting signalling pathways that are unresponsive to androgen control. The proliferation of such clones of cells, like the human PC3 human prostate cancer cell line, may be promoted by the autocrine production and action of TGF-α through the EGF receptor (EGF-R). It is interesting that the PC3 cells fail to respond to the tyrosine-specific protein kinase inhibitor ZM252868 (Zeneca, Macclesfield, UK), which interferes with growth factor receptor activation, whereas growth of the Du145 cell line is restrained.[110,111]

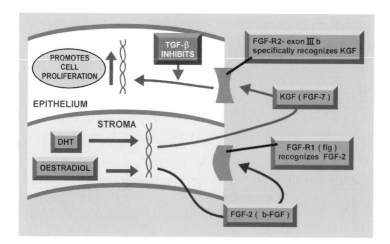

Figure 4.16 Stromal–epithelial interrelationships. The stromally produced KGF specifically binds to the epithelial receptor FGF-R2-exonIIIb. TGF-β regulates this effect of KGF on epithelial proliferation. FGF-2 appears to regulate stromal cell proliferation through the FGF-R1 (flg) receptor.

Enhanced growth factor production through oncogene activation, dysfunctional growth factor receptor expression, autocrine signalling pathways and the inexorable loss of suppressor gene products such as p53 and the retinoblastoma (Rb) proteins, are the very basis of androgen-independent prostatic cancer progression.[62,78,79,107] TGF-α, a growth factor that associates with and activates the EGF-R, is recognized as an important mitogen in androgen-independent prostate cancer phenotypes.[112] An increased level of EGF-R is associated with prostatic cancer de-differentiation and increased grade,[113] and also with an enhanced expression of the *myc* oncogene products.

DIETARY COMPONENTS AND THE PATHOGENESIS OF PROSTATE CANCER

Earlier in this chapter, reference was made to the significant differences in the incidence of prostate cancer between Asian people and their counterparts in the USA and northern Europe.

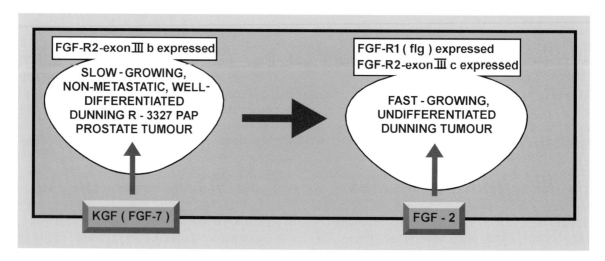

Figure 4.17 A less specific receptor, the FGF-R2-exonIIIc is expressed by the fast-growing undifferentiated Dunning tumour.

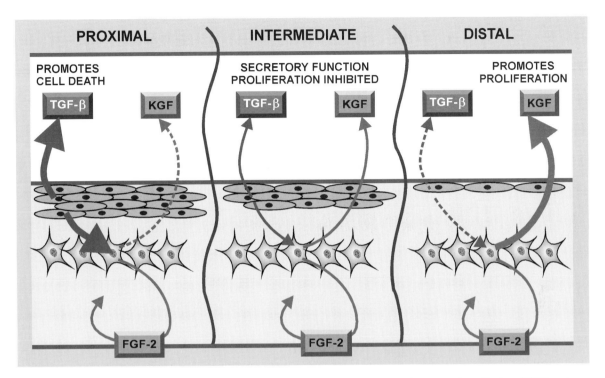

Figure 4.18 Regrowth variation in epithelial and stromal function: a balance between the effects of KGF and TGF-β.

The male population of the Mediterranean countries occupies an intermediate position.[7,10] Over the years, attention has been directed primarily to the high fat content of the Western diet as a potential *causal* agent.[114] More recently, however, the concept has been emphasized[10] that certain components of the Asian diet and, to some extent, that of the Mediterranean people may *restrain* the development of cancer of the prostate.

With regard to prostate cancer, the concept relates to the possibility that these dietary components may restrain the initiation and early progression of the small, latent or slowly growing foci of prostate cancer, to the malignant phenotype.[7,30–33] Attention is directed[10] to the constituents of soya, whole grain, fruit and vegetables that are metabolized by the normal gut microflora to generate body fluids, particularly compounds referred to as isoflavonoids, flavonoids and lignans (Figure 4.19). Of particular interest are the isoflavonoids genistein and daidzein, and the lignan enterolactone.

Some of these polyphenolic compounds possess weak oestrogenic activity and, as such, like the drug tamoxifen, can act as an antioestrogen. In particular tissues and biological systems, such weak oestrogens can elicit agonistic as well as antagonistic properties.[10] Soya, a major component of the Japanese and Chinese diet, is a particularly good source of isoflavonoids. Unlike the isoflavonoids, however, the flavonoids are ubiquitous in nature, and high concentrations exist in many vegetables and fruits. Many flavonoids, e.g. apigenin, which is found in various leaves but particularly in tea leaves, are also weakly oestrogenic.[115] The lignans[116,117] are also widely distributed, with the precursors found in cereals, grains, fruits and vegetables, but particularly linseed (flaxseed).

The concentration of isoflavonoids is very high[118,119] in the urine and plasma of Japanese and Chinese people (Figure 4.20), and the levels of lignans are high[120] in the urine of vegetarians.

As weak oestrogens, these polyphenolic compounds increase SHBG synthesis and

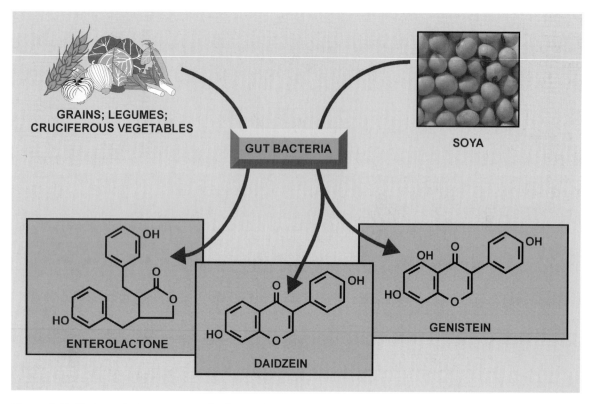

Figure 4.19 Various phyto-oestrogens (isoflavonoids and lignans) that are produced from food components by the gut microflora, and which appear in biological fluids.

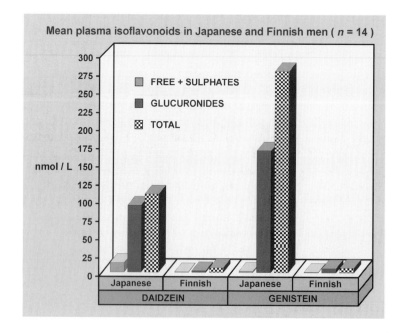

Figure 4.20 Plasma levels of isoflavonoids and lignans.

secretion,[121] enterolactone inhibits the aromatase enzyme system,[122,123] and isoflavonoids and lignans inhibit 5α-reductase and 17β-hydroxysteroid dehydrogenase enzyme systems[124] and have long been recognized as antioxidants.[125]

Tyrosine-specific protein kinases, constituents of the intracellular domain of receptors for EGF, KGF and FGF, for example, and essential for signal transduction pathways activated by such growth-stimulatory factors, are reported to be inhibited by genistein.[126] Tyrosine kinase (TK) inhibitors are currently being developed as anti-cancer agents,[127,128] and the Zeneca TK inhibitor ZM252868 inhibits the growth of LNCaP and Du145 prostate cancer cell lines in culture.[110,111]

In addition, genistein is reported to promote programmed cell death in human breast cancer cells,[129] inhibits invasion of murine mammary cancer cells,[130] and enhances adhesion of endothelial cells.[131] The sophisticated and exciting investigations by Folkman and coworkers[132–134] indicate that angiogenesis, the generation of new blood capillaries through the proliferation and migration of endothelial cells, is required for foci of cancer cells to grow beyond 2 mm in size. The process is probably invoked by the production of growth factors by the cancer, and members of the FGF family have been identified as angiogenic agents. Angiogenesis is a prerequisite for cancer progression, and reports suggest that genistein inhibits the process in vitro.[135]

In a wide variety of animal model systems for cancer, isoflavonoids and lignans have inhibited experimental carcinogenesis.[136] Moreover, isoflavonoids and flavonoids inhibit the bioactivation of potent chemical carcinogens such as benzo[a]pyrene,[137] with the flavonoid catechins from green and black tea inhibiting the activation of certain tobacco carcinogens that induce lung cancer in A/J mice.[138]

When the large amount of information on these exciting 'phyto-oestrogens' was compiled,[10] the conclusion drawn was that the accumulated evidence provided a substantive case for actively pursuing the concept that certain of the isoflavonoids, flavonoids and lignans could well exercise an important role in the prevention of prostatic cancer and breast cancer. Certainly, in the absence of other chemopreventive agents, the possibility of using such phyto-oestrogens as preventive health care offers a major challenge. It would seem that, taken in the appropriate amounts, the enhanced daily intake of such dietary components can do little harm, and may well provide a considerable health advantage.

REFERENCES

1. Silverberg E, Boring CC, Squires TS, Cancer statistics, 1990. *CA* 1990; **40**: 9–26.
2. World Health Organization, Trends in prostate cancer 1980–1988. *WHO Weekly Epidemiol Rec* 1992; **67**: 281–8.
3. Boyle P, The evolution of an epidemic of unknown origin. In: *Prostate Cancer 2000* (Denis L, ed). Springer-Verlag: New York, 1994: 5–11.
4. Zaridze DG, Boyle P, Cancer of the prostate: epidemiology and aetiology. *Br J Urol* 1987; **59**: 493–502.
5. Carter HB, Coffey DS, Prostate cancer: the magnitude of the problem in the United States. In: *A Multidisciplinary Analysis of Controversies in the Management of Prostatic Cancer* (Coffey DS, Resnick MI, Dorr FA, Karr, JP, eds). Plenum Press: New York, 1988: 1–7.
6. Huland H, Ackermann R, Adolfsson J et al, Treatment of localised disease: treatment of clinically localised prostate cancer T1/T2. In: *First International Consultation on Prostatic Cancer* (Murphy G, Griffiths K, Denis L et al, eds). SCI: Paris, 1997: 227–58.
7. Boyle P, Napalkov P, Barry MJ et al, Epidemiology and natural history of prostatic cancer. In: *First International Consultation on Prostatic Cancer* (Murphy G, Griffiths K, Denis L et al, eds). SCI: Paris, 1997: 1–29.
8. Parkin DM, Pisani P, Ferlay J, Cancer statistics. In: *Biennial Report 1994–1995.* IARC: Lyon, 1995: 14–15.

9. Brody J, Prospects for an aging population. *Nature* 1985; **315**: 463–6.

10. Griffiths K, Adlercreutz A, Boyle P, Denis L, Nicholson RI, Morton MS (eds), *Nutrition and Cancer*. Isis Medical Media: Oxford, 1996.

11. Haenszel W, Kurihara M, Studies of Japanese migrants. I. Mortality from cancer and other diseases among the Japanese in the United States. *J Natl Cancer Inst* 1968; **40**: 43–68.

12. Parkin DM, Muir CS, Whelan S, Gao YT, Ferlay J, Powell J, *Cancer Incidence in Five Continents*, Vol. VI, IARC Scientific Publication No. 120. IARC: Lyon, 1992.

13. McNeal JE, Age related changes in prostatic epithelium associated with carcinoma. In: *Some Aspects of the Aetiology and Biochemistry of Prostatic Cancer* (Griffiths K, Pierrepoint CG, eds). Alpha Omega Press: Cardiff, 1970: 23–32.

14. McNeal JE, The zonal anatomy of the prostate. *Prostate* 1981; **2**: 35–49.

15. McNeal JE, Anatomy of the prostate and morphogenesis of BPH. In: *New Approaches to the Study of Benign Prostatic Hyperplasia* (Kimball FA, Buhl AE, Carter DB, eds). AR Liss: New York, 1984: 27–53.

16. Armenian HK, Lilienfeld AM, Diamond EL, Bross IDJ, Relation between benign prostatic hyperplasia and cancer of the prostate: a prospective and retrospective study. *Lancet* 1974; **ii**: 115–17.

17. Greenwald P, Kirmass V, Polan AK, Dick VS, Cancer of the prostate among men with benign prostatic hyperplasia. *J Natl Cancer Inst* 1974; **53**: 335–40.

18. Bostwick DG, Balcells FS, Cooner WH et al, Benign prostatic hyperplasia and cancer of the prostate. In: *The First International Consultation on BPH* (Cockett ATK et al, eds). SCI: Paris, 1992: 139–59.

19. Griffiths K, Akaza H, Eaton CL et al, Regulation of prostatic growth. In: *The Second International Consultation on BPH* (Cockett ATK et al, eds). SCI: Paris, 1993: 49–75.

20. Griffiths K, Coffey DS, Cockett ATK et al, The regulation of prostatic growth. In: *The Third International Consultation on BPH* (Cockett ATK, Khoury S, Aso Y et al, eds). SCI: Paris, 1996: 71–115.

21. McNeal JE, Price HM, Redwine EA, Freiha FS, Stamey TA, Stage A versus stage B adenocarcinoma of the prostate; morphological comparison and biological significance. *J Urol* 1988; **139**: 61–5.

22. Epstein JI, Paull G, Eggleston JC, Walsh PC, Prognosis of untreated stage A1 prostatic carcinoma: A study of 94 cases with extended follow-up. *J Urol* 1986; **136**: 837–9.

23. Cantrell BB, de Klerk DP, Eggleston JC, Boitnott JK, Walsh PC, Pathological factors that influence prognosis in stage A prostatic cancer: the influence of extent versus grade. *J Urol* 1981; **125**: 516–20.

24. Stamey TA, Cancer of the prostate. *Monogr Urol* 1982; **3**: 1–10.

25. Kovi J, Mostofi FK, Atypical hyperplasia of prostate. *Urology* 1989; **34**(suppl): 23–7.

26. McNeal JE, Bostwick DG, Intraductal dysplasia: a premalignant lesion of the prostate. *Hum Pathol* 1986; **17**: 54–71.

27. Kastendieck H, Correlations between atypical primary hyperplasia and carcinoma of the prostate: a histological study of 180 total prostatectomies. *Pathol Res Pract* 1980; **169**: 366–87.

28. McNeal JE, Bostwick DG, Kindrachuk RA, Redwine EA, Freiha FS, Stamey TA, Patterns of progression in prostate cancer. *Lancet* 1986; **i**: 60–3.

29. Bostwick DG, Brawer MK, Prostatic intraepithelial neoplasia and early invasion in prostate cancer. *Cancer* 1987; **59**: 788–94.

30. Baba S, Epidemiology of cancer of the prostate: analysis of countries of high and low incidence. In: *Prostate Cancer. International Perspectives in Urology*, Vol. 3 (Jacobi GH, Hohenfellner R, eds). Williams & Wilkins: Baltimore, 1982: 11–28.

31. Oota K, Misu Y, A study on latent carcinoma of the prostate in Japanese. *GANN* 1958; **49**: 283–93.

32. Breslow NE, Cahn CW, Dhom G et al, Latent carcinoma of the prostate at autopsy in seven areas. *Int J Cancer* 1977; **20**: 680–8.

33. Yatani R, Shiraishi T, Akazaki K et al, Incidental prostatic carcinoma: morphometry correlated with histological grade. *Virchows Arch A Pathol Anat Histopathol* 1986; **409**: 395–405.

34. Office of Technology Assessment (OTA), Costs and effectiveness of prostate cancer screening in elderly men. *OTA-BPH-145*. Washington, DC: US Government Printing Office, May 1995: Table 2.5.

35. Huggins C, Hodges CV, Studies on prostatic cancer. I. The effect of castration, of estrogen and of androgen injection on serum phosphatases in metastatic carcinoma of the prostate. *Cancer Res* 1941; **1**: 293–7.

36. Huggins C, Stevens RE, Hodges CV, Studies on prostatic cancer. *Arch Surg* 1941; **43:** 209–23.

37. Bruchovsky N, Lesser B, VanDoorn E, Craven S, Hormonal effects on cell proliferation in rat prostate. *Vitamin Hormone* 1975; **33:** 61–102.

38. Lee C, Physiology of castration-induced regression in rat prostate. In: *The Prostatic Cell: Structure and Function* (Murphy GP, Sandberg AA, Karr JP, eds). AR Liss: New York, 1981: 145–59.

39. Isaacs JT, Antagonistic effect of androgen on prostatic cell death. *Prostate* 1984; **5:** 545–57.

40. Sensibar JA, Liu X, Patai B, Alger B, Lee C, Characterisation of castration-induced cell death in the rat prostate by immuno-histo-chemical localisation of cathepsin D. *Prostate* 1990; **16:** 263–76.

41. Furuya J, Isaacs JT, Differential gene regulation during programmed cell death (apoptosis) versus proliferation of prostatic glandular cells induced by androgen manipulation. *Endocrinology* 1993; **133:** 2660–6.

42. Huggins C, Endocrine-induced regression of cancers. In: *Les Prix Nobel, Imprimerie Royale.* PA Norstedt & Soner: Stockholm, 1967: 172–82.

43. Weinberg RA, Oncogenes, antioncogenes and the molecular basis of multistep carcinogenesis. *Cancer Res* 1989; **49:** 3713–21.

44. Sager R, Tumor suppressor genes: the puzzle and the promise. *Science* 1989; **246:** 1406–12.

45. Baird DT, Uno A, Melby JC, Adrenal secretion of androgens and oestrogens. *J Endocrinol* 1969; **45:** 135–6.

46. Lipsett MB, Steroid secretion by the human testis. In: *The Human Testis* (Rosemberg E, Paulsen CA, eds). Plenum Press: New York, 1970: 407–21.

47. Santen RJ, Bardin CW, Episodic luteinizing hormone secretion in man. Pulse analysis, clinical interpretation, physiological mechanisms. *J Clin Invest* 1973; **52:** 2617–28.

48. Longcope C, Widrich W, Sawin CT, The secretion of estrone and estradiol-17β by human testis. *Steroids* 1972; **20:** 439–48.

49. Baird DT, Galbraith A, Fraser IS, Newsam JE, The concentration of oestrone and oestradiol-17β in spermatic venous blood in man. *J Endocrinol* 1973; **57:** 285–8.

50. McDonald PC, Origin of oestrogen in man. In: *Benign Prostatic Hyperplasia, NIAMDD Workshop* (Grayhack JT, Wilson JD, Scherbenske MJ, eds). NIH Publication No. 76-1113. DHEW: Bethesda, 1976: 191–3.

51. Vermeulen A, Rubens R, Verdonck L, Testosterone secretion and metabolism in male senescence. *J Clin Endocrinol Metab* 1972; **34:** 730–5.

52. Vermeulen A, Van Camp A, Mattelaer J, De Sy W, Hormonal factors relating to abnormal growth of the prostate. In: *Prostate Cancer* (Coffey DS, Isaacs JT, eds). UICC Technical Report Series, Vol. 48. UICC: Geneva, 1979: 81–92.

53. Vermeulen A, Testicular hormone secretion in aging in males. In: *Benign Prostatic Hyperplasia, NIAMDD Workshop* (Grayhack JT, Wilson JD, Scherbenske MJ, eds). NIH Publication No. 76-1113. DHEW: Bethesda, 1976: 177–82.

54. Rubens R, Dhont M, Vermeulen A, Further studies on Leydig function in old age. *J Clin Endocrinol Metab* 1974; **39:** 40–5.

55. Rittmaster RS, Androgen conjugates: physiology and clinical significance. *Endocr Rev* 1993; **14:** 121–32.

56. Mooradian AD, Morley JE, Korenman SG, Biological actions of androgens. *Endocr Rev* 1987; **8:** 1–28.

57. Ito T, Horton R, The source of plasma dihydrotestosterone in man. *J Clin Invest* 1971; **50:** 1621–7.

58. Rennie PS, Bruchovsky N, Studies on the relationship between androgen receptors and the transport of androgens in rat prostate. *J Biol Chem* 1973; **248:** 3288–97.

59. Hryb DJ, Kahn MS, Romas NA, Rosner W, Solubilization and partial characterization of the sex hormone-binding globulin receptor from human prostate. *J Biol Chem* 1989; **264:** 5378–83.

60. Bruchovsky N, Wilson JD, The intranuclear binding of testosterone and 5α-androstan-17β-ol-3-one by rat prostate. *J Biol Chem* 1968; **243:** 5953–60.

61. Bruchovsky N, Wilson JD, The conversion of testosterone to 5α-androstan-17β-ol-3-one by rat prostate in vivo and in vitro. *J Biol Chem* 1968; **243:** 2012–21.

62. Griffiths K, Eaton CL, Harper ME, Weir AMK, Evans BAJ, Some aspects of the molecular endocrinology of prostatic cancer. In: *Antiandrogens in Prostatic Cancer* (Denis L, ed.). Springer-Verlag: Heidelberg, 1995: 3–30.

63. Beato M, Gene regulation by steroid hormones. *Cell* 1989; **56:** 335–44.

64. Truss M, Beato M, Steroid hormone receptors: interaction with deoxyribonucleic acid and

transcription factors. *Endocr Rev* 1993; **14:** 459–79.

65. Yamamoto KR, Steroid receptor regulated transcription of specific genes and gene networks. *Annu Rev Genet* 1985; **19:** 209–52.

66. Gronemeyer H, Transcription activation by estrogen and progesterone receptors. *Annu Rev Genet* 1991; **25:** 89–123.

67. Evans RM, Hollenberg SM, Zinc fingers: gilt by association. *Cell* 1988; **52:** 1–3.

68. Rhodes D, Klug A, Zinc fingers. *Sci Am* 1993; **Feb:** 32–9.

69. Ham J, Thomson A, Needham M, Webb P, Parker M, Characterization of response elements for androgens, glucocorticoids and progestins in mouse mammary tumour virus. *Nucleic Acid Res* 1988; **16:** 5263–76.

70. Riegman PHJ, Vlietstra RJ, van der Korput JAGM, Brinkmann AO, Trapman J, The promoter of the prostate-specific antigen gene contains a functional androgen-responsive element. *Mol Endocrinol* 1992; **5:** 1921–30.

71. Ohara-Nemoto Y, Stromstedt P-E, Dahiman-Wright K, Nemoto Y, Gustafsson JA, Carlstedt-Duke J, The steroid binding properties of recombinant glucocorticoid receptor: a putative role for heat shock protein hsp90. *J Steroid Biochem Mol Biol* 1990; **37:** 481–90.

72. Schowalter DB, Sullivan WP, Maihle NJ et al, Characterization of progesterone receptor binding to the 90- and 70-kDa heat shock proteins. *J Biol Chem* 1991; **266:** 21 165–73.

73. Cadepond F, Schweizer-Groyer G, Segard-Maurel I et al, Heat shock protein 90 as a critical factor in maintaining glucocorticoid receptor in a nonfunctional state. *J Biol Chem* 1991; **266:** 5834–41.

74. Picard D, Khursheed B, Garabedian MJ, Fortin MG, Lindquist S, Yamamoto KR, Reduced levels of hsp90 compromise steroid receptor action in vivo. *Nature* 1990; **348:** 166–8.

75. Smith DF, Toft DO, Steroid receptors and their associated proteins. *Mol Endocrinol* 1993; **7:** 4–11.

76. Kumar V, Chambon P, The estrogen receptor binds tightly to its responsive element as a ligand-induced homodimer. *Cell* 1988; **55:** 145–56.

77. Imperato-McGinley J, Guerrero L, Gautier T, Peterson RE, Steroid 5α-reductase deficiency in man: an inherited form of male pseudohermaphroditism. *Science* 1974; **186:** 1213–15.

78. Aaronson S, Growth factors and cancer. *Science* 1991; **254:** 1146–53.

79. Griffiths K, Davies P, Eaton CL, Harper ME, Turkes A, Peeling WB, Endocrine factors in the initiation, diagnosis and treatment of prostatic cancer. In: *Endocrine Dependent Tumors* (Voigt KD, Knabbe C, eds). Raven Press: New York, 1991: 83–130.

80. Berredge MJ, Inositol triphosphates and diacyl glycerol: two interacting second messengers. *Annu Rev Biochem* 1987; **56:** 159–93.

81. Bishop JM, The molecular genetics of cancer. *Science* 1987; **235:** 305–11.

82. Weinberg RA, The action of oncogenes in the cytoplasm and nucleus. *Science* 1983; **230:** 770–6.

83. Rohr HP, Bartsch G, Human benign prostatic hyperplasia: a stromal disease? New perspectives by quantitative morphology. *Urology* 1980; **16:** 625–33.

84. Franks LM, Riddle PN, Carbonell AW, Gey GO, A comparative study of the ultrastructure and lack of growth capacity of adult human prostate epithelium mechanically separated from its stroma. *J Pathol* 1970; **100:** 113–19.

85. Cunha GR, Chung LWK, Shannon JM, Taguchi O, Fujii H, Hormone-induced morphogenesis and growth: role of mesenchymal–epithelial interactions. *Recent Prog Hormone Res* 1983; **39:** 559–95.

86. Cunha GR, Donjacour AA, Cooke PS et al, The endocrinology and developmental biology of the prostate. *Endocr Rev* 1987; **8:** 338–62.

87. Chung LWK, Cunha GR, Stromal-epithelial interactions: II. Regulation of prostatic growth by embryonic urogenital sinus mesenchyme. *Prostate* 1983; **4:** 503–11.

88. Kim IY, Ahn HJ, Zelner DJ, Park L, Sensibar JA, Lee C, Expression and localisation of transforming growth factor-β receptors type I and type II in the rat ventral prostate during regression. *Mol Endocrinol* 1996; **10:** 107–15.

89. Lee C, Kozlowski JM, Grayhack JT, Etiology of benign prostatic hyperplasia. *Urol Clinics North Am* 1995; **22:** 124–8.

90. Sherwood ER, Fong CJ, Lee C, Kozlowski JM, Basic fibroblast growth factor: a potential mediator of stromal growth in the human prostate. *Endocrinology* 1992; **130:** 2955–63.

91. Yan G, Fukabori Y, Nikolaropoulos S, Wang F, McKeehan WL, Heparin-binding keratinocyte growth factor is a candidate stromal to epithelial cell andromedin. *Mol Endocrinol* 1992; **6:** 2123–8.

92. Yan G, Fukabori Y, McBride G, Nikolaropoulos S, McKeehan WL, Exon switching and activa-

tion of stromal and embryonic fibroblast growth factor (FGF) – FGF receptor genes in prostate epithelial cells accompany stromal independence and malignancy. *Mol Cell Biol* 1993; **13**: 4513–22.

93. Miki T, Bottaro DP, Fleming TP et al, Determination of ligand-binding specificity by alternate splicing: two distinct growth factor receptors encoded by a single gene. *Proc Natl Acad Sci USA* 1992; **89**: 246–50.

94. Yan G, Wang F, Fukabori Y, Sussman D, Hou J, McKeehan WL, Expression and transforming activity of a variant of the heparin-binding fibroblast growth factor receptor (flg) gene resulting from splicing of the alpha exon at an alternate 3'-acceptor site. *Biochem Biophys Res Commun* 1992; **183**: 423–30.

95. Sugimura Y, Cunha GR, Hayword S, Hayashi N, Arima K, Kawamura J, Keratinocyte growth factor (KGF) is a mediator of testosterone induced prostatic development. *J Urol* 1994; **151**: 381A.

96. Berry SJ, Coffey DS, Walsh PC, Ewing LL, The development of human benign prostate hyperplasia with age. *J Urol* 1984; **132**: 474–9.

97. Isaacs JT, Coffey DS, Etiology and disease process of benign prostatic hyperplasia. *Prostate* 1989; (suppl 2): 33–50.

98. Lee C, Sensibar JA, Dudek SM, Hiipakka RA, Liao S, Prostatic ductal system in rats: regional variation in morphological and functional activities. *Biol Reprod* 1990; **43**: 1079–86.

99. Sensibar JA, Griswold MD, Sylvester SR et al, Prostatic ductal system in rats: regional variation in localisation of an androgen-suppressed gene product, sulfated glycoprotein-2. *Endocrinology* 1991; **128**: 2091–102.

100. Wong P, Pineault J, Lakins JN et al, Genomic organisation and expression of the rat TRPM-2 (clusterin) gene, a gene implicated in apoptosis. *J Biol Chem* 1993; **268**: 5021–31.

101. Ichihara I, Kallio M, Pelliniemi LJ, Light and electron microscopy of the ducts and their subepithelial tissue in the rat ventral prostate. *Cell Tissue Res* 1978; **192**: 381–90.

102. Nemeth J, Lee C, The prostatic ductal system in rats: regional variation in stromal organization. *Prostate* 1996; **28**: 124–8.

103. Kyprianou N, Isaacs JT, Expression of transforming growth factor-β in the rat ventral prostate during castration-induced programmed cell death. *Mol Endocrinol* 1989; **3**: 1515–22.

104. Martikainen P, Kyprianou N, Isaacs JT, Effect of transforming growth factor-β on proliferation and death of rat prostate cells. *Endocrinology* 1990; **127**: 2963–8.

105. Kassen A, Kozlowski JM, Lee C, Role of basic fibroblast growth factor in the autocrine regulation of LNCaP proliferation induced by dihydrotestosterone. In: *77th Annual Meeting Endocrine Society*, Abstract P1-639.

106. Lee C, Sutkowski DM, Sensibar JA et al, Regulation of proliferation and production of prostate-specific antigen in androgen-sensitive prostatic cancer cell line LNCaP, by dihydrotesterone. *Endocrinology* 1995; **137**: 991–9.

107. Lee C, Cellular interactions in prostate cancer. *Br J Urol* 1997; **79**(suppl 1): 21–7.

108. Veldscholte J, Ris-Stalpers C, Kuiper GGJM et al, A mutation in the ligand binding domain of the androgen receptor of human LNCaP cells affects steroid binding characteristics and response to antiandrogens. *Biochem Biophys Res Commun* 1990; **173**: 534–40.

109. Vogelstein B, Fearon ER, Hamilton SR et al, Genetic alterations during colon rectal tumor development. *N Engl J Med* 1988; **319**: 525–32.

110. Griffiths K, Morton MS, Nicholson RI, Androgens, androgen receptors, antiandrogens and the treatment of prostate cancer. *Eur Urol* 1997; **32**: 24–40.

111. Jones HE, Dutkowski CM, Barrow D, Harper ME, Wakeling AE, Nicholson RI, A new EGF-R selective tyrosine kinase inhibitor reveals variable growth responses in the prostate carcinoma cell lines PC-3 and Du145. *Int J Cancer* 1997; **71**: 1010–18.

112. Hofer D, Sherwood E, Bromberg W, Mendelsohn J, Lee C, Kozlowski JM, Autonomous growth of androgen-independent prostatic carcinoma cells: Role of TGF-α. *Cancer Res* 1991; **51**: 2780–5.

113. Davies P, Eaton CL, France TD, Phillips MEA, Growth factor receptors and oncogene expression in prostate cells. *Am J Clin Oncol* 1988; **11**(suppl 2): S1–7.

114. Miller AB, Berriono F, Hill M, Pietinen G, Riboli E, Wahrendorf J, Diet in the aetiology of cancer: a review. *Eur J Cancer* 1994; **30A**: 207–20.

115. Miksicek RJ, Commonly occurring plant flavonoids have estrogenic activity. *Mol Pharmacol* 1993; **44**: 37–43.

116. Price KR, Fenwick GR, Naturally occurring oestrogens in food: a review. *Food Add Contam* 1985; **2**: 73–106.

117. Rao CBS (ed), *The Chemistry of Lignans*. Andra University Press: Waltair, India, 1978: 1–377.

118. Adlercreutz H, Honjo H, Higashi A et al, Urinary excretion of lignans and isoflavonoid phytoestrogens in Japanese men and women consuming traditional Japanese diet. *Am J Clin Nutr* 1991; **54**: 1093–100.

119. Adlercreutz H, Markkanen H, Watanabe S, Plasma concentrations of phyto-oestrogens in Japanese men. *Lancet* 1993; **342**: 1209–10.

120. Adlercreutz H, Fotsis T, Bannwart C et al, Determination of urinary lignans and phyto-estrogen metabolites, potential antiestrogens and anticarcinogens, in urine of women on various habitual diets. *J Steroid Biochem* 1986; **25**: 791–7.

121. Adlercreutz H, Hockerstedt K, Bannwart C et al, Effect of dietary components, including lignans and phytoestrogens on enterohepatic circulation and liver metabolism of estrogens and on sex hormone binding globulin (SHBG). *J Steroid Biochem* 1987; **27**: 1135–44.

122. Adlercreutz H, Bannwart C, Wahala K et al, Inhibition of human aromatase by mammalian lignans and isoflavonoid phytoestrogens. *J Steroid Biochem Mol Biol* 1993; **44**: 147–53.

123. Evans BAJ, Personal communication.

124. Evans BAJ, Griffiths K, Morton MS, Inhibition of 5α-reductase and 17β-hydroxysteroid dehydrogenase in genital skin fibroblasts by dietary lignans and isoflavonoids. *J Endocrinol* 1995; **147**: 295–302.

125. Rice-Evans CA, Miller NJ, Bolwell PG, Bramley PM, Pridham JB, The relative antioxidant activities of plant-derived polyphenolic flavonoids. *Free Radical Res* 1995; **22**: 375–83.

126. Akiyama T, Ishida J, Nakagawa S et al, Genistein, a specific inhibitor of tyrosine-specific protein kinases. *J Biol Chem* 1987; **262**: 5592–5.

127. Schlessinger J, Schreiber AB, Levi A, Lax J, Liberman T, Yarder Y, Regulation of cell proliferation by epithelial growth factor. *Crit Rev Biochem* 1983; **14**: 93–111.

128. Kenyon GL, Garcia GA, Design of kinase inhibitors. *Med Res Rev* 1987; **7**: 389–416.

129. Kiguchi K, Glesne D, Chubb CH, Fukiki H, Huberman E, Differential induction of apoptosis in human breast cells by okadaic acid and related inhibitors of protein phosphatases 1 and 2A. *Cell Growth Differentiation* 1994; **5**: 995–1004.

130. Scholar EM, Toews ML, Inhibition of invasion of murine mammary carcinoma cells by the tyrosine kinase inhibitor genistein. *Cancer Lett* 1994; **87**: 159–62.

131. Tiisala S, Majuri MI, Carpen O, Renkonen R, Genistein enhances the ICAM-mediated adhesion by inducing the expression of ICAM-1 and its counter receptors. *Biochem Biophys Res Commun* 1994; **203**: 443–9.

132. Folkman J, Watson K, Ingber D, Hanahan D, Induction of angiogenesis during the transition from hyperplasia to neoplasia. *Nature* 1989; **339**: 58–61.

133. Folkman J, Towards an understanding of angiogenesis: search and discovery. *Persp Biol Med* 1985; **29**: 10–36.

134. Weidner M, Semple JP, Welch WR, Folkman J, Tumour angiogenesis and metaplasia – correlation in invasive breast cancer. *N Engl J Med* 1991; **324**: 1–8.

135. Fotsis T, Pepper M, Aldercreutz H, Fleischmann G, Hase T, Montesano R, Schweigerer L, Genistein, a dietary-derived inhibitor of an in vitro angiogenesis. *Proc Natl Acad Sci USA* 1993; **90**: 2690–4.

136. Messina MJ, Persky V, Setchell KDR, Barnes S, Soy intake and cancer risk: a review of the in vitro and in vivo data. *Nutr Cancer* 1994; **21**: 113–30.

137. Chae YH, Ho DK, Cassady JM, Cook VM, Marcus CB, Baird WM, Effects of synthetic and naturally occurring flavonoids on metabolic activation of benz[*a*]pyrene in hamster cell cultures. *Chem Biol Int* 1992; **82**: 181–93.

138. Shi ST, Wang ZY, Smith TJ et al, Effects of green tea and black tea on 4-(methylnitrosoamino)-1-(3-pyridyl)-1 butanone bioactivation, DNA methylation and lung tumorigenesis in A/J mice. *Cancer Res* 1994; **54**: 4641–7.

5

Prostate immunology

Taz J Harmont, Timothy L Ratliff

The field of immunology has blossomed from an infant into a healthy child during the last three decades. A better understanding of the immune system has led to better graft survival in organ-transplant recipients, treatment for autoimmune diseases, immune dysfunction (in patients with acquired immune deficiency syndrome (AIDS)), and further insight into cancer, including novel immune therapy. This chapter is not intended to provide a detailed description of the immune system, but only a brief overview, concluding with a review of the current status of the immunology of the prostate.

CELLS OF THE IMMUNE SYSTEM

The immune system is composed of a functional network of cells. These cells are subgrouped based on their specific structure and function. For our purposes the important functional cells of the immune system can be divided into three groups: lymphocytes, monocytes/macrophages, and plasma cells.

Lymphocytes

Several lymphocyte subsets have been identified based on specific cell-surface markers and functional capacity. T cells, B cells, and natural killer (NK) cells form the lymphocyte population of the immune system that will be discussed in this review.

T cells

T cells differentiate in the thymus. The thymic-derived T cells considered here are the cytotoxic T lymphocyte (CTL) and the T-helper lymphocyte (Th).

The cluster of differentiation (CD) nomenclature defines cell-surface proteins on eukaryotic cells.[1] In immunological literature, CD designations are used to identify functional lymphocyte populations. For example, Th cells express the CD4 marker, whereas CTLs express CD8. The CD4 marker is a 55-kDa cell-surface glycoprotein that binds to major histocompatibility complex (MHC) class II molecules. CD8 is a disulfide-linked heterodimer glycoprotein (34 kDa) that binds MHC class I molecules.[1]

The CD markers conveniently segregate T cells into their respective functional categories.

CD4$^+$ Th cells function in the initiation and amplification of antigen-specific immune responses. Th cells are subdivided into two main functional subgroups, Th1 and Th2, based on cytokine production profiles.[2] Th1 cells produce cytokines that support delayed-type hypersensitivity responses and CTLs, while Th2 cells support antibody production.

The CD8$^+$ T cells function primarily as cytotoxic T cells. These cells are activated when presented with antigen complexed to the MHC class I molecule. Cytotoxic T cells mediate their cytolytic effects through a process called apoptosis.[3]

B cells
B cells are bone-marrow-derived lymphocytes that reside in the marginal zone of the spleen, the cortex of lymph nodes, and the Peyer's patches of the intestine. These cells have a life-span of several months. B cells express cell-surface immunoglobulin (Ig) complexed to the Ig-α, Ig-β heterodimer.[4] These cell-surface receptors, known as B-cell receptors (BCRs), allow the B cell to bind whole antigen. The antigen–receptor complex is phagocytosed and the antigen is processed within the cytoplasm of the cell. The processed antigen is presented on the cell surface in association with specific antigen-presenting molecules to Th cells, which produce the cytokines that support the differentiation of B cells into plasma cells.

Plasma cells
Plasma cells are derived from activated B cells, through a maturation process activated by antigen.[1,3] These changes lead to terminal differentiation of the B cell into antibody-forming cells called plasma cells. Plasma cells comprise a very small portion of the lymphocyte system and are not found in circulating pools of lymphocytes, but reside in secondary lymphoid tissues and organs. Plasma cells have a very short life-span (approximately 3–7 days). During this short life-span, they produce antibodies of only one specificity and Ig class.

Natural killer cells
Natural killer (NK) cells are a distinct group of lymphocytes that are separated functionally and phenotypically from T and B lymphocytes.[5] NK cells mediate the lysis of target cells in an antigen-independent manner. They do not express CD4, CD8, immunoglobulins or T-cell antigen receptor.[6] Therefore, NK cells do not recognize antigen via the TCR, nor is their cytotoxic activity subject to the MHC class I or class II restrictions of CTLs or Th cells, respectively.

The NK-cell recognition of the target cell is via an unknown mechanism. The NK cell attaches to the target cell, releasing perforins from its cytoplasmic granules. Perforins create holes in the target-cell membrane. This is followed by the influx of granzymes through the perforin channels, which induce apoptosis.[7] NK-cell activity is stimulated via interleukin-2 (IL-2) and interleukin 4 (IL-4).[8] Stimulated NK cells produce interferon-γ (IFN-γ), which acts as positive feedback to enhance NK-cell activity further by promoting rapid differentiation of precursor cells.

Monocytes and macrophages

Macrophages are bone-marrow-derived cells that have two main functions: (1) to remove particulate antigen; and (2) to function as antigen-presenting cells.[9] These cells mature from monocytes, which migrate into the circulation and subsequently back through the capillaries and into tissues and various organs, where they mature into tissue histocytes or macrophages.

Macrophages serve many functions, including phagocytosis of apoptotic cells and bacteria, and the lysis of tumor cells.[9] Other receptors expressed by monocytes/macrophages include receptors for IL-2, IL-4 and IFN-γ. Thus macrophages are responsive to T-cell-derived cytokines at inflammatory sites. It also should be noted that, during phagocytosis, macrophages secrete numerous cytokines, including IL-2, which promotes Th1 immune responses.[2] Macrophages also function as antigen-presenting cells and appear to be necessary for the activation of previously unstimulated lymphocytes.

MAJOR HISTOCOMPATIBILITY COMPLEX AND ANTIGEN PRESENTATION

The major histocompatibility molecules are specialized glycoprotein receptors inherent in a gene complex called the major histocompatibility complex (MHC).[10] All mammals contain within their genome a major histocompatibility complex region. In humans, the MHC genes have been localized to the short arm of chromosome 6.[11] The MHC region is composed of three classes of genes, referred to in humans as human leukocyte antigens (HLAs).

MHC class I genes code for MHC proteins that are present on the surface of most nucleated cells, but not on red blood cells.[12] MHC class I genes present antigen peptides to CD8[+] CTL, as described below.

Class II genes code for surface molecules on dendritic cells, B cells and macrophages, and in some cases epithelial cells.[13] MHC class II genes present antigen peptides to Th lymphocytes.

Foreign antigens must be recognized by the cellular defense system in association with MHC. Immune recognition of antigen requires the antigen to be internalized and degraded, and the degraded portions of the antigens (peptides) must be linked to MHC, forming a peptide–MHC complex.[14]

MHC class I

Class I molecules are composed of two subunits, a heavy chain of 42 kDa and a smaller chain of 12 kDa.[10,11]. The smaller subunit does not vary with MHC type, and is known as β_2-microglobulin when found free in serum. The heavy chain, or α-subunit, traverses the cell membrane. The α-subunit is divided structurally into the α_3 domain, which has a transmembrane, and a cytoplasmic domain that is highly conserved. The extracellular surface domains are α_1 and α_2, which are polymorphic in structure. The α_1 and α_2 molecules form a trough with closed ends to create a long groove. Within this groove, peaks and valleys are created by amino acid variability, allowing for highly diversified binding specificity for anti-

gen peptides. The function of MHC molecules is to present the MHC–peptide complex to CTLs.

Class I molecules associate with antigens produced intracellularly. Endogenous antigens are degraded into short peptides of approximately nine amino acids and are transported into the endoplasmic reticulum where the peptides associate with MHC class I.[12,13] The complex is transported to the cell surface where it is stably expressed. MHC not linked to antigen peptides is unstable and is rapidly endocytosed by the cell.

MHC class II

The human MHC class II region, referred to as HLA-D, is subdivided into five loci (HLA-DN, -DO, -DP, -DQ, and -DR) on chromosome 6.[13] The structures of MHC class I and II molecules are similar. The class II molecules are glycoproteins composed of two α-chains (31–34 kDa) and two β-chains (25–29 kDa) non-covalently linked in a heterodimer fashion. This extracellular portion is connected via a short transmembrane sequence to a cytoplasmic domain. The outermost domains fold over to create an extended groove, similar to MHC class I. However, this trough is open-ended, so that longer peptides can be accommodated. The large number of alleles, both functional and non-functional, in the HLA-D sequence allows for a vast array of structural conformations at this binding site. The ability to diversify sequencing creates a high degree of polymorphism for the MHC class II molecules.

The expression of class II molecules is limited to specialized antigen-presenting cells of the immune system, including B cells, macrophages, dendritic cells of skin, and epithelial cells at sites of inflammation.[13,15]

MHC class II molecules primarily associate with antigen peptides internalized from the external environment.[14] Exogenous antigen is phagocytosed and fragmented within cytoplasmic lysosomes of the macrophage. The fragmented antigen binds to the MHC class II receptor and is transported to the cell surface where the complex is stably expressed. This complex on the cell's surface is recognized by the T-cell receptor of Th cells. Th cells can only recognize a foreign antigen if it is bound to a MHC class II molecule, and hence they are MHC class II-restricted cells.

CYTOKINES OF THE IMMUNE SYSTEM

As a result of appropriate stimulation and activation, the cells of the immune system secrete a vast array of proteins that function to signal certain cells to react and cause others to be inhibited, thus allowing control over the immune response. Generally, these proteins are called cytokines. Lymphokines are secreted specifically by lymphocytes. The plethora of cytokines secreted by the immune cells have many overlapping functions, creating a complex, interwoven cytokine network. For simplicity, we review here the most important cytokines in reference to urologic immunology.

Cytokines can be subdivided into several classes: interleukins, interferons, and tumor necrosis factors (growth factors and chemokines are two others, but these are not discussed here). In general, interleukins regulate the interactions between lymphocytes and other leukocytes. Interferons are glycoproteins synthesized in response to immune stimulation and many chemical stimulators, especially viral infections. IFN-γ is the only interferon that is truly a cytokine, although other interferons exist. Tumor necrosis factors are produced by macrophages and T cells and possess the ability to kill tumor cells. The cytokines are reviewed on the basis of their cells of origin.

Cytokines produced from macrophages

Interleukin-12
Macrophages produce many cytokines, including IL-12 and tumor necrosis factor-α (TNF-α).[16–18] IL-12 stimulates the Th1 response by promoting the secretion of IL-2 and IFN-γ. IFN-γ production functions as a positive feedback loop, which further enhances IL-12 pro-

duction by macrophages.[19] This not only further stimulates macrophages, but also causes NK-cell activation. IL-12 also induces lymphokine-activated killer (LAK) cell activation.

In addition to its stimulatory role, IL-12 possesses inhibitory effects. It inhibits Th2 functions, such as IgE production from stimulated B cells.[16]

Tumor necrosis factor-α
Macrophages also produce TNF-α, a 17-kDa protein. TNF-α functions as an inflammatory mediator and a growth factor.[20–22] It may also function as an integral membrane protein, imparting cytotoxic activity when the expressing cell comes into contact with the target cell.[20] Hence TNF-α can directly kill tumor cells. The proliferation of T and B cells, especially cytotoxic-T-cell activity, is stimulated by TNF-α. NK-cell activity is also enhanced by this cytokine.

TNF-α acts as a growth factor by stimulating the transcription factors *myc*, *jun*, and *fos*. It also functions as a fibroblast growth factor.[20,21] TNF-α stimulates vascular endothelial cells to produce leukocyte adhesion molecules, procoagulants, and MHC class I molecule expression. MHC class II molecule expression can also be induced by TNF-α.

Cytokines produced from T cells

T cells also produce cytokines; some are specific to Th1 cells and others to Th2 cell lineages.[2] The Th1 activities tend to counteract the Th2 activities, and thus a control mechanism exists between the two groups of effector cells.

Th1-produced cytokines
As noted previously, CD4[+] Th cells are subdivided into Th1 and Th2 subclasses, based on their cytokine-production profiles. The cytokines produced by each subset drives the development of functionally distinct immune responses.

IL-2 is a glycoprotein synthesized by Th1 cells in response to appropriately presented antigen and stimulation with IL-12.[2,23] It is produced by CD4[+] and some CD8[+] cells. IL-2 is the most potent T-cell growth factor and activator in the immune system. This lymphokine not only functions as a T-cell growth factor, but also mediates the activation of both B and NK cells. The production of IgG2a from B cells is stimulated by IL-2.[23] It should be noted that, like IL-12, IL-2 also stimulates the production of LAK cells, which lyse tumor cells in a manner similar to NK cells.[16]

Interferon-γ

IFN-γ is a glycoprotein produced by Th1 cells, CD8[+] T cells and NK cells.[19] IFN-γ stimulates T cells to produce IL-2 and assists IL-2 in initiating cytotoxic-T-cell proliferation. IFN-γ also acts as a positive feedback and further enhances NK-cell lytic activity. IFN-γ also activates macrophages and boosts antibody-mediated phagocytosis, as well as antibody-dependent cell-mediated cytotoxicity reactions. The expression of MHC class I and II molecules is also enhanced by IFN-γ, which enhances T-cell recognition of antigen.

IFN-γ plays a paradoxical role in the immune milieu. While IFN-γ functions to stimulate the immune system as noted above, it may also be immunosuppressive and enhance target-cell resistance to cell-mediated lysis. Cell growth is inhibited by the ability of IFN-γ to synchronize dividing cells into one phase of the cell cycle and increase the time spent in that phase. IFN-γ enhances the expression of TNF-α receptors on target-cell surfaces, thus conferring vulnerability to TNF-α and its mode of cell lysis.

Th2-produced cytokines

IL-4, previously known as B-cell activating or differentiating factor 1, functions as its name implies.[2,23] IL-4 stimulates B-cell activation, which promotes the production of immunoglobulins, especially IgG1 and IgE. MHC class II expression by B cells is enhanced by IL-4, but it inhibits the production of IL-1 and TNF-α.

IL-4 is the key cytokine in inducing the differentiation of Th2 cells. IFN-γ abrogates the functions of IL-4, except that both of these lymphokines stimulate MHC class II expression in macrophages.

Interleukin-10

IL-10 is a cytokine synthesis inhibitory factor secreted by Th2, B cells, and activated macrophages.[24] While functioning primarily as an inhibitory factor, IL-10 stimulates B-cell activation, induces MHC class II expression and promotes B-cell growth. The inhibitory effects of IL-10 are broad. IL-10 inhibits IFN-γ and IL-12 production, the ability of macrophages to present antigen, and the expression of delayed-type hypersensitivity responses. IL-10 also inhibits IL-4-induced IgE synthesis by B cells.[24] The immune system is a complex entity that is driven by the production of inflammatory cytokines, antigen activation of T cells, and their subsequent cytokine production. While there is functional overlap in cytokine activities, specific cytokines are linked to identifiable cell types and the differentiation and expression of either a cell-mediated or antibody response. Thus, characterization of the infiltrating cell types and cytokine profiles in organ-specific inflammation provides insight into the character of the immune response.

HISTOLOGICAL CHARACTERIZATION OF PROSTATE INFLAMMATION

Histological and immunohistochemical analysis of prostate specimens reveals that virtually 100% of specimens contain foci of chronic inflammation.[25,26] Our studies in men with benign prostates (documented by three negative multicore biopsies) with no prostatitis symptoms showed 98.6% (145/147) with chronic mononuclear inflammation.[26] Steiner and associates[27,28] characterized the mononuclear infiltrate in benign prostatic hyperplasia (BPH), and reported a predominance of CD3[+] T lymphocytes expressing the α,β T-cell receptor. The inflammatory infiltrate was observed in periglandular stroma.[28] Epithelial cells associated with the inflammatory sites expressed HLA-DR but not other class II haplotypes.[28] Mononuclear infiltration of the epithelial cells was reported in about 20% of glands evaluated; however, epithelial cell degeneration was not observed. Instead, squamous metaplasia was observed at inflammatory sites.[29] In our analysis, basal epithelial cell hyperplasia was more often seen.

FUNCTIONAL CHARACTERIZATION OF PROSTATIC INFLAMMATION

There is a paucity of data characterizing the functional aspects of the inflammatory infiltrate of the prostate. Steiner and associates[27,30] extended their immunohistochemical observations to include a functional analysis of infiltrating lymphocytes. These investigators isolated infiltrating lymphocytes via a series of density gradients and determined activation state and cytokine profiles. Flow cytometric analysis revealed that the infiltrating T cells were almost exclusively activated cells expressing CD45RO (94% for CD8$^+$ for CD4$^+$). In addition, the T cells were shown to produce IL-2 and IFN-γ after in vitro stimulation.[30] Immunohistochemical analysis for IL-2 and IFN-γ showed elevated expression of IFN-γ in BPH tissue compared to control and carcinoma specimens, but no detectable IL-2. Other cytokine levels were not reported.

A spontaneous model of chronic prostatic inflammation in rats has also been reported.[31] It was demonstrated that three strains of rats (Wistar, Lewis, and Sprague–Dawley) were susceptible to the development of prostatic inflammation. Histologically, the disease was characterized by mononuclear infiltration in the prostate. Interestingly, the inflammatory process was shown to be age-dependent, hormonally modulated, and, based on our independent review of the histology, to induce stromal and epithelial cell hyperplasia.

The incidence of spontaneous prostatic inflammation was increased from 30% in untreated Wistar rats to 100% in estrogen-treated rats. Estrogen (17β-estradiol) was administered for 30 days to 10- to 13-month-old rats at a dose of 0.25 mg/kg daily. While testosterone blocked the effects of estrogens, dihydroxytestosterone did not. A similar enhancement of prostate inflammation was observed with castration. Interestingly, the

treatment of rats on days 3 and 5 of life with 100 µg 17β-estradiol followed by testosterone (2 mg/day) for 14 days induced chronic prostatic inflammation in young rats (aged 84 days at sacrifice). These data show that inflammation in the prostate can be modulated by steroidal hormones. Either the absence of testosterone or the addition of estrogen enhances the development of chronic prostatic inflammation. The mechanisms by which this occurs and the effects of such modulation on prostate function are not known.

Induction of prostate inflammation using autologous antigen as an immunogen was first shown in 1981 by Pacheco-Rupil et al.[32] In animals immunized once with prostate protein in Freund's complete adjuvant, only 30% of the rats developed inflammation, while inflammation was observed in 90% of animals after multiple immunizations.[33,34] The inflammatory response was characterized by mononuclear infiltration of cells into the interstitium primarily surrounding blood vessels and close to the epithelium. The reported pattern of inflammation is similar to that observed in histological studies on clinical prostate specimens by us and others.[25,28] In some animals the inflammatory process induced fibrosis with enlargement of the acini and epithelial flattening in the parenchyma. We adapted this model for use in mice, and obtained similar results.[35] In our model the chronic inflammatory process was characterized by perivascular inflammation, lymphocytic infiltration of the stroma and periglandular region, edema, and occasional degeneration of epithelial cells. The induction of the inflammatory response was specific for the prostate.

IMMUNOTHERAPY OF PROSTATE CANCER

Prostate cancer is a high incidence cancer in men. No adequate treatment for invasive, hormone-insensitive cancer is available. Several studies have suggested that immunotherapy may provide an approach to the development of effective therapy for this disease.[36,37]

However, clinical trials are in their early stages and additional preclinical testing is needed.

Previous animal studies using retrovirus-transduced Dunning rat prostate cancer cells showed antitumor activity that was limited to local antitumor mechanisms.[38,39] These investigators observed inhibition of tumor growth after immunization with the cytokine-secreting tumor cells, but did not observe protection against secondary tumor challenge or CTL activity. We observed similar results using the pox virus gene delivery system, ALVAC (Virogenetics, Inc., Troy, New York).[40] In contrast to these studies, Vieweg et al[41] reported the development of CTL activity after multiple (three) immunizations with IL-2-secreting Dunning Mat/LyLu tumor cells. These investigators showed inhibition of tumor growth which was associated with the CTL activity but did not determine whether rats were protected against secondary tumor challenge. The reason for the contradictory CTL results is not known.

It is clear from previous reports that the mechanism by which a viable tumor inoculum is rejected varies with the tumor model system.[42–44] Fearon et al,[42] using the B16 melanoma model, showed inhibition of tumor growth only by IL-2 recombinants. No other cytokine-transduced cell line was rejected when viable tumor cells were injected. Although the initial inoculum of IL-2-producing cells was rejected, no protection against a secondary challenge was observed. This was true for both live and irradiated IL-2-transduced B16 cells. Similarly, Connor et al[45] observed inhibition of the growth of viable cytokine-transduced bladder carcinoma tumor growth that was independent of tumor-specific immunity. However, in the mammary tumor model, long-term protection against secondary tumor challenge was observed. These data suggest that the mechanisms by which primary tumor cells are killed differ from the traditional CTL-dependent mechanisms often associated with tumor rejection, regardless of whether long-term immunity mediated by CD8[+] CTL is observed. As suggested by the data for prostate tumors, an important antiprostate tumor mechanism is independent of B and T cells. Further unpublished data from our laboratory suggest an important role for NK-mediated effector mechanisms.

Taken together, these data suggest that the delivery of cytokines to the prostate may be an effective non-surgical therapy for localized prostate cancer. We believe that the canarypox virus, ALVAC, which is restricted to avian species for productive replication, provides a means of safely implementing local therapy of prostate cancer. While ALVAC replication is restricted, its ability to induce expression of an engineered gene in mammalian cells is excellent.[46] Thus, the inability of ALVAC to productively replicate in non-avian species provides an excellent safety barrier against the occurrence of vaccine-associated or vaccine-induced complications such as those seen with replicating vaccinia virus in the vaccination for smallpox.[47]

REFERENCES

1. Tizard I, Lymphocytes. In: *Immunology: An Introduction* (Tizard I, ed), 4th edn. WB Saunders: Philadelphia, 1995: 125–38.

2. Romagnani S, Human TH1 and TH2 subsets: doubt no more. *Immunol Today* 1991; **11:** 256–7.

3. Roitt I, Brostoff J, Male O, *Immunology*, 4th edn. Mosby: St Louis, MO, 1996.

4. Amigorena S, Drake JR, Webster P, Mellman I, Transient accumulation of new class II MHC molecules in a novel endocytic compartment in B lymphocytes. *Nature* 1994; **369:** 113–20.

5. Westermann J, Pabst R, Distribution of lymphocyte subsets and natural killer cells in the human body. *Clin Invest* 1992; **70:** 539–44.

6. Trinchiell G, Biology of natural killer cells. *Adv Immunol* 1989; **47:** 187–376.

7. Heusei JW, Wesselschmidt RL, Shresta S et al, Cytotoxic lymphocytes require granzyme B for

the rapid induction of DNA fragmentation and apoptosis in allogenic target cells. *Cell* 1994; **76:** 977–87.

8. Brooks CG, Georgiou A, Jordan RK, The majority of immature fetal thymocytes can be induced to proliferate to IL-2 and differentiate into cells indistinguishable from nature natural killer cells. *J Immunol* 1993; **151:** 6645–56.

9. Johnston RB, Current concepts: immunology monocytes and macrophages. *N Engl J Med* 1988; **318:** 747–52.

10. Steinmetz M, The major histocompatibility complex: organization and evolution. *Clin Immunol News* 1986; **7:** 134–7.

11. Bodmer JG, Marsh SE, Albet ED et al, Nomenclature for factors of the HLA system. *Tissue Antigens* 1994; **46:** 1–18.

12. Salter RD, Benjamin RJ, Wesley PK et al, A binding site for the T cells co-receptor CD8 on the α_3 domain of HLA-A2. *Nature* 1990; **345:** 41–6.

13. Brown JH, Jardetzky TS, Gorga JC et al, Three-dimensional structure of the human class II histocompatibility antigen HLA-DR1. *Nature* 1993; **364:** 33–9.

14. Stern LJ, Wiley DC, Antigenic peptide binding by class I and class II histocompatibility proteins. *Structure* 1994; **2:** 245–51.

15. Clevers H, Alarcon B, Wileman T, Terhorst C, The T cell receptor/CD3 complex: a dynamic protein ensemble. *Annu Rev Immunol* 1988; **6:** 629–62.

16. Teinchier G, Function and clinical use of interleukin-12. *Curr Opin Hematol* 1997; **4:** 59–66.

17. Scott P, IL-12: initiation cytokine for cell-mediated immunity. *Science* 1994; **260:** 496–7.

18. Smith CA, Farrah T, Goodwin RG, The TNF receptor superfamily of cellular and viral proteins: activation costimulation and death. *Cell* 1994; **76:** 959–62.

19. Young HA, Hardy KJ, Role of interferon-gamma in immune cell regulation. *J Leukocyte Biol* 1995; **58:** 373–81.

20. Rine L, Kitchnor H, Recent progress in the TNF-α field. *Int Arch Allergy Immunol* 1996; **14:** 199–209.

21. Riches DW, Chan ED, Winston BW, TNF-α-induced regulation and signalling in macrophages. *Immunobiology* 1996; **195:** 477–90.

22. Barbara JA, Van Ostads X, TNF: the good, the bad, and time-potentially very effective. *Immunol Cell Biol* 1996; **74:** 434–43.

23. Rebollo A, Gomez J, Martinez AC, Lessons from immunological, biochemical and molecular pathways of the activation mediated by IL-2 and IL-4. *Adv Immunol* 1996; **63:** 127–96.

24. Howard M, O'Garra A, Biological properties of IL-10. *Immunol Today* 1992; **13:** 198–200.

25. McClinton S, Miller ID, Eremin O, An immuno-histochemical characterisation of the inflammatory cell infiltrate in benign and malignant prostatic disease. *Br J Cancer* 1990; **61:** 400–3.

26. Nadler RB, Humphrey PA, Smith DS et al, Effect of inflammation and benign prostatic hyperplasia on elevated serum prostate specific antigen levels. *J Urol* 1995; **154:** 407–13.

27. Steiner G, Gessl A, Kramer G et al, Phenotype and function of peripheral and prostatic lymphocytes in patients with benign prostatic hyperplasia. *J Urol* 1994; **151:** 480–4.

28. Theyer G, Kramer G, Assmann I et al, Characterization of infiltrating leukocytes in benign prostatic hyperplasia. *Lab Invest* 1992; **66:** 96–107.

29. Smith CJ, Gardner A, Inflammation–proliferation: possible relationships in the prostate. In: *Current Concepts and Approaches to the Study of Prostate Cancer* (Coffey D, Bruchovsky N, Gardner W et al, eds). AR Liss: New York, 1987: 317–25.

30. Steiner GE, Knerer B, Dorfinger K et al, Increased expression of interferon-γ in benign prostatic hyperplasia. *J Urol* 1996; **155:** 465A.

31. Naslund MJ, Strandberg JD, Coffey DS, The role of androgens and estrogens in the pathogenesis of experimental nonbacterial prostatitis. *J Urol* 1988; **140:** 1049–53.

32. Pacheco-Rupil B, Depiante-Depaoli M, Ronero O et al, Experimental autoimmune damage to rat male accessory glands (MAG). *Am J Reprod Immunol* 1981; **1:** 255–61.

33. Depiante-Depaoli M, Pacheco-Rupil B, Casakio B, Experimental autoimmune damage to rat male accessory glands. I. Transfer of autoimmune response by spleen cells. *Am J Reprod Immunol* 1984; **5:** 9–14.

34. Pacheco-Rupil B, Depiante-Depaoli M, Casakio B, Experimental autoimmune damage to rat male accessory glands. II. T cell requirement in adoptive transfer of specific tissue damage. *Am J Reprod Immunol* 1984; **5:** 15–19.

35. Keetch DW, Humphrey PA, Ratliff TL, Development of a mouse model for nonbacterial prostatitis. *J Urol* 1994; **152:** 247–50.

36. Hock H, Dorsch M, Kuzendorf U et al, Vaccinations with tumor cells genetically engineered to produce different cytokines: effectively

not superior to a classical adjuvant. *Cancer Res* 1993; **53:** 714–16.

37. Moss B, Replicating and host-restricted non-replicating vaccinia virus vectors for vaccine development. *Dev Biol Stand* 1994; **82:** 55–63.

38. Yoshimura I, Heston WDW, Gansbacher B, Fair WR, Cytokine mediated immuno-gene therapy in rat prostate cancer model. *J Urol* 1996; **155:** 510A.

39. Sanda MG, Ayyagari SR, Jeffer EM et al, Demonstration of a rational strategy for human prostate cancer gene therapy. *J Urol* 1994; **151:** 622–8.

40. Kawakita M, Rao GS, Richey JK et al, Effect of canarypox virus (ALVAC)-mediated cytokine expression on murine prostate tumor growth. *J Natl Cancer Inst* 1997; **89:** 428–36.

41. Vieweg J, Rosenthal FM, Bannerji R et al, Immunotherapy of prostate cancer in the Dunning rat model: use of cytokine gene modified tumor vaccines. *Cancer Res* 1994; **54:** 1760–5.

42. Fearon ER, Pardoll DM, Itaya T et al, Interleukin-2 production by tumor cells by passes T helper function in the generation of an antitumor response. *Cell* 1962; **60:** 397–403.

43. Townsend SE, Allison JP, Tumor rejection after direct costimulation of CD8$^+$ T cells by B7-transfected melanoma cells. *Science* 1993; **259:** 368–70.

44. Pagador A, Bannerji R, Watanabe Y et al, Antimetastatic vaccination of tumor-bearing mice with two types of IFN-gamma gene-inserted tumor cells. *J Immunol* 1993; **150:** 1458–70.

45. Connor J, Bannerji R, Saito S et al, Regression of bladder tumors in mice treated with interleukin-2 gene-modified tumor cells. *J Exp Med* 1993; **177:** 1127–34.

46. Tartaglia J, Perkus ME, Taylor J et al, NYVAC: a highly attenuated strain of vaccinia virus. *Virology* 1992; **188:** 217–32.

47. Baxby D, Paoletti E, Potential use of non-replicating vectors as recombinant vaccines. *Vaccine* 1992; **10:** 8–9.

6

Gene therapy

Warren DW Heston

Gene therapy is defined as the transfer of genetic material into the cells of an organism in order to treat a disease. In a recent article in *Time Magazine* it was stated that in 20 years all diseases will be treatable by gene therapy.[1] That may be a little overly optimistic, but reflects the rosy outlook being engendered by the enthusiasts who are applying these new technologies for the treatment of disease.

INBORN ERRORS OF METABOLISM: ADA DEFICIENCY

The easiest disease to treat with gene therapy would be one in which there is a known gene deficiency, wherein all that is required is to insert a gene that is functional when expressed. A strong initial effort has focused on diseases such as adenosine deaminase deficiency (ADA). This disease will be inherited as ADA$^{-/-}$ in less than 1 per 100 000 live births.[2] In some children with this disease a single point mutation out of 30 000 in each copy of the gene is enough to result in a failure of the immune system to protect against persistent viral and fungal infections, repeated bacterial infections, and early

cancer. This category of immune deficiency disease is called *severe combined immune deficiency* (SCID). ADA deficiency has been treated successfully by inserting the message for adenosine deaminase into bone marrow progenitor cells of the young patients with this disease.[2] The restoration of the ability to live a normal life and not be forced to live a life confined to a sterile environmental support bubble is a dramatic reflection of what can be achieved by gene therapy approaches.

Treatment of ADA deficiency is considered optimal for a gene therapeutic approach, in that one has a disease in which the specific problem (i.e. a functionless protein) is known, and this can be corrected by insertion into the genome of a gene which can be expressed in the stem cells of the patient and be permanently expressed in the patient's cells, and thus the condition can be 'cured'.[2] The gene can be inserted under controlled conditions using cells ex vivo, and these cells reinserted back into the patient. This is what can be achieved in a specific targetable correctable deficiency. In the instance of ADA deficiency, there is no attempt to correct the faulty DNA, but rather a functional DNA is inserted to correct the loss of active protein.

This is accomplished outside the body, by obtaining the 'stem cell' population and transfecting with retroviral vectors. Retroviral vectors incorporate into the DNA of the cell and provide the best chance of giving the cell a 'permanent' ability to produce the new protein. While there are problems and limitations associated with this form of gene therapy, they are less than those associated with the treatment of other diseases such as cancer.

Problems arise because the inserted gene may be silenced over time, with further gene therapy being required later.[2] With some forms of gene therapy in which attenuated viral vectors such as retroviral vectors are used, there is always the possibility of a subsequent recombination event leading to a restoration of a functional retrovirus, with the attendant risk of infection and potential for cancer induction in future years. Most viral vectors are now attenuated in such a manner that it is highly unlikely that the virus could become reactivated. To avoid this problem, viral vectors are being developed which, even if reactivated, would not be able to cause infection in humans or to use non-viral vectors for transfection. A constant concern is that long-term expression requires that the gene be inserted into the cell's DNA. Because such insertion is random, it is always possible that the gene might insert into an oncogene suppressor region, and thus end up being oncogenic. Vectors are being developed that enter into defined regions of the genome, thus reducing the likelihood of insertional mutagenesis. In terms of corrective gene therapy for disorders such as ADA deficiency, gene therapy can prove to be effective.[2]

GENE THERAPY FOR CANCER

The development of gene therapy for diseases such as cancer will be a much more demanding task.[1,2] Cancer is the result of massive genetic damage. Once a cancer has become a clinical problem, it has undergone many genetic hits in critical regions. In order to correct this genetic damage, theoretically we would have to insert corrective DNA into each and every cancer cell.

Cancers are notoriously heterogeneous, and so different tumor regions might require different corrective DNA. In the future the selective correction of host cells in situ may be possible, but at present we lack the technology to deliver corrective DNA to each and every cancer cell. A further problem is the nature of the action of the corrective gene. Corrective gene therapy can be used both for suppressor genes and for oncogenes. Suppressor genes are associated with a loss of function, similar to the ADA model, and reinsertion of the suppressor gene is corrective. Positive-acting oncogenes provide a gain of function in action, and are a problem because their abnormal function needs to be eliminated. In the case of the oncogenes such as *ras*, often a single nucleotide has been mutated. This presents a real challenge for 'corrective gene therapy'. One approach is to use a 'ribozyme' that selectively cuts the specific mutated RNA, thus eliminating the mutant product. However, such esoteric approaches to eliminating the specific expression of an oncogene require substantial work before they are readily translatable to use in patients.[2]

Gene therapy for cancer is currently being pursued along approaches that have certain strategies in common. These strategies include the insertion of genes for activation of prodrugs at the tumor site, for imparting drug resistance to bone marrow stem cells for use in high-dose regimens, for replacement of lost suppressor genes or inactivation of oncogenes, and for enhancement of tumor recognition by the immune system, with subsequent tumor rejection.[2]

GENE THERAPY DELIVERY SYSTEMS

In gene therapy the delivery system is critical in getting the genes to the target. Many systems involve the use of viral vectors for gene delivery, because Nature has already provided the virus with all the proteins necessary for binding and injecting DNA into the cell, with the foreign DNA being able to gain access to the nucleus in order to use and subvert the host's transcriptional machinery. There are a number

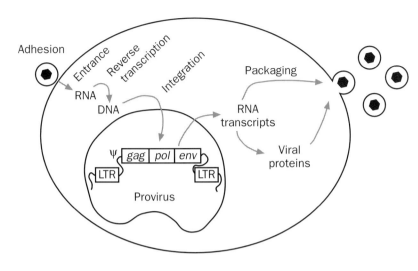

Figure 6.1 The retrovirus life cycle. The retrovirus binds to the cell surface, and the viral RNA and protein are injected into the cell, where the retroviral reverse transcriptase transcribes it into cDNA. The cDNA is then integrated into the host DNA at random sites of integration, following which the viral DNA is transcribed into mRNA, which codes for the viral proteins involved in packaging the viral mRNA and associated proteins such as the viral reverse transcriptase. The packaged viral particles then bud from the cell and are infectious and ready to infect another cell.

of viral vectors currently in use: retroviral vectors, adenoviral vectors, the herpes simplex viral vector, and others such as vaccinia and adeno-associated viral vectors. Viral vectors that are unable to reinfect cells and are thus incapable of infectious spread, such as baculovirus and avian pox virus, are also being investigated.[3–5]

One of the first viral vectors used was the retroviral vector. These vectors are well understood and a number of packaging cell lines are available for use. The retrovirus life cycle is illustrated and discussed in Figure 6.1. Briefly, the retrovirus binds to the cell membrane and then enters the cell. Inside the cell a unique polymerase, reverse transcriptase, converts the viral RNA to DNA, and the DNA migrates to the nucleus where it integrates into the cell's DNA. This is a key feature of retroviruses and represents an important aspect for consideration in gene therapy; that is, integration into the host's DNA provides for 'long-term' expression of the transfected DNA. If one wishes to achieve long-term gene expression, retroviral vectors provide a useful approach. A minor problem with the insertion of a retrovirus into the DNA is that the retrovirus inserts into random sites within the host-cell DNA, and there-fore could integrate into the site of a suppressor gene, the loss of expression of which could lead to the development of uncontrolled growth. This is an unlikely occurrence, but one that needs to be considered.

For gene therapy, the retrovirus is engineered such that the DNA-coding regions for *gag*, *pol*, and *env* are removed and are replaced with the gene of interest in a plasmid construct (Figure 6.2). The plasmid is then transfected into a packaging cell line that has been transfected with a crippled virus such that the viral coat proteins are made but cannot combine with the viral DNA to form infectious virus. When transfected with the re-engineered virus that expresses the DNA of interest, the genetically engineered shuttle vector has a proper packaging signal and so becomes incorporated in the viral coat protein and forms infectious viral particles. The engineered retrovirus is excreted from the cell, which can then be harvested from the tissue culture supernatant. This supernatant can then be added to the cells into which one wants to insert the gene of interest. Most of the retroviral vectors used are amphotropic in their host range, i.e. they will infect a wide range of cells. In this way it is possible to make a new gene but not retroviral

Retrovirus

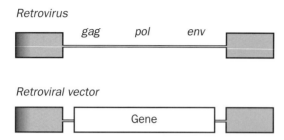

Retroviral vector

Figure 6.2 Retroviral vector. The retroviral genome is fairly simple in structure, containing three main coding regions that can be totally replaced by another gene product. Thus in a retroviral vector the *gag*, *pol*, and *env*-coding regions are replaced by a gene of interest, say a cytokine such as interleukin-2 or granulocyte–macrophage colony-stimulating factor (GM-CSF). The region that is not replaced contains the packaging signal. These constructs are made in a plasmid vehicle, which can then be transfected into a packaging cell in order to generate infectious viral particles that will express the novel gene but not the viral gene.

proteins, and thus the retrovirus is not infectious (Figure 6.3). In the viral vectors currently being considered for use in gene therapy, the amount of DNA that can be packaged into the retrovirus is less than 10 kb. For most genes currently being used, such as cytokine genes being inserted singly, this amount of DNA is adequate. However, for large genes or multiple genes, one would have to consider some of the larger viral vectors such as herpes simplex virus or vaccinia.

Following infection, the reverse transcriptase produces the engineered cDNA, which then integrates into the host DNA and is expressed. Gene therapy with retroviral vectors is usually performed in vitro. There are three reasons for this. First, the cells must be undergoing cell division for the retrovirus to incorporate in the cell DNA. Secondly, complement inactivates retroviruses, and thus it is unlikely that in vivo transfection will work. Thirdly, for in vivo therapy one requires a fairly high number of viral particles, but most of the retroviral production

schemes produce a low yield of retroviral particles. Some of the advantages and disadvantages of some viral vectors are listed in Table 6.1.

An undesirable aspect of viral vectors is that they exhibit little specificity when infecting cells.[6,7] In addition, the promoters for viral vectors are strongly expressed in most cells, and thus there is no specificity of infection once the vector is inside the cell. In order to achieve specificity, methods are being developed to increase the targeting specificity of vectors by coupling to antibodies or by genetically engineering the coat protein to express a ligand that will bind to the cell surface protein of the target cell. One recent example of increasing the specificity of retroviruses is to modify the coat protein to express erythropoietin (EPO) for uptake into EPO-positive cells. This is a complex issue because the machinery for binding and insertion of the retroviral DNA cannot be interfered with in order to maintain infectious particles.

In the case of retroviruses, they are integrated only into the DNA of dividing cells. Retroviruses would not therefore incorporate into non-dividing normal tissues (which are non-dividing), but would incorporate into tumor tissue (which is dividing), thus offering some selective advantage. Other viral vectors have different advantages and disadvantages. A major advantage with most is that they do not integrate into the DNA of the host and do not require a dividing cell for expression. However, expression will not be prolonged and thus not useful for strategies calling for long-term expression. Some other vectors produce much greater amounts of protein, such as adenoviral, herpes, and pox vectors. Pox vectors have the additional advantage that they do not need to reside in the nucleus for transcriptional activation to occur. Most other gene delivery systems must reach the nucleus in order that the mRNA be generated and expressed. Unusual vectors such as the insect cell baculovirus are also being investigated.

Non-viral vector systems have the appeal that there is no possibility of reactivation of a virus by recombination with endogenous host viruses, and thus there is a very low likelihood

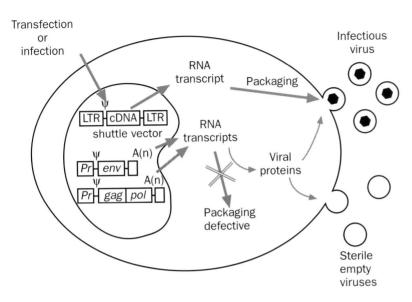

Figure 6.3 The packaging cell at work. The plasmid vector described in Figure 6.2 is transfected into a packaging cell line. These are cell lines that have been infected with crippled retrovirus such that they are incapable of making all of the viral proteins and are unable to package the viral mRNA. They are thus packaging defective. The plasmid gene construct shuttle vector contains the packaging signal so that the mRNA it generates has the packaging signal, and the gene for gene therapy is packaged into the viral particle. The particles are taken and used to infect cells with the retroviral vector.

Table 6.1 Advantages and disadvantages of retroviral, adenoviral, and herpes simplex viral (HSV) vectors[3]

Virus	Advantages	Disadvantages
Retrovirus	Non-pathogenic	Low virus titers
	DNA integration	Limited capacity (10 kb)
	Simple design	Inefficient in vivo
	Known biology	Requires dividing cells
		Expression may not be prolonged
Adenovirus	Non-pathogenic mutants available	Virus does not integrate into host genome
	Humans are hosts	Vector design complex
	High virus titers	May recombine with naturally occurring viruses
	Excellent in vivo	<7.5 kb of DNA
	Non-dividing cells OK	
	Infects cells refractory to viral infection	
HSV	Replication mutants and packaging plasmid available	Plasmids package with low efficiency
	High virus titers	Plasmids recombine with helper virus
	30 kb of foreign DNA	Replication defective virus still cytotoxic
	Broad host-cell range	Viral genome difficult to manipulate
	High infection efficiency	Gene regulation is complex
	Infects cell refractory to retrovirus infection	

of the vector being infectious or having any viral protein expression that would be recognized and immunologically destroyed by the host. Non-viral systems often use DNA in the form of a plasmid that is composed of naked double-stranded DNA. Like the surface of the cell, the DNA is negatively charged. Therefore, a coating must be put onto the naked DNA so that it can attach to and be taken up by the cell. The DNA can be coated with cationic liposomes so that the positive charge on the cation masks the negative charge of the DNA and the lipid of the liposome allows the combination to diffuse into the cell. A generic type of plasmid construct is depicted in Figure 6.4.

Plasmid DNA, which is negatively charged,

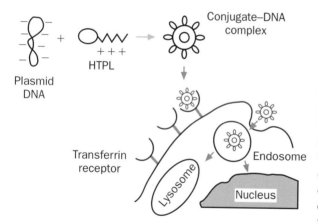

Figure 6.4 Plasmids (naked DNA) as a gene therapy vehicle. Plasmids are simple double-stranded DNA constructs that can be used as transfection cells. Because the DNA is negatively charged, the charges are masked by binding to a cationic counterion such as polylysine. To enhance the targeting and uptake of the DNA, a transportable protein such as transferrin is bound covalently. The lysine masks the negative charges and the transferrin is transported into the cell following binding of the transferrin receptor. Once in the endosome some of the DNA is able to gain entry into the cell cytoplasm and migrate to the nucleus where the transcription factors activate its expression of its encoded DNA.

may be bound to positively charged molecules such as polylysine. The polylysine itself is coupled to a protein, such as transferrin or asialoprotein, which will be transported to the inside of a cell. These plasmids have demonstrated some cell targeting efficiency. Here again, however, the difficulty is that, once inside the cell, the DNA must be freed so that it can gain access to the nucleus where the transcription factors will read the encoded message. Therefore, in some cases, a nuclear localization signal is included in the targeting package.

Normal drug delivery relies on adequate blood flow to a diseased tissue and diffusion of the drug into the diseased site for long enough and in sufficiently high concentration for the drug to exert its biologic activity. It has been known since the days of Paul Ehrlich that small diffusible drugs are likely to be able to reach the diseased site, while large molecules such as proteins do not penetrate diseased sites very well. Indeed, this is one reason why antibody therapy in the form of selective and specific in vitro assay systems has not yet become available for clinical use. Because they are so large, antibodies have difficulty in penetrating the vascular tissues and reaching the site of disease. The use of gene therapy poses a similar problem – genes are very large molecules and thus will have trouble diffusing into the treatment area. It should be noted at this point that an underexplored approach to gene therapy and cancer treatment is one that exploits the neovascularity of tumors. Tumors induce angiogenesis, and it has been found that the new blood vessels have unique features. The preliminary evidence obtained by Folkman's research group, regarding the unique features and therapeutic responsiveness of the neovascularity of tumors, suggests that this would be an excellent subject for future research.[11]

Jain and colleagues have demonstrated that tumors lack lymphatic drainage, and because of this will often lead to a build-up of intratumoral pressure to a level that is very high relative to the blood pressure. This pressure differential further decreases the ability of molecules, especially large molecules, to diffuse into the tumor.[8] Tumors also develop an abnormal and tortuous vascular supply. Cells near the vascular supply tend to be better oxygenated and viable, but cells more interior and distant from the blood supply tend to be hypoxic and dying, thus generating areas of necrosis. Cell lysis associated with lysosomal disintegration can provide for the proteolysis of administered proteins and the digestion by RNAase and DNAase of administered nucleic acids. Another problem in gene therapy is the ongoing evolution of a tumor, which becomes progressively more heterogeneous. In addition, solid tumors lie in contact with supporting stromal elements, and these different stroma can provide different growth factors and microenvironments that can change the phenotypic expression of the tumor cells. This leads to very high heterogeneity within tumors and their resultant metastasis, making any therapeutic option targeted at the tumor difficult to achieve.[9]

The biology of the solid tumor therefore presents an incredible challenge in gene therapy. However, it is worth noting that in the early phase of prostate cancer the majority of the cells are thought to be dispersed as single cells or located at metastatic sites in clumps containing only a few cells.[10] The tumor cells may reside in such a loosely attached state for some time. Thus, in the early stages, the tumor at metastatic sites may be very treatable, even by means of therapy with large molecules such as DNA and RNA. The suggestion that metastatic prostate cancer is present in these small clumps or individual cells is based on assumptions made about growth following definitive radiation therapy for the primary cancer. Folkman[11] has reported that metastatic deposits of cancer are kept to a small size because they cannot develop a blood supply and grow as long as the primary tumor is in place and molecules such as vasostatin and angiostatin are being produced by the action of the primary tumor.

THERAPEUTIC VACCINES

As described above, there are a number of basic approaches towards treating cancer by using gene therapy. These include the addition of a pro-drug-activating enzyme, the insertion of a tumor suppressor gene, and immunostimulation. These approaches have potential for the development of an antitumor vaccine. We would call this a 'therapeutic vaccine', because it would be given when the patient already has a tumor, not before.

Bladder cancer

Initially we investigated a murine model of bladder cancer, the MBT-2 model.[12,13] Transfection with interleukin-2 (IL-2) so that the tumor cells themselves produce significant quantities of bioactive IL-2, and the administration of these genetically engineered cytokine-producing cells, generated an antitumor response in animals. Thus the engineered cells either would not take and grow in the animals, or they would take but would subsequently regress. The findings were totally different in animals with an unmodified tumor or with a modified control tumor that received an empty vector. Both these MBT-2 tumors took and grew, and eventually overwhelmed the animal. The animal exposed to the cytokine-expressing cells exhibited long-term immunologic memory, i.e. if the same animals were given an unmodified tumor after they had rejected the IL-2-producing MBT-2 tumor, the animal would reject the unmodified tumor. However, this is not the way it happens in the clinic. Subsequently, we observed that if we administered the therapeutic vaccine (IL-2 transfected tumor cells) after the tumor had been implanted orthotopically into the bladder and was growing, as would occur in the clinical setting, we still saw cures. This was very encouraging and raised our enthusiasm for this approach.

Basically we only saw 'cures' of established tumors if the tumor burden being treated was fairly small, and only if we gave multiple treatments. This finding is not unexpected, because most immunotherapeutic strategies recognize that it is unlikely that the immune system will be able to eliminate large tumor burdens. What limits the immune response is not clear. Some of the postulated reasons are that the tumor produces immunosuppressive proteins such as transforming growth factor-β (TGF-β), or that the tumor growth rate is such that it has too much of a head start on the immune response and the immune cell proliferation cannot keep pace with the tumor division, etc. However, it is encouraging that an immune response against the tumor can be generated. In our studies we observed that the immune activation was indeed tumor specific, in that the animals did not demonstrate any protection against another type of tumor such as a lymphoma. What is really dramatic, though, is that this antitumor activity is accomplished without any observable toxicity to the host animal.[12,13]

One can ask whether IL-2 production within a tumor might be achievable with other systems, such as a continuous-release method, releasing IL-2 at the site of the tumor, or IL-2-producing fibroblasts inoculated into the tumor site, etc. In some systems it appears that this might indeed be the case. The initial hypothesis of transfecting tumor cells with cytokines such as IL-2 was that this would bypass the need for antigen-presenting cells and helper T cells (see Figure 6.7). Some evidence is accumulating that such a concept is oversimplified, and that what in fact occurs is that IL-2 encourages the killing of the tumor cells by natural killer (NK) cells and the released tumor antigens are presented by antigen-presenting cells. Recent investigations performed by Larchian (unpublished) have also shown that, while cytokine-expressing therapeutic vaccines have an effect, their activity is enhanced tremendously by the addition in an ordered sequence of modified tumor cells that express selected immune-activating adhesion molecules. This being the case, it would be unlikely that such cells could be mimicked in constant-release devices or by other cell types such as fibroblasts. Regardless of the mechanism, therapeutic vaccines are dramatic when they work. We have never observed MBT-2 cells that have been irradiated or transfected with an empty vector to have any activity. Optimized tumor vaccines result in cures and immunologic memory.

Prostate cancer

Dunning tumors

We have performed similar experiments on prostate cancer, using the very aggressive and metastatic tumor MAT-LyLu. Vieweg et al[14] have developed an orthotopic tumor model for studying the role of cytokine engineered therapeutic vaccines. As in the bladder, there are localized influences in the pancreas that may differ substantially from those experienced by tumors implanted to grow subcutaneously. Indeed, while it is easier to follow the course of growth of subcutaneously implanted tumors, subcutaneous metastases are rare occurrences and the results obtained from such studies may be misleading. The MAT-LyLu tumor cells are non-immunogenic in the sense that treatment with irradiated tumor cells did not alter the growth of subsequently implanted tumor cells. In animals that received the therapeutic vaccine cells cytokine transfected with IL-2, we observed a specific lysis of the tumor cells. The tumor cells were either the anaplastic MAT-LyLu, or another member of the Dunning prostate cancer family, the androgen-sensitive R3327G tumor, which shares a common tumor history with the R3327MAT-LyLu; both these tumors derive from the original R3327 tumor.[15] No effect was observed in animals implanted with a breast-derived tumor and treated with the MAT-LyLu therapeutic vaccines. In these studies, it was observed that there was a dramatic difference in antitumor response depending on whether the tumor was implanted subcutaneously or orthotopically, with cures observed with the subcutaneous tumor implants but not in animals implanted orthotopically (Figure 6.5).

In studies that have compared IL-2 and granulocyte–macrophage colony-stimulating factor (GM-CSF) producing cytokine vaccines, GM-CSF appeared to be the better cytokine. However, IL-2 and GM-CSF appeared to have similar effects on MAT-LyLu, with IL-2 appearing to have the better antitumor effect in animals in which the prostate had been surgically removed and that were followed for subsequent recurrence. We plan to repeat this study

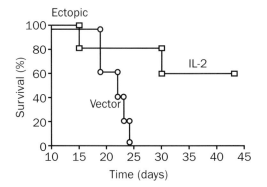

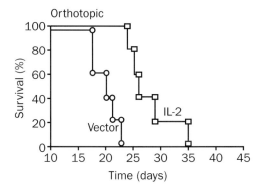

Figure 6.5 Therapeutic vaccine strategy using retroviral cytokine gene-transfected prostate cancer cells. Non-transfected or control transfected metastatic R3327MAT-LyLu cells were inoculated either ectopically into the flank or orthotopically into the prostate of male Copenhagen rats. Therapeutic immunizations were performed by injecting 5×10^6 irradiated IL-2 cytokine-secreting transfected cells on days 3, 6, and 9. The retroviral control (empty vector or irradiated non-transfected 'control cell' treated) animals all died by 24 days following transfection. The animals with tumor growing ectopically in the flank had a prolonged survival, and 40% were apparently cured. Those in which the tumor was implanted orthotopically and which were then treated with the therapeutic regimen described had all prolonged survival, but there were no cures. (Data adapted from Vieweg et al.[15])

and to examine the role of adhesion proteins and the administration of therapeutic vaccines in specific sequences to determine whether the effect will be as dramatic as it was in the bladder cancer model.

We also have investigated the effect of cytokine gene transfection on the R3327 G tumor. We examined this tumor because of its slower growth rate, with the simplistic expectation that it would be easier for the immune response to 'overtake' this slower growing tumor and produce immunotherapeutic cures.

We found that tumor cells transfected to generate either IL-2 or GM-CSF enabled the animal to reject the cytokine-producing tumor, regardless of whether the cytokine-modified tumor was placed orthotopically.[16] However, when control non-transfected tumors were implanted first and the genetically engineered cytokine-producing cells administered later as a therapeutic vaccine, GM-CSF had a significant antitumor effect only in the animals in which the primary tumor was growing subcutaneously, not orthotopically.[16] It was also observed that the GM-CSF transfectant resulted in stimulation of the humoral immunity, in that a significant titer of antitumor antibody was generated.[16]

A problem encountered in clinical trials of this form of therapy is that the most effective gene transfer is via transfection in vitro. This requires that the tumor be: removed from the patient; identified; freed of all non-tumor elements; made to grow and then infected; and the transfected cells expanded and injected back into patients. This is obviously a problem in prostate cancer patients. Prostate cancer is notoriously difficult to grow in vitro. When one examines primary prostate cancers grown in vitro for markers of prostate function such as prostate-specific antigen, prostate-specific acid phosphatase, or prostate-specific membrane antigen, their expression is found to be virtually non-existent when compared to the level found in the cells of the tissue when it was removed. Markers such as keratin may have some meaning with regard to the presence of an epithelial cell population, but not with regard to the identification of the functional prostate cell. It is important that the markers of prostate function be expressed, as it has often been found that what is activating the cellular response is a peptide fragment from a tissue-specific antigen, such as tyrosinase in melanoma. Dunning rat tumors have been repeatedly passaged for a number of years and no longer express the known tissue-specific proteins such as DP-1 or DP-2. Thus it is obviously possible that there may be a response against other unknown proteins. In the human the known prostate antigens have been demonstrated to have regions of peptides that could activate a cellular immune response. Thus, to go to all the trouble of growing prostate cells in vitro and then not having cells that express these prostate antigens is pointless.

LNCaP human prostate cancer cells

Prostate tumors are difficult to grow and what does grow does not express tissue-specific antigens. The tumorous region itself can be difficult to identify, and normal cellular constituents, such as fibroblasts and endothelial cells, may be present. Thus non-epithelial cells may be transfected, resulting in less specificity.

We take the approach of using tumor cell lines that express tumor-specific antigens (Figure 6.6). In this way one has a pure population of cells that are known entities and have no admixed normal cells of any type. The prostate cancer cell we have chosen to use in clinical investigations is the LNCaP cell line. LNCaP cells are notable for a number of reasons. They were first established in tissue culture by Horoszewicz et al[17] at Roswell Park Memorial Institute, and were derived from a patient with hormone refractory prostate cancer that had metastasized to the supraclavicular lymph node. The cells maintained expression of prostate-specific markers such as prostatic acid phosphatase (PAP) prostate-specific antigen (PSA), prostate-specific membrane (PSM) antigen, etc. In most cases, if something is found to be expressed in prostate cancer, it will likewise be found to be expressed in the LNCaP cells. They have proven to be an excellent tumor model.[18]

Because LNCaP cells express all the known antigens, and because of our prior success in obtaining growth delays or cures in animals in the Dunning prostate tumor model system, our collaborator, Bernd Gansbacher, decided to use his and Gilboa's patented N2 retroviral

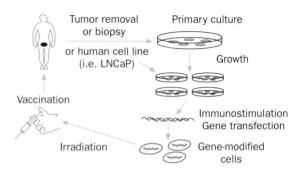

Figure 6.6 Retroviral tumor vaccine strategy. Because the retrovirus constructs so far available for clinical use suffer from the drawback of a lack of efficacy in vivo, most therapeutic regimens call for removal of the tumor, growing the tumor in vitro, transfecting it with the retroviral vector of interest, and expanding the transfected cells (under good manufacturing practice conditions as laid down by the US Food and Drugs Administration), irradiating the cells, and then giving them back to the patient. Some tumors, such as those of the prostate, are notoriously difficult to grow in vitro and there is a loss of expression of known prostate function, such as prostate-specific antigen expression. In light of this, an alternative strategy is to take a known cell line such as LNCaP, which expresses all the prostate biomarkers, and use it as a therapeutic vaccine.

system to transfect LNCaP cells with a double cytokine expression vector.[19] In brief, LNCaP cells that were in logarithmic phase growth were overlaid with a supernatant containing NCIFNγ/TIL2 and 8 μg/ml of polybrene. The supernatant containing the virus was left overnight and changed the next morning. After 48 hours, 0.5 mg/ml G418 was added and the cells grown in this selective medium for 10–14 days. The cells were expanded, assayed for bioactive IL-2 and interferon-γ (IFN-γ) secretion, proviral integration, and helper virus production. After it had been ascertained that the infected cells had appropriate proviral integration and were free of mycoplasma and helper virus, they were frozen in liquid nitrogen. The transfected cells have been generated and expanded under good manufacturing practice (GMP) conditions by Magenta Corporation. They are frozen down and are provided as frozen stock ready for use in patients.[19]

It is planned that patients who are HLA-A2 will receive at least four vaccinations. The vaccine will consist of 10×10^6 allogeneic LNCaP cells, which have been found to be HLA-A2 also. One vaccination will be given on each of days 1, 15, and 29. If a patient shows a major clinical response, boosters will be given every 3 months for 1 year. On the day of the vaccination, the cells will be thawed in MSKCC's Gene Therapy facility, resuspended in 1 ml of sterile phosphate-buffered saline, and placed into a sterile syringe. The syringe and its contents will be irradiated with 10 000 rad and delivered to the outpatient department for subcutaneous injection.[19]

During the study the response to the therapeutic vaccine will be monitored using the blood chemistry evaluations. In addition, blood will be drawn for assays of serum PSA, and for measurement of circulating cells by means of reverse-transcriptase polymerase chain reaction (RT-PCR) for PSA and PSM antigen. Enzyme-linked immunosorbent assays (ELISAs) will be performed to determine the number of T cells that have been specifically activated against known prostate antigens, and the serum examined for the presence of anti-LNCaP antibodies. As usual with any procedure utilizing retroviral transfected cells, a Mus-duni co-cultivation assay will be performed to test for the presence of helper virus, and the serum tested for the presence of antibodies against the murine Maloney virus.[19]

The use of an allogeneic tumor vaccine circumvents the problems associated with growing the patient's own tumor cells. However, the technique has a number of other problems. First, even though the allogeneic cell is HLA matched, it still has other minor histocompatibility regions that do not match and will thus generate a non-specific immune response. Secondly, the technique has the same drawback as the autologous vaccine, in that one is asking a patient to receive a dose of 10×10^6 live tumor cells – even if these have been killed by irradiation, the patient is bound to be concerned.

Another aspect of the problem is related to the hypothesis around which the therapeutic-vaccine strategy was built. It was considered (Figure 6.7) that the cell's lack of ability to recognize tumors was because the antigens are in the wrong location to be presented, or there is a flawed expansion of CD4 helper cells, or there is active suppression of cytotoxic CD8 cells, or some combination of all three. Thus it made theoretical sense to bypass the need for antigen presentation and CD4 activation by having the tumor itself present the antigen by expressing IL-2.[20] However, this has not proven to be straightforward. Cells transfected with granulocyte–macrophage colony-stimulating factor (GM-CSF) have often outperformed IL-2 in therapeutic vaccines, even though GM-CSF would not be expected to activate cytotoxic T cells. Recently it has been postulated that IL-2 recruits NK cells to the vaccine site. The NK cells lyse the tumor-releasing antigen for processing by antigen-presenting cells (APCs), which then teach the immune system to recognize the tumor. GM-CSF recruits dendritic cells to the site, and these then use the antigens released by the tumor for antigen presentation and to teach antitumor recognition. If the initial hypothesis is wrong, then it will not matter much whether or not the patient matches the HLA of the tumor allogeneic vaccine. Because evidence is accumulating to suggest that the vaccine cell may still require antigen presentation, other approaches are also being considered. Other cytokines and vectors are being prepared for use in patients, e.g. a vaccinia vector is already in use[21] and an avian pox virus is being prepared for clinical use.[22]

An approach that is currently under intense investigation is the use of dendritic cells.[23] Dendritic cells can be pulsed with the peptide from a tissue-specific antigen such as PSA or PSM antigen, and the dendritic cells will then present the antigen to the T cells. Using PSM antigen and dendritic cells, Murphy et al[23] have demonstrated that this is possible in patients. Dendritic cells can be difficult to grow, which raises one drawback to the procedure. Another

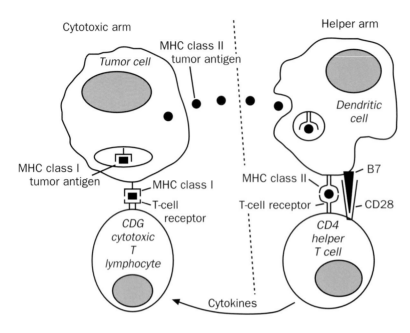

Figure 6.7 Cytotoxic T-cell activation pathway. It is currently felt that tumor cells release antigens, which are taken up and processed by antigen-presenting cells such as dendritic cells and macrophages. These antigens are processed by proteolytic degradation into smaller fragments and become bound to MHC II molecules. Helper T cells (CD4$^+$) have a T-cell receptor that recognizes the small peptide antigen lodged in the MHC II receptor pocket and binds to both it and the B7 adhesion molecule, and is 'activated' to secrete cytokines such as IL-2. IL-2 expands cytotoxic T cells (CD8$^+$), which have a T-cell receptor that recognizes antigens being processed within the tumor on the MHC I receptor cleft, and with that recognition kills the tumor cell. It was hoped that transfection of the tumor itself with cytokines would bypass the need for the helper arm.

problem is the need to use specific peptides from the tissue-specific antigens. There are computer programs that will identify which amino acid sequence is likely to fit into the antigenic site associated with a particular major histocompatibility complex (MHC) molecule, but one really needs to ascertain which peptides will activate an immune recognition and response for all the different potential peptide molecules.

A potential approach in gene therapy is that, rather than using peptides, one could genetically engineer the dendritic cell to express the tissue-specific antigen. The dendritic cell would then continually express, process, and present the activating peptide of interest. Because dendritic-like cells can be grown from an individual's peripheral blood cells, this is much less problematic than trying to grow an individual patient's tumor (see Figure 6.7).[24,25] Furthermore, dendritic cells are the most efficient cells for teaching immune recognition. Indeed, some

have suggested that what is absent in the patient's response to a tumor is that tumors grow in areas where there are few dendritic cells, and this fact, rather than an invoked deficient immune surveillance, is responsible for allowing tumors to escape and grow.

T BODIES

An approach which would bypass the need for antigen presentation is the use of T bodies. An interesting gene therapy approach is to modify the T cell so that it recognizes the tumor by another mechanism. One way to do this is to generate a T body (Figure 6.8).[26] In this case the T-cell receptor is modified so that the intracellular domain and part of the extracellular domain are the same, but the most distal part of the receptor (i.e. that part which would normally recognize the peptide antigen in the MHC cleft) is replaced with a single-chain monoclonal anti-

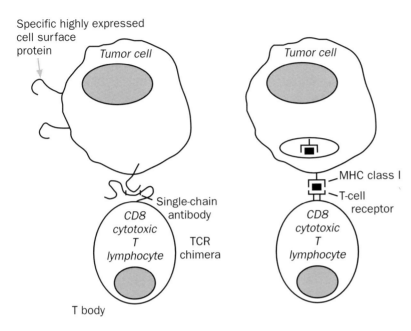

Specific highly expressed cell surface protein

Tumor cell

Tumor cell

Single-chain antibody

CD8 cytotoxic T lymphocyte

TCR chimera

MHC class I

T-cell receptor

CD8 cytotoxic T lymphocyte

T body

Figure 6.8 Single-chain antibody T-cell receptor chimeras (T bodies). As described in Figure 6.7, a cytotoxic T cell recognizes a specific small peptide sitting in an MHC I receptor, and destroys the antigen-presenting tumor cell. A drawback of this approach is that many cells, particularly those that are poorly differentiated, have greatly reduced or no expression of MHC I molecules on their cell surface. A recent advance in this strategy is to make a cytotoxic T cell with a chimeric T-cell receptor. This moiety has a high-affinity single-chain antibody that recognizes a unique cell-surface molecule that is highly expressed on the tumor cell surface, e.g. PSM antigen.

body (Figure 6.8). In this way a T cell could be activated to attack a tumor using an antibody to a tumor-specific antigen on the surface of the tumor. For instance, the majority of prostate cells express PSM antigen. One can thus take a monoclonal antibody that produces a hybridoma, alter the gene of the monoclonal antibody in order to generate a single-chain antibody, and attach the DNA encoding that single-chain antibody to the external part of the T-cell receptor. This process can be repeated for many different antibodies. Rather like a socket and ratchet set, one can change the target specificity by changing the type of single-chain antibody that is inserted.

PROMOTER-DRIVEN PRO-DRUG-ACTIVATING ENZYMES

Obviously, it is important to avoid toxicity to patients from cytotoxic antitumor agents. One means of doing this is to deliver to the tumor a gene encoding an enzyme that is not normally expressed in the mammalian system, and which will act on substrates that are not toxic to the patient but will produce an intratumoral conversion of the non-toxic drug to a toxic drug within the confines of the tumor. There are a number of therapeutic approaches using cytotoxic drug activation. Most of these strategies are based on the use of pro-drugs, with the gene for the activation of the pro-drug being expressed behind a tissue of tumor-specific promoter (Figure 6.9). Huber and coworkers[27] have used such an approach for carcinoma of the colon, with carcinoembryonic antigen (CEA) as the promoter and cytosine deaminase. Similarly, Belldegrun and coworkers[28] have used PSA as the promoter and herpes DNA polymerase activation of ganciclovir. This method gives specificity for the tumor, because the tissue-specific or tumor-specific promoter is most active in the tumor. Thus CEA drives expression in colon cancer that has metastasized to the liver, and the PSA promoter drives

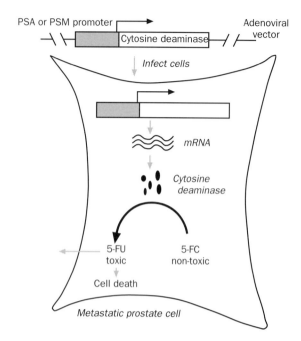

Figure 6.9 Promoter-driven gene therapy. Most viral vectors rely on viral promoters to drive expression of the therapeutic gene upon transfection of a cell. There is no specificity to this expression, and often the vector is non-specific; thus there is no specificity of the vector. One way to provide some specificity of expression is to use tissue- or tumor-specific promoters to drive gene expression of the transfected cell such as tyrosinase in melanoma, CEA in colon tumors, and PSA or PSM antigen in prostate tumors. The diagram shows PSA or PSM promoter driving cytosine deaminase. Inside a metastatic prostate cell the cytosine deaminase protein would be produced. Cytosine deaminase is a pro-drug-converting enzyme that converts the non-cytotoxic 5-fluorocytosine (5-FC) to 5-fluorouracil (5-FU) and kills the prostate cell. Normal cells at the metastatic site do not make cytosine deaminase because they lack the transcription factors for PSA or PSM antigen, and are thus spared toxicity.

expression most highly in tumor that has metastasized to the bone. Chung and colleagues[29] have identified factors produced by bone that tend to drive the progression of prostatic bone metastatic deposits to increase PSA expression in the absence of androgens, which makes such a target even more attractive.

In these approaches it is critical that the pro-drug is activated, so that it can be useful in killing via a bystander effect; that is, the pro-drug is activated by the cells expressing the transfected gene protein product, but the activated drug can diffuse and be toxic to surrounding cells. Obviously there are trade-offs. If expression is too high and there is extensive tumor in the bone marrow, substantial bone marrow toxicity may occur. Again gene therapy could be used – one could isolate the bone marrow stem cells, transfect them with a resistance gene to the therapy being used, and reinject the resistant cells that can be subjected to more intensive chemotherapy. However, one should focus on tumor-specific strategies and make every attempt to limit toxicity to the patient.

GENE CORRECTION

In gene correction approaches, an attempt is made to correct the underlying problem. For instance, regulatory genes such as *RB* or *p53* may become lost or inactivated, and antiapoptosis genes such as *bcl-2* may become overexpressed. The idea is to insert and have expressed the suppressor gene. Theoretically, the gene must be inserted into every tumor cell in order to correct the defect. However, early work with *p53* suggests that this may in fact not be the case, the fixing of only a fraction of the damaged cells translating into modified behavior of other tumor cells or other mechanisms such as immunological recognition and destruction.

A number of groups have investigated the role of transfection of *p53* in prostate cancer tumor models.[29–32] Adenoviral vectors have frequently been used. These have a high transduction efficiency, are able to infect many cell types, and infection does not require cell division. On the negative side, this vector does not integrate into the host DNA and thus there is a limited time of expression, there is a lack of specificity in targeting, there is a limited amount of DNA insertion of 4.5 kb, and there is a potential for immunogenicity of the viral infected cells. Thompson and coworkers used the adenoviral vectors Ad5CMV-*p53* and Ad5CMV-*p21* to drive the expression of either of two tumor suppressor proteins following transfection of 148-1PA, a metastatic derivative of the *his* recombinant mouse prostate tumor model. In this model *p21* had a greater tumor suppressive effect than did *p53*, both in vitro and in vivo.[32]

Srivasta et al[30] have transfected the available prostate cell lines, PC-3 Du-145, TSU-Pr1, and LNCaP with wild-type *p53* using an adenoviral vector. All lines were inhibited in growth, both in vitro and in vivo. What is interesting in this regard is that the LNCaP cells were inhibited as well, and yet they supposedly have normal *p53*. The reason for the different response of these cells from that in the mouse tumor model-derived cells just described is unknown. The results obtained by transfection with *p53* in the TSU-Pr1 prostate cells were replicated by Yang et al,[31] who used an adenoviral *p53* expression vector. These workers also observed that *p53*-transfected cells died both in vitro and in vivo. However, they transfected the cells in vitro before inoculating them in vivo, which is less realistic than the approach of transfection in vivo.[31] Chung and colleagues[29] used a *p53* adenovirus and an aggressive hormone-independent variant of the LNCaP cell line that they had developed and designated C4. This variant was killed both in vitro and in vivo. In this case the tumor was inoculated with the adenoviral vector in vivo as well, and was effective in curing these aggressive prostate tumors. That they treated the tumors while they were growing in the animal is encouraging. However, the problem of inoculating metastatic bony tumor deposits in patients, at each and every site, remains. It would be more practically realistic to inject the vector intravenously. Theoretically, infection with a crippled adenovirus should not prove to be infectious, and the overexpression of *p53* would not be expected to be toxic to normal cells. Although not stated by the authors, the lack of *p53* antibody staining of the non-infected C4 cells is an indication that they have a normal *p53* like the parental LNCaP. The growth of the C4 line was also inhibited, but the line was not killed by the in vitro transfection

by *p53*. The authors state that they do not know why they found extensive necrosis in vivo following *p53* therapy, but suggest it may be the result of NK-cell activity.[29]

Roth and coworkers[3] have used the same adenoviral *p53* vector to treat patients. Of nine patients with advanced lung cancer, they have observed one complete response, two partial responses, and three stable responses. It is not clear why the therapy is working as it is unlikely that all the tumor cells are being infected, but it appears to have sufficient merit to continue to move the effort forward.[3]

The above-described gene correction strategies revolve around increasing the expression of an absent suppressor gene. Other strategies utilize an antisense strategy.[33] In this strategy one wants to knock out gene expression. In theory, one can express a gene in a reverse orientation so it will be the 'antisense' message of the gene which one wants to eliminate. The antisense message will pair with the sense message and the double-stranded RNA will be unable to bind to the ribosomal complex and thus will not be translated. In practice the strategy does not necessarily reduce expression to zero. Genes such as the antideath gene *bcl-2* are frequently used target genes for elimination, other targets including telomerase and vascular endothelial growth factor receptor. Antisense strategies are currently undergoing clinical trials involving phosphorothioate oligodeoxynucleotides against *bcl-2* in patients with follicular lymphoma, *PKC*-α for solid tumors, and *c-myb* for acute myelogenous leukemia.[33] Another strategy for gene inactivation involves the use of hammerhead ribozymes. These RNA molecules are designed to bind to a region of the mRNA of the molecule that one wants to inactivate. When properly designed they bind to and enzymatically destroy the unwanted gene product by cleaving it in two.[34]

SUMMARY

All strategies involving gene transfer have drawbacks. A major problem is how one can get the gene to the target and to express in the target tissue. Despite this, Roth[3] has stated that: 'The first clinical protocols began just five years ago, gene transfer and expression into tumors is possible and appears to be relatively safe.'

Indeed, tumor regression has been observed, and Roth feels that this is a very promising area for the future.

REFERENCES

1. Jarie L, Gene therapy. *Time Magazine*, Fall (Special Edition: The Frontiers of Medicine) 1996.
2. Culver KW, *Gene Therapy*. Mary Ann Liebert: New York, 1994.
3. Roth JA, Cristiano RJ, Gene therapy for cancer: What have we done and where are we going? *J Natl Cancer Inst* 1997; **89:** 21–39.
4. Crystal RG, Transfer of genes to human: early lesson on and obstacles to success. *Science* 1995; **270:** 404–10.
5. Herrmann F, Cancer gene therapy: principles, problems, and perspectives. *J Mol Med* 1995; **73:** 157–63.
6. Roemer K, Friedmann T, Concepts and strategies for human gene therapy. *Eur Biochem* 1992; **208:** 211–25.
7. Miller N, Vile R, Targeted vectors for gene therapy. *FASEB J* 1995; **9:** 190–9.
8. Jain RK, Barriers to drug delivery in solid tumors. *Sci Am* 1994; **270:** 58–65.
9. Fair WR, Heston WDW, Cordon-Cardo C, Overview of cancer biology. In: *Campbell's Urology* (Walsh PC, Retik AB, Vaughan DE, Wein AJ, eds). WB Saunders: Orlando, FL, 1997: 2259–82.
10. Yorke ED, Fuks Z, Norton L, Whitmore W, Ling CC, Modeling the development of metastases from primary and locally recurrent tumors: comparison with a clinical data base of prostatic cancer. *Cancer Res* 1993; **53:** 2987–93.
11. Folkman J, Fighting cancer by attacking its blood supply. *Sci Am* 1996; **275:** 150–4.
12. Connor J, Bannerji R, Saito S, Heston WDW, Fair WR, Gilboa E, Regression of bladder tumors in mice treated with interleukin 2 gene modified tumor cells. *J Exp Med* 1993; **177:** 1127–34.
13. Saito S, Bannerji R, Gansbacher B et al, Immunotherapy of bladder cancer with cytokine gene modified tumor vaccines. *Cancer Res* 1994; **54:** 3516–20.
14. Vieweg J, Heston WDW, Gilboa E, Fair WR, An experimental model simulating local recurrence and pelvic lymph node metastasis following orthotopic induction of prostate cancer. *Prostate* 1994; **24:** 291–8.
15. Vieweg J, Rosenthal FM, Bannerji R et al, Immunotherapy of prostate cancer in the Dunning rat model: use of cytokine gene modified tumor vaccines. *Cancer Res* 1994; **54:** 1760–5.
16. Yoshimura I et al, submitted.
17. Horoszczewicz JJ, Leong SS, Kawinski E et al, LNCaP model of human prostate carcinoma. *Cancer Res* 1983; **43:** 1809–18.
18. Heston WDW, Biologic implications for prostate function following identification of prostate specific membrane antigen as a novel folate hydrolase, neuro-carboxypeptidase. In: *Prostate: Basic and Clinical Aspects* (Naz RK, ed). CRC Press: Boca Raton, FL, 1997: 267–98.
19. Gansbacher B, A pilot study of immunization with HLA-class I matched allogeneic prostate carcinoma cells engineered to secrete IL-2 and gamma interferon given in patients with progressive prostate cancer. *Memorial Sloan–Kettering Clinical Protocol No. 94-134*, 1996.
20. Pardoll D, Immunotherapy with cytokine gene transduced tumor cells: the next wave in gene therapy for cancer. *Curr Opin Oncol* 1992; **4:** 1124–9.
21. Lee SS, Eisenjohr LC, McCue PA, Mastrangelo MJ, Lattime EC, Intravesical gene therapy: In vivo gene transfer using recombinant vaccine viral vectors. *Cancer Res* 1994; **54:** 3325–8.
22. Kawakita M, Rao GJ, Ritcher JK et al, Effect of canary pox virus (ACMC) mediated cytokine expression on murine prostate tumor growth. *J Natl Cancer Inst* 1997; **89:** 428–36.
23. Murphy G, Tjoa B, Ragde H, Kenny G, Boynton A, Phase I clinical trial: T-cell therapy for prostate cancer using autologous dendritic cells pulsed with HLA-A0201-specific peptide from prostate-specific membrane antigen. *Prostate* 1996; **29:** 371–80.
24. Song ES, Lee V, Surh D, Antigen presentation in retroviral vector mediated gene transfer in vivo. *Proc Natl Acad Sci USA* 1997; **94:** 1943–8.
25. Aicher A, Westermann J, Caseux S et al, Successful retroviral mediated transduction of a reporter gene in human dendritic cells: feasibility of therapy with gene modified antigen presenting cells. *Exp Hematol* 1997; **25:** 35–44.

26. Hekele A, Dall P, Moritz D et al, Growth retardation of tumors by adoptive transfer of cytotoxic and lymphocytes reprogrammed by CD446-specific scf:zeta-chimera. *Int J Cancer* 1996; **68:** 232–8.

27. Richards CA, Austin EA, Huber BE, Transcriptional regulatory sequences of carcinoembryonic antigen: Identification and use with cytosine deaminase for tumor-specific gene therapy. *Hum Gene Ther* 1995; **6:** 881–93.

28. Pang S, Taneja S, Dardashti K et al, Prostate tissue specificity of the prostate specific antigen promoter isolated from a patient with prostate cancer. *Hum Gene Ther* 1995; **6:** 1417–26.

29. Ko SC, Gotoh A, Thalmann GN et al, Molecular therapy with recombinant p53 adenovirus in an androgen independent metastatic human prostate cancer model. *Hum Gene Ther* 1996; **7:** 1683–91.

30. Srivastara S, Katayose D, Tong Y et al, Recombinant adenovirus vector expression wild-type *p53* is a potent inhibitor of prostate cancer cell proliferation. *Urology* 1995; **46:** 843–8.

31. Yang C, Cirielli C, Capogrossi MC, Pasanti A, Adenovirus-mediated wild-type *p53* expression induces apoptosis and suppressed tumorigenesis of prostate tumor cells. *Cancer Res* 1995; **55:** 4210–13.

32. Easthan SA, Hall SJ, Schhal I et al, In vivo gene therapy with *p53* or *p21* adenovirus for prostate cancer. *Cancer Res* 1995; **55:** 5151–5.

33. Narayanan R, Akhtar S, Antisense therapy. *Curr Opin Oncol* 1996; **8:** 509–15.

34. Li M, Lonial H, Citrella R, Lindl D, Colina L, Kramer R, Tumor inhibitor activity of anti-*ras* ribozymes delivered by retroviral gene transfer. *Cancer Gene Ther* 1996; **3:** 221–8.

7

Prostate cancer screening

Baudouin Standaert, Louis Denis

CONTENTS • **Evaluation of cancer screening programmes** • **Studies of prostate cancer screening** • **Additional research** • **Conclusion**

Unlike for breast and cervical cancer, screening remains a controversial issue in the early detection of prostate cancer.[1] The disease is prevalent among elderly men in the Western World, with estimated new cases per year in the USA and Europe currently being 200 000 (145/100 000) and 85 000 (65/100 000), respectively. It is the second most important tumour in men after lung cancer.[2,3] Mortality rates are about the same for both the USA and Europe, with estimated rates ranging from 20 to 30 deaths per 100 000 men per year (between 35 000 and 40 000 deaths per year).[4,5] The huge discrepancy observed between incidence and mortality rates in the USA results partly from the greater use of cancer detection techniques there than in Europe and from the ethnic mix because black people make up a high-risk group for this cancer.[6]

There will be an increase in incidence and mortality data for prostate cancer over the next few decades as a result of several factors such as age of the male population, greater usage of tests that could detect the cancer and a real increase in prostate cancer risk.[7]

Prostate cancer affects mainly the ageing man who is more likely to die with than from his tumour. It has been estimated that a man aged 85 years old has a life-time risk of developing prostate cancer of 13.5 whereas at the age of 65 that risk is only 4.5.[8] However, these numbers are subject to some variation depending on how aggressively the prostate cancer is searched for.

Despite these impressive numbers there is still the controversy about why prostate cancer screening has not yet been accepted as a general health care rule, because of the unproved benefit of any screening programme tested to date on hard clinical outcome measures, including survival benefit, specific mortality reduction or increased quality of life.[9]

To understand the problem caused by this screening – whether screening should be refrained from or promoted – the issue is tackled from three points of view: the first looks at the benefits and the rules that need to be endorsed before any screening activity is accepted as a global health care prevention strategy; the second is a review of what has already been achieved in prostate cancer screening research; and the final one tackles such proposals as what should also be done in order to come up with credible answers to the

Table 7.1 The principles of screening
1. The condition sought should be an important health problem
2. There should be an accepted treatment for the patients with recognized disease
3. Facilities for diagnosis and treatment should be available
4. There should be a recognizable latent or early symptomatic stage
5. There should be a suitable test or examination
6. The test should be acceptable to the population
7. The natural history of the disease, from latent phase to declared disease, should be adequately understood
8. There should be an agreed policy about whom to treat as patients
9. The cost of case finding (including diagnosis and treatment of patients diagnosed) should be economically balanced in relation to possible expenditure on medical care as a whole
10. Case finding should be a continuing process and not a once-for-all activity

From Wilson et al.[11]

question: 'Should we screen or not screen for prostate cancer?'

EVALUATION OF CANCER SCREENING PROGRAMMES

Cancer screening is a process by which a healthy or asymptomatic population is encouraged to come forward to try to detect pre-cancerous lesions.[10] After the application of a simple screening test the group is subdivided into groups of suspect individuals dependent on the risk of having a pre-cancerous lesion. The goal of early detection of cancer is to try to stop the natural history of cancer development, which could cause morbidity or mortality, by the application of efficient treatment. Cancer screening is therefore perceived as a method of controlling spread of a prevalent cancer type. If primary cancer prevention fails, it is a second-order 'control' approach.

As the asymptomatic population is actively contacted about a medical intervention strategy, the benefits of screening must clearly out-weigh the potential harm caused by the whole screening process. For ethical reasons, in order to be proposed screening must result in important, net benefits. Some basic principles therefore have to be met or satisfied before any screening programme could be generally promoted. These basic principles are reported in Table 7.1,[11] and the benefits and disadvantages of a screening programme are given in Table 7.2.[12]

A screening project is first evaluated using the two quantitative variables of sensitivity and specificity of the screening test(s) used. The sensitivity measures how the test classifies those people who have the disease, whereas the specificity measures classification by testing against those who do not have it. As both measures are independent of disease prevalence, other variables need to be defined in order to evaluate the usefulness of any test proposed for use in a screening setting. Moreover, it is important to note that sensitivity and specificity cannot be improved concomitantly. If one tries to increase specificity by changing the cut-off point of a screening test, its sensitivity is auto-

---

Table 7.2 Benefits and disadvantages of screening

Benefits
Improved prognosis for some cases detected by screening
Less radical treatment which cures some early cases
Reassurance for those with negative test results

Disadvantages
Longer morbidity for cases whose prognosis is unaltered
Overtreatment of questionable abnormalities
False reassurance for those with false-negative results
Anxiety and sometimes morbidity for those with false-positive results
Unnecessary medical intervention for those with false-positive results
Hazards of screening test (for example, venepuncture, radiation)
Diversion of scarce resources to screening programme

From Chamberlain.[12]

matically decreased. What is most important to work with in a screening setting: using a more sensitive or a more specific test?[13] The answer is simple if one looks at the following equation, which depicts the index of misclassification (I_m) of a screening test for a disease of a certain prevalence (p_d): the lower the prevalence, the more important is the role of the specificity value in limiting I_m:

$$I_m = [(1 - \text{Sensitivity}) \times p_d] \\ + [(1 - \text{Specificity}) \times (1 - p_d)].$$

An overview of all the definitions used here is given in Table 7.3. Predictive values are determined from the test results, for example, they indicate what proportion of the people with a positive test result will effectively have the disease under study. This value is the first value to be measured easily in any pilot screening trial. An important and undervalued problem

Table 7.3 Definitions of performance measures of a screening test

Screening test	Disease	
	Present	Absent
Positive	a	b
Negative	c	d

Screen-positive rate	$(a + b)/(a + b + c + d)$
Detection rate	$a/(a + b + c + d)$
Sensitivity	$a/(a + c)$
Specificity	$d/(b + d)$
Positive predictive value of a positive test result	$a/(a + b)$
Negative predictive value of a positive test result	$b/(a + b)$
Positive predictive value of a negative test result	$d/(d + c)$
Negative predictive value of a negative test result	$c/(d + c)$

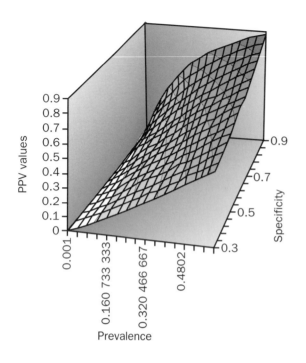

Figure 7.1 PPV values with changing prevalence rate (0.1–60%) and changing specificity values (30–90%), but fixed sensitivity at 50%.

■	0.8–0.9
■	0.7–0.8
■	0.6–0.7
□	0.5–0.6
□	0.4–0.5
□	0.3–0.4
□	0.2–0.3
□	0.1–0.2
□	0–0.1

related to predictive values is their dependence on the prevalence of the disease being screened;[14] a simple example should clarify this statement.

If we consider a disease that has a true prevalence in the target population of 2%, then, when a sample of 1000 individuals is screened using a test that has a sensitivity and a specificity of 80%, only 16 of the 20 people who have the disease in that sample will be detected by the screening, whereas 196 participants will be misclassified as possibly having the disease. The positive predictive value (PPV) is therefore $16/(196 + 16) = 7.5\%$; that is, the disease is present in less than 1 in 10 of those with a positive test result. The PPVs obtained for different values of a test's sensitivity, specificity and prevalence rate are shown in Figures 7.1 and 7.2. The PPVs reach limits that are determined by disease prevalence and the test's specificity if the disease has a low prevalence rate. This is not improved by the test's sensitivity. From these figures it can be seen that, when the reported

validity values of a screening test are set, the screening effectiveness can be improved only by more careful selection of the target population with a higher cancer risk. This can be achieved through use of questionnaires or genetic research.

Two other factors also contribute to the difficulties in interpreting screening benefits correctly: lead time and length–time bias.[15,16] Lead time bias is defined as early diagnosis of a cancer that will result in an increase in the time interval between diagnosis and death of a screened person, although not necessarily leading to a survival benefit. The longer it takes to detect pre-cancerous lesions, the greater the risk of having lead time bias.

Length–time bias is the tendency towards selective detection of a disproportionate number of slowly progressive cancers. The most aggressive tumours are missed and these are often the only ones to cause real harm such as metastasis or death. Under such conditions, early detection and treatment of just non-

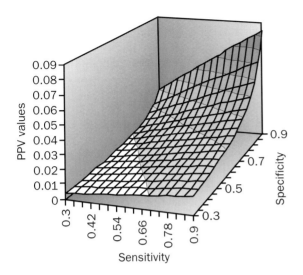

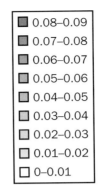

Figure 7.2 PPV values with changing sensitivity values (30–90%) and changing specificity values (30–90%), but fixed prevalence rate at 10%.

- 0.08–0.09
- 0.07–0.08
- 0.06–0.07
- 0.05–0.06
- 0.04–0.05
- 0.03–0.04
- 0.02–0.03
- 0.01–0.02
- 0–0.01

aggressive cancers do not result in clinical benefits for those screened; indeed they cause overdiagnosis and overtreatment.

Thus screening as a medical activity is a delicate balance in which not only must clear clinical benefit be proven, but also potential disadvantages should be restricted as much as possible. The latter could be mental or physical problems resulting from the screening procedure itself, or from the waiting time until a result is received. In addition, a positive screening result means that the screened person will have to undergo additional diagnostic tests which could be quite invasive, and lead to additional problems. If the screening test is not very specific, many will experience unnecessary anxiety or fear. If the new results do confirm the suspected screening findings, however, treatment used is sometimes less aggressive than if the disease would have been discovered at a later clinical stage, although not necessarily free of problems. Finally, if the test validity is insufficient, showing false-negative results, this causes suffering that could have been avoided with a more sensitive test.

A final point to tackle here is a non-medical one.[17] Cancer screening engenders extra costs to society that could have been devoted to other priorities within health care. To date, no cancer screening programmes have shown any cost savings and this issue is discussed much more now because health care budgets are being cut as a result of overall budget constraints together with the search for greater efficiency. Any new proposed screening activity therefore has to be evaluated for its cost-effectiveness, demonstrating the cost per unit of effectiveness gained. This can be analysed at two levels: one relates to detection of the number of relevant cancers;[18] the other relates to the overall effect of the screening process showing, for example, an increased survival benefit expressed in years, months or days. In the case of prostate cancer, because of the competing causes of death among elderly people, the overall effectiveness is preferentially expressed as a specific reduction in mortality rather than a survival benefit.

STUDIES OF PROSTATE CANCER SCREENING

The recently conducted screening studies on prostate cancer can be subdivided into two groups: demonstration projects and randomized trials.[19] Both types of studies try to prove whether screening of early prostate cancer is meaningful, by assessing its benefit through specific mortality reduction. The development of such studies is a necessary step before screening can be generally recommended as an appropriate prevention; this needs to be endorsed by the target group at regular intervals. The results and pitfalls of the most important studies conducted so far are summarized here.

Demonstration projects have been undertaken preferentially in the USA; they differ from the other group of studies because they do not include a randomization process of the target population.[20,21] Randomization should normally be introduced once the participant has agreed to participate in the screening project. If this process occurs before asking for consent, selection bias among the participants may occur which cannot be corrected for later.

Randomized trials are the golden standard for precise evaluation of the benefit of a screening programme on specific mortality reduction.[22] Demonstration projects show their effects by historical comparison of the impact of their screening activity on mortality rates through close monitoring of local cancer and mortality registers. They can show an impact, but not the precise amount caused by their specific intervention because they do not control what happens in the unscreened population. Demonstration projects are, however, an appropriate alternative if the randomization procedure could not take place as a result of, for example, a high contamination rate of the potential control group with screening tests.

Arguments currently used against screening of prostate cancer are twofold:[23,24] one concerns the validity of the screening tests used, associated with the unnecessary pain caused by the diagnostic procedures; the other concerns the clinical benefit achieved and the high rate of side effects experienced with the treatment strategies proposed for detection of early cancers.

The screening tests

The screening tests selected so far in research trials are digital rectal examination (DRE) of the prostate gland, transrectal ultrasonography (TRUS) and prostate-specific antigen (PSA), a serum marker in blood. Specific questionnaires could also be stressed here as an opportunity to identify subgroups in which the risk for developing prostate cancer is higher, as seen among familial clusters or black people in the USA.[25] Screening of these subgroups will enhance better predictive values as expected (see above). New tumour markers, such as prostate-specific membrane antigen (PSMA), prostate inhibin peptide (PIP), prostate cancer antigen-1 (PCA-1) and others, are currently under investigation in clinical settings, but are not discussed here. The appropriate review literature should be referred to.[26]

Prostate-specific antigen is a glycol protein produced mainly by the prostate. It was first characterized in seminal fluid and in prostate tissue in 1979.[27] Monoclonal as well as polyclonal essays are available to measure levels of PSA in serum and the test was initially used for several years to monitor patients for disease recurrence. In 1991, Catalona reported the use of PSA as a screening test in about 1600 healthy men at risk for prostate cancer.[28] Other studies have been reported at the same time by Labrie et al in Québec and Brawer et al in Seattle.[29,30] The conventional upper limit for the normal monoclonal PSA essay is 4 µg/ml. Such an elevation often occurs when benign prostatic hyperplasia is present. Values of more than 10 µg/ml are more often indicative of cancer.

TRUS is used to image the contents of the prostate glands with the development of the 5–7 MHz multiplanner transducer.[31] Ultrasonography is also helpful in guiding automatic biopsy systems. It is used to measure gland and tumour volumes, but it can also determine the extent of disease in those patients who have had prostate cancer diagnosed. In 1988, Lee et al used TRUS first as a screening method to detect 22 cancers in 784 men.[32] The study of Cooner, on urological patients, also included

TRUS.[33] Compared with DRE, TRUS has shown a superiority in sensitivity but not in specificity. Therefore it has a poor predictive value in men with normal PSA and normal DRE.

In general, the population that is most often targeted in screening trials is men aged 50–74 years (Table 7.4).[34–38] Within that specific group of asymptomatic men, the prevalence of cancer detectable by currently used screening tests ranges from 1% to a maximum of 6%. The first screening round will yield the highest prevalence rate. If annual screening is proposed the rate will drop to a level of 1% after a few screening rounds. Also a shift is observed in the type of cancers detected over the different screening rounds: from a mixture including aggressive cancers (stage T3 with Gleason score >5) during the first screening round, to the presence of more latent cancers after a few years (stage T1c with Gleason score <5).

The most frequently used test is the PSA with a cut-off value of 4 ng/ml, followed by DRE and TRUS. Comparing the three tests separately for their predictive values, it can be deduced that they all have comparable data in the range of 25–40%. The measurable sensitivity, assuming prevalence rate to be the number

of cancers found in a screening round, varies from 45% for DRE to 91% for TRUS, with PSA being in the middle at 75%. The specificity, which for ethical reasons is more difficult to measure but is more important in screening settings, could also vary widely from 65% for TRUS to 98% for DRE. The PSA specificity has been measured retrospectively in a database including more than 20 000 men over a period of 10 years and accounts for 91% over that period.[39]

Taking these numbers as a reference with a prevalence rate that varies from 1% to 6%, a specificity value for PSA of between 85% and 95%, while keeping the sensitivity fixed at 75%, it is possible to calculate the range of PPV that could be obtained for PSA alone. These values are depicted in Figure 7.3, which shows how, by increasing the specificity to 95%, it will dramatically improve the PPV to 48%; 50% of the PPV values will, however, range between 10% and 38%. The same exercise could be repeated, varying the sensitivity from 70% to 80%, while keeping the same variation in specificity, but fixing the prevalence rate to 2.5%. The results in Figure 7.4 show a range of variability of PPV values for 50% of the data of between 11% and

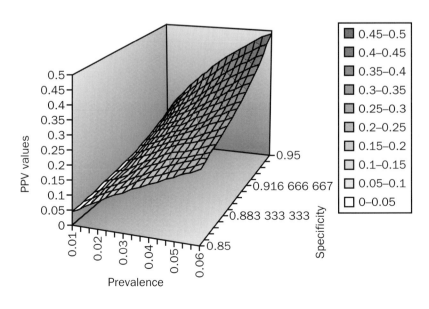

Figure 7.3 PPV values with changing prevalence rate (1–6%) and changing specificity values (85–95%), but fixed sensitivity values at 75%.

Table 7.4 Summary of the most important screening studies conducted to date

Trial	Sort	Starting year	Age group (years)	No.	Tests used	Rescreen period	Detection rate, first year (%)	PVV–PSA, first year (%)
ACS-NPCD*	Demonstration	1987	55–70	2 999	PSA, DRE, TRUS	Annual	2.8	15.9
Washington†	Demonstration	1989	>50	10 248	PSA	Every 6 months	2.8	30
Washington†	Demonstration	1991	>50	18 608	PSA, DRE	Every 6 months	3.3	19.4
PCAW‡	Demonstration	1992	>50	50 000	PSA	Annual	4.7	31.6
Tyrol§	Demonstration	1993	45–74	21 078	PSA	Once	1.2	25
ERSPC¶	Randomized	1995	50–74	180 000	PSA, DRE (TRUS)	Every 4 years	2.1–3.5	28–36

*American Cancer Society, National Prostate Cancer Detection Project.[34] †St Louis, MO.[38] ‡Prostate Cancer Awareness Week.[37] §Tyrol Trial, Austria.[35] ¶European Randomized Screening on Prostate Cancer.[36]

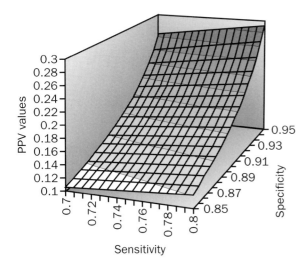

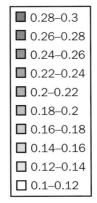

Figure 7.4 PPV values with changing sensitivity values (70–80%) and changing specificity values (85–95%), but fixed prevalence rate at 2.5%.

24%. This is much lower compared with the previous run. It can be concluded that it is sensible to increase the specificity of PSA in order to improve the PPV. In this respect PSA is an interesting cancer screening test because it has a continuous value scale that could be adapted to improve its specificity.

Many researchers have searched to obtain better PPV results by adjusting the PSA values to: a density function of the prostate volume;[40] a velocity function with changes over time;[41] an age-dependent function;[42] a prostate volume-specific function;[43] or by combining it with a more specific test, such as DRE,[44] or looking for more specific PSA values such as free and total PSA.[45] Some sensitivity may be lost when increasing the specificity, but a small specificity gain may ultimately increase the PPV value which compensates sufficiently for the loss in sensitivity when annual screening is considered. Among the different suggestions proposed to increase the specificity of PSA, no definite answer has as yet been found. It does become clear, however, that prostate volume is a more influential factor than age for the exact interpretation of PSA results as a risk marker for cancer.[46]

In conclusion it has been argued that cur-rently used screening tests for prostate cancer detection were not sufficiently valid, causing a rate of false-positive results that was too high, which resulted in a lot of unnecessary diagnostic harm. It can, however, be observed that the current screening setting may produce reliable data with acceptable PPV values that are not inferior to other cancer screening programmes, taking into account the prevalence rate of the disease under study and the acceptability of the screening method proposed. Moreover, the screening study in Rotterdam has recently made extensive reports about the complications of the diagnostic, transrectal-guided biopsies performed, subdividing them into haemor-rhagic and infectious complications.[47] On the 1687 sextant biopsies accomplished, haem-atospermia was the most prevalent symptom in 45%, followed by haematuria for more than 3 days in 23%. Pain was only reported by 8% of those who had a biopsy, whereas fever occurred in 4.2% of the cases and less than 0.5% needed hospitalization and follow-up. The authors compared their results with what had been reported in the literature about referred patient populations. They did not observe any significant differences from their study results. They concluded that the procedure of diagnostic transrectal-guided sextant biopsies is safe. An important preventive measure is, however, to give counselling about possible problems to anyone undergoing such a biopsy.

Another argument employed against the selection of the currently used screening tests is that these tests have low prognostic power for clear differentiation among the more or less aggressive cancers.[48] When performing biopsies, it is ideal to detect those cancers that could be harmful for the patient, through causing a later stage metastatic disease and/or death. A great deal of research has shown doubt that the screening process and biopsies will identify these cancers.[49] It has, however, been proved, by demonstration projects and randomized trials, that by using the screening strategy only 1–6% of the target population have cancers that are detectable; this is a much lower percentage compared with postmortem results, showing a positive rate of 34%. Could the 1–6% of cancers detected be latent forms discovered by accident when biopsies are performed in the outer regions of the prostate gland? Here again the answer to date is that the group of cancers detected by screening belong to the TNM (tumour, node, metastasis) classification that is appropriate for early detection and treatment.[50] The spread of cancers found in the Rotterdam

screening trial after the TNM classification system is shown in Figure 7.5.[51] The demonstration project of the American Cancer Society National Cancer Detection Project (ACS-NPCDG) has shown that, through their annual evaluation of the prostate gland, the initial large prevalent cancer rate is followed in subsequent screening rounds by much lower detection rates, which mainly discover cancers of stage II type (Figure 7.6).[52]

One problem that can result from this biopsy strategy is that the 'at random' number of biopsies taken must be proportional to the prostate volume in order to obtain an equivalent cancer yield among small versus large prostate glands.[53]

Treatment of early prostate cancer

The life-time risk of prostate cancer in a group of men aged over 50 is more than 10%.[54] The risk of dying of prostate cancer is less and could be between 3% and 5%.[55] After the cancer has spread beyond the prostate gland, it usually moves to the bones before a first diagnosis will be made. If the cancer is confined to the prostate gland, the 10-year relative survival rate is 75%, compared with 55% in those with regional metastasis beyond the prostate capsule

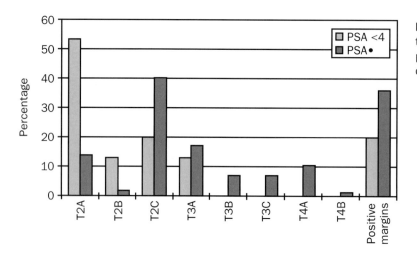

Figure 7.5 Distribution of cancer types found in the screening programme of Rotterdam, dependent on PSA values.

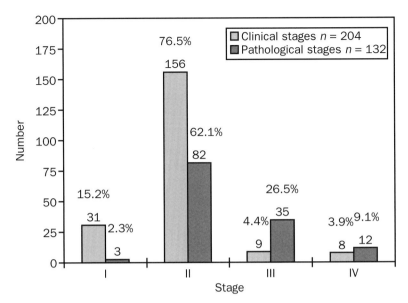

Figure 7.6 Clinical and pathological American Joint Committee on Cancer staging shown for cancers detected in the ACS-NPCOP.

and 15% in those with distant metastases.[56] Favourable survival is thus restricted to those who are diagnosed at the early stages of the disease. However, the most promising method of controlling the cancer and reducing its specific mortality should be via early detection and treatment. The fear of overdiagnosis and subsequent overtreatment play an important role in the dilemma of screening for prostate cancer. Related to this is the slow progression of this cancer. If it is diagnosed before it has metastasized, it often takes more than 10 years to progress and kill a patient. In this period, the patient could die from cardiovascular disease or from causes other than prostate cancer.[57] In 70% of the cases cancers found through screening are locally confined. They are clinically important in 85–90% of these, and they do form a potential threat. Do we need to treat them or should we monitor them by 'watchful waiting'?

High survival rates at 10–15 years after treatment by radical open prostatectomy or radiotherapy have been repeatedly described.[58] In particular, the results are favourable for poorly differentiated, locally confined tumours. Although these findings do not prove that treat-

ment improves survival, the conclusion is that a cure is possible.

Side-effects in radical prostatectomy include preoperative mortality of about 0.2–1.1%, with severe or mild incontinence in 5–30% and impotence in up to 60% of treated patients.[59] These effects jeopardize the quality of life of these patients as recently reported.[60,61] However, it should be mentioned that nerve-sparing operations of the prostate gland may yield encouraging results with regard to impairment of impotence and this technique may have a beneficial impact on the quality of life of the treated patients compared with other operative interventions.

Moreover, more experienced centres report lower percentages of side-effects, certainly when younger patients are treated. Radiotherapy of the prostate gland in general incurs fewer side-effects compared with radical open prostatectomy (Table 7.5).[62]

In conclusion it can be said that treatment of localized prostate cancer is not risk free, although it can cure the cancer. The latter should be balanced in an overall evaluation of total benefit, including screening and treatment,

Table 7.5 Reported complication rates for radical prostatectomy and external-beam radiation therapy

Complication	Percentage
Radical prostatectomy	
Impotence	20–85
Incontinence	1–27
Urethral stricture	10–18
Thromboembolism	2–30
Permanent rectal injuries	1–3
Peroperative death	0.3–2
Radiation therapy	
Acute gastrointestinal or genitourinary complications	3–67
Chronic complications requiring surgery or prolonged hospitalization	1–2
Anorectal complications	2–23
Impotence	40–67
Urethral or bladder complications	3–17
Incontinence	1–3
Death	0.2–0.5

with its potential side-effect risks versus no screening and palliation treatment of cancers diagnosed at a later stage.

ADDITIONAL RESEARCH

Widespread implementation of population screening for prostate cancer cannot be recommended yet. It is still unclear whether screening, by whatever modality, will lead to a reduction in the mortality rate of prostate cancer. Moreover the screening could be quite expensive and consume a large percentage of available health resources. Collection of adequate information about sensitivity and specificity of the screening tests used, together with the cost figures of organizing the screening, are a prerequisite for any screening trial conducted now. Much of the workload of the screening programmes developed to date arises from

false-positive test results which are determined by the sensitivity of the tests used. At present, it appears from the Rotterdam randomized screening study in Europe and the ACS demonstration trial in the USA, that DRE with PSA, subspecified as a PSA-density function, have the best yield of relevant cancers found per biopsy taken. However, these data need further confirmation with additional results.[63,64] Besides the serious problem of reducing the level of false-positive screening results, other issues need also to be stressed here and tackled correctly for the global evaluation of screening studies that have been conducted, especially randomized trials:[65]

- In randomized trials the treatment management of prostate cancer should not differ for the screened and unscreened groups, because this would make it difficult to assess the separate benefits of treatment and screening.

- The main end-point for the evaluation of screening of prostate cancer is a significant reduction in prostate cancer mortality in the screened population compared with a control group. All other clinical end-points are susceptible to lead time, length–time or selection bias.[66]

- To avoid biases it is essential that randomized screening trials should be analysed on an 'intention to treat' basis. Thus an intervention group receiving screening should be compared with a control group not receiving screening. Mortality of the two groups from the date of randomization should be compared. To maximize the statistical power of the trial, as many men as possible in the intervention group should be screened and as many men in the control group should be discouraged from undergoing screening outside the trial, because this can lead to a dramatic decrease in the power of the study. Suitable follow-up systems of both treatment arms should be established in order to obtain notification of the deaths, the causes of death and the cancers diagnosed between two screening rounds in the case arm. For an open-ended study rules for stopping must also be agreed on in advance.

- The period of follow-up should at least encompass the period of the natural history of the cancer causing death when detected locally (estimated follow-up of 10 years).

- To compare the results with other cancer screening programmes, costs should be related to effectiveness measures. The best measure for prostate cancer as specified above is specific mortality reduction. However, as a result of the long observation period needed to obtain reliable data, intermediate effectiveness measures are sometimes used such as cost per detected cancer or screening cost per patient receiving curative treatment. It is important to stress here that the latter type of cost-effectiveness analysis reflects only the programme efficiency. Such analysis does not provide any guidance for determining whether the total benefit of the programme outweighs its total cost.

- The importance of evaluating marginal cost-effectiveness in prostate cancer screening by comparing different cancer detection strategies has been demonstrated by Littrup and colleagues.[67,68] He showed that the cost per detected prostate cancer increased exponentially with repeated screening rounds because fewer cancers are discovered after each round. His study of annual screening found that DRE had the lowest marginal cost during the first 2 years, although the low sensitivity of DRE created a rapid increase in the marginal cost during the third screening round. In contrast PSA demonstrated the lowest marginal cost per cancer detected during the third year.

- It became clear from participation data of the Antwerp screening trial that not all the men in the age group 55–74 years old would attend the screening.[69] That specific age group is confronted with many different 'life' problems, whether or not related to health. Men in this group therefore put a priority scale on the importance of being screened for prostate cancer when confronted with the issue. Any screening programme developed to date using an invitation letter is a self-selecting programme of people willing to participate. The results therefore need to be adjusted before general conclusions can be made for the whole population.

- No prospective assessment or other scientific evidence has to date been published which shows that mortality from prostate cancer can be reduced or that quality of life can be improved by curative treatment after screening. Quality of life of the target population during screening, and treatment where applicable, should be assessed adequately. It could be that mortality reduction and survival benefit are achieved through screening by randomized trials, but at the expense of some lower quality of life which does not justify the screening procedure.[70]

- The potential impact of screening programmes could be studied using analytical decision models in order to identify which variables should prospectively be measured and in which way.[71] Several models have been developed to date. One interesting study is a Swedish project modelled on the comparison of expected quality-adjusted life years among men who have had prostate cancer screening versus none. The results showed that the choice of the benefit values played a relatively minor role, whereas the choice of screening strategy was important. Two main factors affecting the overall results were the high frequency of non-cancer-related deaths such as cardiovascular events and the relatively slow rates of growth of prostate tumours. Many patients die with the disease rather than from the disease. Consequently, age of the patient and his general medical condition became key determinants of the treatment decision – to treat or not to treat – especially for locally confined prostate cancers.

CONCLUSION

It is far from conclusive that prostate cancer screening should now generally be recommended using any method of early detection. However, it cannot be denied that tests are available on the market that could identify those at higher risk for this cancer. It should be recommended that people willing to undergo these tests are informed about what currently is and is not known about the screening used for this cancer.[72]

Those men who are offered or receive screening should be given full information about the consequences of having a positive test result and being treated. Moreover, initiatives should be undertaken to conduct population-based studies in order to augment the knowledge about the natural history of this cancer, about screening and its early treatment, and about the benefits and costs. These studies should be developed and guided by international supervision and by agreement of governmental ethical committees.

REFERENCES

1. Woolf SH, Screening for prostate cancer with prostatic-specific antigens. An examination of the evidence. *N Engl J Med* 1995; **333:** 1401–5.
2. Wingo PA, Landis S, Ries LAG, An adjustment to the 1997 estimate for new prostate cancer cases. *CA Cancer J Clin* 1997; **80:** 1810–13.
3. Black RJ, Bray F, Ferlay J, Parkin DM, Cancer incidence and mortality in the European Union: cancer registry data and estimates of national incidence for 1990. *Eur J Cancer* 1997; **33:** 1075–107.
4. Haas GP, Sakr WA, Epidemiology of prostate cancer. *CA Cancer J Clin* 1997; **47:** 273–87.
5. Boyle P, Maisonneuve P, Napalkov P, Geographical and temporal patterns of incidence and mortality from prostate cancer. *Urology* 1995; **46:** 47–55.
6. Alexander FE, The risk in prostate cancer: myth or reality? In: *Epidemiology of Prostate Diseases.*

(Garraway WM, ed). Springer-Verlag: Berlin, 1995: 192–226.
7. Boyle P, Prostate cancer 2000: Evolution of an epidemic of unknown origin. In: *Prostate Cancer 2000* (Denis L, ed). Springer-Verlag: Berlin, 1994: 6–11.
8. Coeberg J, Van der Heyden L, Janssen-Heijen M, Cancer incidence and survival in the Southeast of the Netherlands 1955–1994. Integrale Kankerstichting Zuid: Eindhoven, 1995.
9. Graham SD Jr, Screening for prostate cancer. *Cancer* 1994; **74:** 3077–9.
10. Austoker J, Current controversies in cancer screening. Balancing benefit and harm. *Eur Cancer News* 1997; **6:** 4–11.
11. Wilson JMG, Jungen G, *Principles and Practice of Screening for Disease.* World Health Organization: Geneva, 1968.
12. Chamberlain J, Screening for early detection of

cancer. *Oncol Nurses Health Care Profess* 1988; **1:** 155–73.

13. Roulston JE, Limitations of tumour markers in screening. *Br J Surg* 1990; **77:** 961–2.

14. Thompson IM, Screening for carcinoma of the prostate. *AUA Update Series* 1990; **9:** 226–32.

15. Smart CR, The results of prostate carcinoma screening in the U.S. As reflected in the surveillances epidemiology, and end results program. *Cancer* 1997; **80:** 1835–44.

16. Graham SD Jr, Screening for prostate cancer. *Cancer* 1994; **74:** 3077–9.

17. Optenberg SA, Thompson SA, Economics for carcinoma of the prostate. *Urol Clin N Am* 1990; **17:** 719–37.

18. Gustafsson O, Carlsson P, Norming U, Nyman CR et al, Cost-effectiveness analysis in early detection of prostate cancer; an evaluation of six screening strategies in a randomly selected population of 2,400 men. *Prostate* 1995; **26:** 299–309.

19. Denis LJ, Murphy GP, Schröder FH, Report of the Consensus Workshop on Screening and Global Strategy for Prostate Cancer. *Cancer* 1995; **75:** 1187–207.

20. Schröder FH, Albrecht W, Auvinen A et al, Screening and early detection of prostate cancer. In: *First International Consultation on Prostate Cancer. Proceedings 1* (Murphy G, Griffiths K, Denis L et al, eds). Scientific Communication International: Monaco, 1997: 179–98.

21. Auvinen A, Rietbergen JBW, Denis LJ et al, Prospective evaluation plan for randomised trials of prostate cancer screening. *J Med Screen* 1996; **3:** 97–104.

22. Schröder FH, The European Randomized Study of Screening for Prostate Cancer. *AUA News* 1997; **3–4:** 31–7.

23. Chodak GW, Questioning the value of screening for prostate cancer in asymptomatic men. *Urology* 1993; **42:** 116–18.

24. Gerber GS, Chodak GW, Value of prostate cancer screening. *Eur Urol* 1993; **24:** 161–5.

25. Porter AT, Zimmerman J, Ruffin M et al, Recommendations of the First Michigan Conference on Prostate Cancer. *Urology* 1996; **48:** 519–34.

26. Murphy GP, Maguine RT, Rogers B et al, Comparison of serum PSMA, PSA levels with results of Cytogen-356 Prostascrint scanning in prostatic cancer patients. *Prostate* 1997; **33:** 281–5.

27. Bentvelsen FM, Schröder FH, Modalities available for screening for prostate cancer. *Eur J Cancer* 1994; **29:** 804–10.

28. Catalona WJ, Smith DS, Ratliff L et al, Measurement of prostate-specific antigen in serum as a screening test for prostate cancer. *N Engl J Med* 1991; **324:** 1156–61.

29. Labrie F, Dupont A, Suburu R et al, Serum prostate specific antigen as pre-screening test for prostate cancer. *J Urol* 1992; **147:** 846–52.

30. Brawer MK, Ghetner MP, Beatie J et al, Screening for prostatic carcinoma with prostate specific antigen. *J Urol* 1992; **147:** 841–5.

31. Lee F, Torp-Pedersen S, Littrup PJ et al, Hypoechoic lesions of the prostate: clinical relevance of tumor size, digital rectal examination and prostate-specific antigen. *Radiology* 1989; **70:** 29–32.

32. Lee F, Littrup PJ, Torp-Pedersen ST et al, Prostate cancer: comparison of transrectal US and digital rectal examination for screening. *Radiology* 1988; **168:** 389–94.

33. Cooner WH, Mosley BR, Rutherford CL Jr et al, Prostate cancer detection in a clinical urological practice by ultrasonography, digital rectal examination and prostate specific antigen. *J Urol* 1990; **143:** 1146–54.

34. Mettlin CJ, Murphy GP, Babaian RJ et al, Observations on the early detection of prostate cancer from the American Cancer Society National Prostate Cancer Detection Project. *Cancer* 1997; **80:** 1814–17.

35. Reissigl A, Horninger W, Fink K et al, Prostate carcinoma screening in the County of Tyrol, Austria. *Cancer* 1997; **80:** 1818–29.

36. Standaert B, Denis, L, The European Randomized Study of Screening for Prostate Cancer. *Cancer* 1997; **80:** 1830–4.

37. De Antoni EP, Eight years of 'Prostate Cancer Awareness Week'. Lessons in screening and early detection. *Cancer* 1997; **80:** 1845–51.

38. Smith DS, Humphrey PA, Catalona WJ, The early detection of prostate carcinoma with prostate specific antigen. *Cancer* 1997; **80:** 1852–6.

39. Gann PH, Hennekens CH, Stampfer MJ, A prospective evaluation of plasma prostate-specific antigen for detection of prostatic cancer. *J Am Med Assoc* 1995; **273:** 289–94.

40. Babaian RJ, Miyashita H, Evans RB, Ramirez AI, The distribution of prostate specific antigen in men without clinical or pathological evidence of prostate cancer: Relationship to gland volume and age. *J Urol* 1992; **147:** 837–40.

41. Mettlin C, Littrup PJ, Kane RA et al, Relative sensitivity and specificity of serum PSA level compared to age-referenced PSA, PSA density

and PSA change: Data from the American Cancer Society National Prostate Cancer Detection Project. *Cancer* 1994; **74:** 1615–20.

42. Oesterling JE, Jacobsen SJ, Chute CG et al, Serum prostate-specific antigen in a community-based population of healthy men. Establishment of age-specific reference ranges. *J Am Med Assoc* 1993; **270:** 860–4.

43. Benson MC, Seong Whang IHN, Olsson CA et al, The use of prostate specific antigen density to enhance the predictive value of intermediate levels of serum prostate specific antigen. *J Urol* 1992; **147:** 817–21.

44. Newling DWW, Expert Panel's Guidelines on PSA. After radiation therapy for prostate cancer. Published in ASTRO's Red Journal. *Eur Cancer News* 1998; **April:** 13–14.

45. Lerner SE, Jacobsen SJ, Lilja H et al, Free, complexed, and total serum prostate-specific antigen concentrations and their proportions in predicting stage, grade, and deoxyribonucleic acid ploidy in patients with adenocarcinoma of the prostate. *Urology* 1996; **48:** 240–8.

46. Standaert B, Alwan A, Nielen V, Denis L, Prostate volume and cancer in screening programs. *Prostate* 1997; **33:** 188–94.

47. Rietbergen JBW, Boeken Kruger AE, Kranse R, Schröder FH, Complications of transrectal ultrasound-guided systematic sextant biopsies of the prostate: Evaluation of complication rates and risk factors within a population-based screening program. *Urology* 1997; **49:** 875–80.

48. Schröder FH, Prostate cancer: to screen or not to screen? It's happening, but the case has not been made. *Br Med J* 1993; **306:** 407–8.

49. Ansell JS, An opposing view. *J Family Pract* 1988; **27:** 525–8.

50. Schwartz KL, Severson RK, Gurney JG, Montie JE, Trends in the stage specific incidence of prostate carcinoma in the Detroit Metropolitan Area 1973–1974. *Cancer* 1996; **78:** 1260–6.

51. Rietbergen JBW, Kranse R, Kirkels WJ et al, Evaluation of prostate-specific antigen, digital rectal examination and transrectal ultrasonography in population-based screening for prostate cancer: improving the efficiency of early detection. *Br J Urol* 1997; **79:** 57–63.

52. Mettlin C, Murphy GP, Lee F et al, Characteristics of prostate cancers detected in a multimodality early detection program. *Cancer* 1993; **72:** 1701–8.

53. Karakiewicz PI, Bazinet M, Aprilian AG et al, Outcome of sextant biopsy according to gland volume. *Urology* 1997; **49:** 55–9.

54. Kirkels WJ, Rietbergen JBW, Screening for prostate cancer. *Urol Res* 1997; **25:** 553–6.

55. Brawley OW, Prostate carcinoma incidence and patient mortality. *Cancer* 1997; **80:** 1857–63.

56. Kramer BS, Brown ML, Prorok PC et al, Prostate Cancer Screening: what we know and what we need to know. *Ann Intern Med* 1993; **119:** 914–23.

57. Garnick MB, The dilemmas of prostate cancer. Do the risks of aggressive treatment for early prostate cancer outweigh the benefits? This question is one of several unresolved issues faced by those who treat, and those who have, prostate cancer. *Sci Am* 1994; **4:** 52–9.

58. Gerber GS, Thisted RA, Scardino PT et al, Results of radical prostatectomy in men with clinically localized prostate cancer. Multi-institutional pooled analysis. *J Am Med Assoc* 1996; **276:** 615–19.

59. Fowler FJ Jr, Wennberg JE, Timothy RP et al, Symptom status and quality of life following prostatectomy. *J Am Med Assoc* 1988; **259:** 3018–22.

60. Perez MA, Meyerowitz BE, Lieskowky G et al, Quality of life and sexuality following radical prostatectomy in patients with prostate cancer who use or do not use erectile aids. *Urology* 1997; **5:** 740–6.

61. Pedersen KV, Carlsson P, Rahmquist M, Varenhorst E, Quality of life after radical retropubic prostatectomy for carcinoma of the prostate. *Eur Urol* 1994; **24:** 7–11.

62. Office of Technology, *Assessment, Cost and Effectiveness of Prostate Cancer Screening in Elderly Men.* Government Printing Office: Washington DC, 1995: OTA-BPH 145.

63. Schröder FH, Dambuis RA, Kirkels WJ et al, European Randomized Study of Screening for Prostate Cancer – The Rotterdam Pilot Studies. *Int J Cancer* 1996; **65:** 145–51.

64. Mettlin C, Murphy GP, Ray P et al, American Cancer Society–National Prostate Cancer Detection Project. Results from multiple examinations using transrectal ultrasound, digital rectal examination and prostate specific antigen. *Cancer* 1993; **71:** 891–8.

65. Boyle P, Screening for prostate diseases. *Prospectives* 1992; Special Issue: 1.

66. Prorok PC, Conoor RJ, Baker SG, Statistical considerations in cancer screening programs. *Urol Clinics N Am* 1990; **17:** 698–708.

67. Littrup PJ, Kane RA, Mettlin CJ et al, Cost-effective prostate cancer detection. Reduction of low-yield biopsies. *Cancer* 1994; **74:** 3146–58.

68. Littrup PJ, Future benefits and cost-effectiveness of prostate carcinoma screening. *Cancer* 1997; **80:** 1864–70.

69. Standaert B, Van Oeckel Ph, Dourcy B et al, Determinants of participation to the project 'Early Detection of Prostate Diseases' in Antwerp. Submitted to *Br J Urol.*

70. Krahn MD, Mahoney JE, Eckman MH et al, Screening for prostate cancer. A decision analytic view. *J Am Med Assoc* 1994; **272:** 773–80.

71. Vanrenhorst E, Carlsson P, Pedersen K, Clinical and economic considerations in the treatment of prostate cancer. *PharmacoEconomics* 1994; **6:** 127–41.

72. Hostetler RM, Mandel IG, Marshburn J, Prostate cancer screening. *Med Clin North Am* 1996; **80:** 83–98.

8

Prostate-specific antigen

Justin Siegal, Michael K Brawer

CONTENTS • **Non-malignant PSA elevation** • **Early detection/screening using PSA** • **Defining normal PSA levels** • **Monitoring using PSA**

Prostate-specific antigen (PSA) is the best marker for prostatic carcinoma and probably is the best tumor marker available today. Serum PSA measurements have demonstrated utility in the early detection or screening, staging, and monitoring of prostatic carcinoma. As a result, PSA has revolutionized our approach to prostatic disease.

PSA is a 34-kDa serine protease produced by the prostatic epithelium. The function of this enzyme is lysis of the seminal coagulum. This analyte is detectable in the serum of all men with functioning prostates. In 1982, the Roswell Park group first observed that abnormal serum PSA concentrations are associated with prostate cancer.

NON-MALIGNANT PSA ELEVATION

Benign prostatic hyperplasia

After the development of sensitive assays for PSA detection, considerable enthusiasm was generated concerning the utility of this test for the detection of prostatic carcinoma. However, interest in PSA for the diagnosis of carcinoma was initially thwarted by reports that PSA was elevated in patients with benign prostatic hyperplasia (BPH)[1-4] (Table 8.1). As BPH is almost universally present in men over 50 years of age (the screening population for prostate cancer), investigators theorized that PSA would play a limited role in cancer detection.

These concerns were mitigated by the observation that BPH has a much less profound affect on serum PSA than does prostate cancer. The Stanford group reported that, volume for volume, prostatic carcinoma contributes 10 times more to the serum PSA than does benign prostatic hyperplasia.[5]

The concentration of PSA in the serum is dependent on the rate of PSA production by the prostatic epithelial cells, the ease with which the PSA extravasates into the serum, and the rate at which the PSA is cleared from the circulation. It appears that elevated serum PSA seen with cancer results primarily from increased diffusion from malignant acini to the blood vessels in the stroma. This conclusion follows from the observation that, while on a cell per cell basis individual epithelial cells from BPH or normal prostate tissue produce more PSA than a given prostate cancer cell, the cancer cells

Table 8.1 Serum PSA levels in patients with histologically confirmed benign prostatic hyperplasia

Study	Year	Assay	No. (%) patients	
			PSA >4.0	PSA >10.0
Ercole et al[2]	1987	Tandem-R	75 (21)	10 (3)
Ferro et al[3]	1987	Tandem-R		13 (33)
Hudson et al[4]	1989	Tandem-R	35 (21)	3 (2)
Stamey et al[5]	1987	Pros-Check	70 (88)	

PSA, prostate-specific antigen.

raise the serum PSA 10-fold above that of the histological BPH cells.[5]

In the normal prostate, natural barriers (including epithelial tight junctions, the basal cell layer, and the basement membrane) minimize PSA leakage. A million-fold PSA concentration difference is maintained between the prostatic fluid and plasma. In prostatic carcinoma the basement membrane and the basal cell layer are disrupted,[6] and prostatic epithelial cells lose organization and may infiltrate the surrounding stroma. These changes contribute to the increased passage of PSA into the circulation and explain the relatively higher serum PSA in cancer patients compared with that in men with BPH alone.

In an effort to understand better the association between PSA and BPH, we studied simple prostatectomy specimens from a series of 81 men suffering from bladder outlet obstruction which was believed to be secondary to BPH.[7] The excised tissue was carefully examined to describe the pathology. Thirteen men were found to have prostatic intraepithelial neoplasia, 11 disclosed adenocarcinoma, and 11 had foci of acute inflammation. The remaining 26 had BPH alone. Of this final group, only one of the men had a serum PSA greater than 4.0 ng/ml. These observations indicate that BPH alone is not a frequent source of elevation of the serum PSA level.

Prostatic intraepithelial neoplasia

Prostatic intraepithelial neoplasia (PIN) exhibits dysplasia and proliferation of the luminal cell layer and is believed to be the primary premalignant lesion of the prostate. Higher grades of PIN demonstrate increasing disruption of the basal cell layer.[6] This disruption may cause the increased serum PSA seen with PIN. This disruption is differentiated from that of malignant histology as it is localized; in prostatic carcinoma the disruption of the normal architecture is generalized. PIN is associated with increased serum PSA levels. In our previously described investigation of simple prostatectomy specimens, we found that patients with focal PIN had elevated PSA values of 7.8 ng/ml. As shown in Table 8.2, men with PIN had an intermediate PSA between those men with benign histology and those with invasive carcinoma. Similar observations have been recorded in other investigations. The source of this rise is not clear. The disruption of the basal cell layer may be associated. However, it may also have resulted from the presence of occult carcinoma.

Table 8.2 Serum PSA* and TRUS PNB[77]

	Benign†	PIN	Carcinoma
Number	36	15	34
Mean PSA (ng/ml)	5.8	7.8	18.3
Range PSA (ng/ml)	0.4–24.9	0.2–19.2	0.2–161
No. (%) patients with PSA >4.0 ng/ml	14 (39)	8 (53)	20 (59)
No. (%) patients with PSA >10 ng/ml	8 (22)	5 (33)	13 (38)

PIN, prostatic intraepithelial neoplasia; PNB, prostate needle biopsy; PSA, prostate-specific antigen; TRUS, transrectal ultrasound.
* Hybritech Tandem-R assay.
† Includes normal, hyperplastic, and chronic inflammation.

Other authorities have concluded that PIN is not associated with elevation of serum PSA.[8] However, these investigators used radical prostatectomy specimens, and thus concomitant invasive carcinoma may have masked any small PSA leakage due to PIN.

We reviewed a series of 21 cases for which repeat biopsies were performed after an initial finding of PIN.[9] All men with a PSA greater than 4.0 ng/ml were found to have carcinoma on their subsequent biopsy. This observation suggests that occult carcinoma, not PIN, is probably associated with increased PSA in men with PIN biopsy findings. For patients with elevated PSA values and biopsies demonstrating PIN, secondary biopsies are warranted.

Prostatitis

Acute prostatic infections have been associated with serum PSA elevation. In contrast, men with chronic prostatitis rarely have an elevated PSA level. These conclusions arise from both laboratory and clinical observations. Neal et al[10] demonstrated that serum PSA levels remained elevated in monkeys with *Escherichia coli*-infected prostates until the infections were resolved. Dalton[11] found an association with clinically defined acute prostatitis and elevated serum PSA. Pathologic observations, based on our previously described simple prostatectomy series, support these observations – PSA was elevated in men with acute prostate infection, while patients with histologically defined chronic prostatitis exhibited no elevation.[7]

Manipulation

Prostatic manipulation, including digital rectal examination (DRE), prostate massage, and prostate needle biopsy (PNB), has been investigated with regard to serum PSA concentrations. It is clear that PNB may cause significant increases in serum PSA values.[12] As a result, serum samples for PSA determination should always be taken in advance of a needle biopsy procedure. Similarly, a vigorous prostate massage may result in a significant serum PSA increase. However, a routine DRE should not increase PSA.[13] This is important, as the

Table 8.3 Performance of PSA in screening studies				
Study	**No. of subjects**	**Positive predictive value (%)**	**Detection rate (%)**	
			Observed	**Estimated**
Catalona et al[15]	1563	33.0	2.2	2.7
Brawer et al:				
Year 1[16]	1249	30.5	2.6	4.6
Year 2[59]	701	17.1	2.0	6.7
Year 3[78]	738	18.6	1.8	3.8

PSA, prostate-specific antigen.

clinician may accurately measure serum PSA with a blood sample taken subsequent to an abnormal DRE.

Investigators have recently demonstrated a slight elevation of PSA associated with sexual activity.[14] This transient elevation peaks approximately 1 h after ejaculation, returning to baseline within 24 h. The clinical significance of this rise remains unclear, and further investigation is necessary to determine if sexual abstinence is critical to obtain accurate diagnostic serum PSA values.

EARLY DETECTION/SCREENING USING PSA

The most widespread application of PSA is in the early detection of and screening for prostate cancer. A number of authors have demonstrated that screening with PSA level in conjunction with DRE will identify prostate cancer at a curable stage for the majority of men.[5,15–22] Virtually every study has found PSA to be the best overall diagnostic tool in the diagnosis of prostate cancer. The efficacy of serum PSA as an initial test in an early detection program was first evaluated by Catalona et al[15] in a group of 1653 men aged over 50 years. Using a serum PSA cut-off of 4.0 ng/ml, they demonstrated an overall detection rate of 2.2% and a positive predictive value of 33%. Of the men with a PSA value between 4.0 and 9.9 ng/ml, 22% were found to have prostatic carcinoma on transrectal ultrasound-guided biopsy, while 67% of the men with a PSA level above 10 ng/ml had carcinoma confirmed (Table 8.3).

We conducted a contemporaneous investigation, screening 1249 men aged over 50 years using the Hybritech Tandem-R PSA assay.[16] Our overall detection rate was 2.6% and the positive predictive value was 30.5%.

Table 8.4 demonstrates the rates of detection of cancer using various combinations of diagnostic modalities: PSA > 4.0 ng/ml, abnormal DRE, and a hypoechoic peripheral zone lesion found on transrectal ultrasound (TRUS). In spite of the subjectivity of the DRE and the variability of the TRUS, it is remarkable to note the consistency of findings for any combination of test abnormalities between reports. In particular, both our data and those reported by Catalona et al[15] demonstrate the predictive strength of PSA as a single parameter. Even in the absence of an abnormality on DRE and TRUS, 22% of patients with an elevated PSA were found to have carcinoma when subjected to systematic sector biopsies.

Given the extraordinary performance of PSA

Table 8.4 Detection of pancreatic cancer using various combinations of DRE, TRUS, and PSA (showing cancers detected divided by total number tested, with percentage in parentheses)

Combination of modalities			Catalona et al[15]	Catalona et al[79]	Cooner et al[80]	Lee et al[81]	Mettlin et al[82]	Ellis and Brawer[83]	Total
DRE	**TRUS**	**PSA level**							
−	−	−	0/11 (0)					0/61 (0)	0/72 (0)
−	−	*	6/37 (16)	57/276 (21)				93/417 (22)	156/730 (21)
*	−	−	0/17 (0)	16/233 (7)			5/30 (17)	31/436 (7)	52/716 (7)
−	*	−	2/35 (6)		19/204 (9)	2/44 (5)	9/164 (6)	41/557 (7)	73/1004 (7)
−	*	*	14/63 (22)	57/191 (30)	41/161 (25)	31/92 (34)	9/37 (24)	203/734 (28)	355/1278 (28)
*	−	*	16/49 (33)	26/63 (41)			3/8 (38)	61/221 (28)	106/341 (31)
*	*	−	11/53 (21)	32/232 (14)	33/195 (17)	6/23 (26)	7/48 (15)	177/1159 (16)	266/1710 (16)
*	*	*	49/81 (60)	64/117 (55)	170/275 (62)	63/89 (71)	17/25 (68)	676/1284 (53)	1038/1871 (55)

DRE, digital rectal examination; PSA, prostate-specific antigen; TRUS, transrectal ultrasound.
* Modality used.

in a biopsy population, many clinicians have used the PSA level as a main indication for biopsy. Table 8.5 demonstrates the positive predictive value of a PSA level greater than 4.0 ng/ml in a variety of patient populations. These investigations indicate that system sector biopsies will identify carcinoma in more than one of three men with a serum PSA level greater than 4.0 ng/ml. Table 8.6 demonstrates the overall performance and yield of PSA in several large biopsy series. Again, the extraordinary performance of this tumor marker is demonstrated.

Importance of digital rectal examination

The number of carcinomas identified by means of DRE and PSA were compared by Catalona et al[23] in a multicenter early detection series of 6630 patients. Abnormal findings on either parameter led to TRUS-guided biopsy (1167 men). Of this group, 264 (22.6%) carcinomas were found. PSA detected 216 of these men with pancreatic carcinoma, while DRE identified 146. The PSA level positive predictive value (31.5%) and detection rate (4.6%) were both greater than those for DRE (21.4% and 3.2%, respectively). The detection rate was optimized by combining DRE and PSA findings, thus achieving a detection rate of 5.8%.

We recently investigated a series of men for whom follow-up was indicated by an abnormality at DRE, despite a serum PSA level of less than 4.0 ng/ml. These men were identified from a group of 1473 patients who had undergone systematic sector biopsies at our institution over the last 10 years. In total, 489 men were indicated for further work-up from DRE alone. From this group, 61 men (12.5%) were found to have invasive carcinoma at systematic sector biopsy. This observation emphasized the importance of DRE in addition to serum PSA level measurement in the detection of invasive prostatic carcinoma.

DEFINING NORMAL PSA LEVELS

Defining a normal PSA reference range is problematic. It is impossible to confirm practically that any given man is free of significant prostatic disease that may cause an elevation of the serum PSA levels. Occult prostatic carcinoma occurs in at least a third of men aged over 50 years. The effect these subclinical carcinomas may play on PSA values is unclear.

The methodology first reported by Myrtle et al[24] is widely used in determining a reference range. The Hybritech group defined the 97.5% confidence interval for men aged over 40 years whose serum PSA level was measured with the Tandem-R assay; their findings established the generally accepted reference range of 0–4.0 ng/ml.

This range demonstrates excellent performance: over one in three men with a PSA level above 4.0 ng/ml will exhibit invasive carcinoma on a subsequent biopsy. However, it has been suggested that additional parameters must be considered in establishing a normal PSA range for a given man. Their attempt to define a normal reference range led Oesterling et al[25] to recommend that normal PSA ranges should vary with patient age. Additional patient parameters that may be considered in conjunction with PSA include race and DRE results.

While a PSA cut-off value of 4.0 ng/ml as an indication for further evaluation exhibits excellent sensitivity, two of three patients with a PSA value above this range will have negative initial biopsies.[15–18] This lack of specificity has encouraged significant effort at improving the performance of this tumor marker. Four refinements have been evaluated: PSA density, PSA velocity, age-specific PSA, and free/total PSA.

Improving specificity

PSA density
In an attempt to adjust for the PSA concentration contributed by benign prostatic hyperplasia, the PSA density (PSAD) has been used. A number of authors have reported an improvement in predictive value when using the PSAD rather than the PSA serum level (Table 8.7). Benson et al[26] were the first to report that the specificity of serum PSA concentrations is enhanced if the prostate size is considered also.

Table 8.5 Positive predictive value (PPV) for pancreatic cancer of a PSA level > 4.0 ng/ml

Study	Year	Population	No. of biopsies	PPV (%)
Babaian and Camps[18]	1991	Mixed	67	31.3
Bazinet et al[33]	1994	Referral	565	37.0
Brawer et al[84]	1989	Referral	188	54.2
Brawer et al[16]	1992	Screening	105	30.5
Catalona et al[15]	1992	Screening	112	33.0
Catalona et al[79]	1993	Screening	1325	37.1
Cooner et al[80]	1988	Referral	96	51.2
Cooner et al[17]	1990	Referral	436	35.0
Ellis and Brawer[83]	1994	Referral	541	36.8
Mettlin et al[82]	1991	Screening	70	41.4
Rommel et al[32]	1994	Referral	2020	41.0
Total			5525	38.9

Table 8.6 Performance of a PSA level of > 4.0 ng/ml in diagnosis of prostate cancer

Study	No. of patients	Sensitivity (%)	Specificity (%)	PPV (%)	NPV (%)	Accuracy (%)
Babaian and Camps[18]	362	81	82	33	97	81
Brawer and Chetner[85]	1473	82	47	36	88	56
Catalona et al[86]	333	87	41	37	89	
Cooner et al[80]	1807	80	75	35	96	76
Labrie et al[87]	1002	72	91	33	98	90
Lee et al[88]	240	92	40	52	88	
Mettlin et al[82]	291	58	84	41	91	

NPV, negative predictive value; PPV, positive predictive value; PSA, prostate-specific antigen.

Table 8.7 Significance of PSA, prostate volume, PSAD in TRUS PNB

Study	Biopsy	No. of patients	PSA† (ng/ml)	Prostate volume† (cm³)	PSAD index†
Benson et al[29]	Positive	98	7.0 ± 1.7*	28.9 ± 14.6	0.30 ± 0.15*
	Negative	191	6.8 ± 1.8	40.1 ± 20.2	0.21 ± 0.11
Seaman et al[31]	Positive	115	6.9 ± 1.7	29.2 ± 14.2*	0.29 ± 0.15*
	Negative	311	6.8 ± 1.7	42.2 ± 21.8	0.20 ± 0.11
Brawer et al[34]	Positive	68	10.7 ± 11.4*	40.5 ± 16.6	0.29 ± 0.41*
	Negative	159	5.2 ± 5.0	42.6 ± 25.6	0.14 ± 0.14
Bazinet et al[33]	Positive	217	21.4 ± 29.6*	37.6 ± 21.4	0.63 ± 0.86*
	Negative	317	9.1 ± 8.1	51.6 ± 27.3	0.21 ± 0.25
Rommel et al[32]	Positive	612	15.5 ± 21.6*	42.7 ± 27.2*	0.47 ± 0.11*
	Negative	1394	4.9 ± 4.7	47.0 ± 31.6	0.11 ± 0.09
Mettlin et al[21]	Positive	171	12.0 ± 16.0*	38.9 ± 16.4*	0.35 ± 0.05*
	Negative	650	2.1 ± 2.3	33.5 ± 14.2	0.08 ± 0.09
Ohori et al[36]	Positive	110	9.3 (0.3–1320)‡	28.1 (15.1–228.7)‡	0.21 (0.009–39.3)‡
	Negative	134	4.8 (0.2–64.1)‡	47.3 (13.3–332.6)‡	0.09 (0.007–1.82)‡

PNB, prostate needle biopsy; PSA, prostate-specific antigen; PSAD; PSA density; TRUS, transrectal ultrasound.
* $p < 0.05$.
† Data are mean ± standard deviation.
‡ Data are median (range); $p < 0.05$.

They defined the PSAD as the serum PSA (ng/ml) divided by the volume of the prostate (cm³). Their suggestion is theoretically consistent with an earlier observation by Stamey et al[5] that PSA levels are elevated in proportion to the volume of benign hyperplastic tissue.

Subsequently, Veneziano et al[27] used a PSAD index to evaluate 33 patients ultimately diagnosed with prostate carcinoma, 75 patients with either prostatitis or BPH, and 35 normal controls. Prostate volume was determined using TRUS. The mean PSAD index was found to be 0.090 in normal patients, 0.099 in those with prostatitis or BPH, and 1.73 in those with pro-

static carcinoma. The authors suggested that the PSAD could be used as a means of distinguishing between benign and malignant processes in the prostate.

Benson et al[28] evaluated PSAD in 61 men with prostatic disease: 41 had carcinoma and 20 had BPH. Serum PSA was measured using the Hybritech Tandem-R assay; however, in some cases this measurement was made after prostatic biopsy. The prostate volume in the radical prostatectomy series was assessed by measuring the pathologic specimen. In the BPH patients, magnetic resonance imaging (MRI) was used to obtain the measurements. The mean and standard deviation for PSA in the BPH group was 3.7 ± 3.3 and in the carcinoma group 24.4 ± 36.9. The mean and standard deviation of the PSAD was 0.044 ± 0.027 in the BPH and 0.581 ± 0.739 in the carcinoma groups, respectively. The mean PSAD for prostate cancer was significantly greater than that for BPH ($p < 0.002$; Student's t-test). No patient with BPH had a PSAD greater than 0.117, and only one had a PSAD greater than 0.1. Two of the 41 prostate cancer patients had a PSAD of less than 0.05.

In an additional study, Benson et al[29] evaluated 289 men who were biopsied after finding PSA levels of 4.1–10.0 ng/ml. This represents the range where the added specificity reputed to be offered by PSAD would be of greatest value. Of these men, 98 had biopsy-proven carcinoma and 191 had a negative TRUS-guided biopsy. The mean PSA concentrations and standard deviations for these groups were 7.0 ± 1.73 and 6.8 ± 1.81 ng/ml, respectively. The corresponding PSAD for these two groups were 0.297 ± 0.153 and 0.208 ± 0.114 ng/ml per cm^3, respectively. Using Student's t-test, no significant difference was noted between the PSA levels in patients undergoing biopsy who had positive and negative results ($p = 0.33$). In contrast, the PSAD values in these two groups were significantly different ($p < 0.00001$).

Despite these initial promising findings, the literature on PSAD is confusing. Data from additional investigations by Bangma et al,[30] Seaman et al,[31] Rommel et al,[32] and Bazinet et al[33] all support the utility of PSAD. In contrast, Brawer et al[34] and Mettlin et al[21] could not demonstrate any advantage in using PSAD over use of the PSA level alone.

To ascertain the utility of a PSAD value in the range 4.0–10.0 ng/ml, we retrospectively evaluated a group of 271 men who had PSA values in this range and known biopsy results.[35] The PSAD was successful at differentiating histology (Table 8.7). In fact, the prostate volume alone could be used to differentiate between patients with cancer and those with BPH. However, over the total study population, for which the PSA values were in the range 0.2–220 ng/ml, the PSAD was not of diagnostic

significance. A similar investigation by Ohori et al[36] did not find any predictive significance of a PSAD value in the range 4.0–10.0 ng/ml.

There are several possible explanations for the inconsistent enhancement of the specificity of diagnosis offered by use of the PSAD. One possibility lies in the inconsistent histology of BPH – volume expansion in BPH may result from glandular proliferation, glandular dilatation, or stromal proliferation. The epithelial/stromal ratio varies significantly between BPH patients. Hyperplasia of the benign epithelium will engender a rise in PSA production, which may be related to a corresponding rise in serum PSA.[37] However, in a patient in whom the BPH is largely a stromal proliferation, a volume-adjusted PSA measurement may in fact mask a significant PSA rise that is due to a tumor, not to BPH.

Another consideration is the considerable margin of error in the prostate volume measured using TRUS. Finally, the reliability of a PNB may be diminished for a large prostate. As a result, the reduction in the number of tumors identified in larger prostates may in fact be a result of the increased difficulty in identifying the neoplasms. An equal volume of cancer is less likely to be identified by a random sextant needle biopsy in a large prostate as compared with a small prostate (Figure 8.1). This problem is compounded because prostate cancer tends to develop in the peripheral zone. As BPH enlarges the transition zone, the peripheral zone is compressed and laterally displaced, making it increasingly difficult to obtain a successful sample by means of a biopsy.[38]

PSA velocity

The PSA velocity (PSAV) is the rate of change in the PSA level over time. Carter et al[39] were the first to evaluate the PSAV, based on the proposition that serial PSA measurements would effectively monitor tumor development. Sera from 20 patients with BPH, 18 patients with prostate cancer, and 16 patients with no evidence of prostate disease were evaluated retrospectively. The patients each had at least three PSA samples taken over a minimum

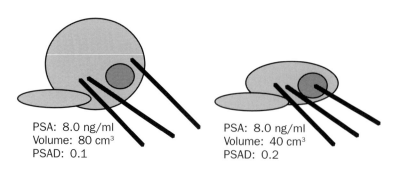

Figure 8.1 Sampling concerns associated with prostate-specific antigen density (PSAD). The carcinoma in the larger prostate (which has a lower PSAD) is more likely to be missed.

PSA: 8.0 ng/ml
Volume: 80 cm³
PSAD: 0.1

PSA: 8.0 ng/ml
Volume: 40 cm³
PSAD: 0.2

interval of 7 years. The data demonstrated significant stratification between benign and malignant histology in those patients who had an annual PSA rise of more than 0.75 ng/ml. Additionally, the specificity of the PSAV (90%) with regard to diagnosis was found to be considerably better than that of PSA alone (60%).

Smith and Catalona[40] also reported that the PSAV was useful in detecting prostate cancer. In this prospective study, 984 men had serum PSA values determined biannually. The men were divided into two groups: those with initial PSA values above 4.0 ng/ml and those with a value below 4.0 ng/ml. For the former group, these investigators also found that an annual PSA increase of 0.75 ng/ml was the optimal cut-off point (79% sensitivity, 66% specificity). For men with an initial PSA level above 4.0 ng/ml, a lower value of 0.4 ng/ml per year was found to offer optimal performance (63% sensitivity, 62% specificity). Littrup et al[41] performed a receiver operator characteristics (ROC) curve analysis to compare the performance characteristics of absolute PSA change with the percentage PSA charge. The percentage change (20% per year increase) did not perform as well as did the absolute change in serum PSA (0.6 ng/ml per year).

In contrast, our group found equivalent performance using a 20% per year PSA increase or a 0.8 ng/ml per year absolute change as an indication for follow-up. In the second year of our PSA screening trial, we performed biopsies on 82 men who demonstrated an increase of more than 20% in the serum PSA level. Carcinoma was detected in 14 (17.1%) of these men (12 of the men with carcinoma (86%) had a second-year PSA of less than 4.0 ng/ml). However, in a subsequent report, neither an absolute nor a relative PSA change stratified men with and without carcinoma.[42] These inconsistent findings may stem from the different time intervals over which the serum samples were obtained.

In a retrospective study, Carter et al[43] attempted to characterize the appropriate number of samples and the interval between measurements necessary to generate useful PSAV data. They determined that the PSAV is most useful if sets of three consecutive measurements are taken over a 2-year period. It does not appear that PSAV values calculated at shorter intervals would increase the chance of predicting cancer.

The lack of utility of short-interval PSA measurements may be explained by day-to-day variations in PSA levels. PSA levels are reported to fluctuate between 20% and 50% on a short-term basis. We recently evaluated serum PSA variations for 24 patients who had their PSA tested daily for 10 consecutive weekdays.[44] We found a mean variation of 8.9%, with a maximum fluctuation of 30%.

Age-specific PSA

Serum PSA values have been shown to generally rise with age. Age-specific PSA cut-off levels are a response to this observation that is, higher PSA values are used with increasing patient age to indicate the need for further work-up. This modification is similar in nature to the PSAD. Both modifications adjust the PSA cut-off values in association with BPH. Age-specific PSA adjustment is believed by many to be the most important single determinant of the PSA level in men without carcinoma. The rise in the PSA level with age is primarily due to the concomitant increase in the prevalence of BPH with age. The use of age-specific PSA values may present an advantage in younger men by providing a higher sensitivity in screening for cancer, while in older men the use of such values provides greater specificity.

Oesterling et al[25] measured the serum PSA concentrations in 471 men without prostate cancer in order to determine age-specific reference ranges that could be used in screening. Age-specific reference ranges were established for 10-year intervals between the ages of 40 and 79 years, using 95% confidence intervals. This group's findings are summarized in Table 8.8. Dalkin et al[45] performed a similar investigation, measuring PSA values in 5220 healthy men in the age range 50–74 years. This group established similar cut-off levels.

Unfortunately, tests of age-specific cut-off values have not established improvements in the predictive value of this quantity. Mettlin et al[46] used data obtained from the American Cancer Society National Prostate Cancer Detection Project to compare age-specific cut-offs with the standard cut-off value of 4.0 ng/ml. Age-specific cut-offs were no more effective than was PSA alone across all groups. However, this study only included patients aged over 55 years, and thus it was not possible to observe any potential improvements in the sensitivity of this measure in younger men. El-Galley et al[47] also compared the normal PSA cut-off of 4.0 ng/ml with age-specific cut-off values. Again, there was not a sufficient number of younger men for significant conclusions to be drawn. However, for the patients aged under 60 years, the age-specific cut-off values would have indicated an additional 17 men for follow-up, two (12%) of whom harbored cancer. In the older population, age-specific cut-offs would have prevented 244 biopsies (12%), missing an additional 18 neoplasms.

Etzioni et al[48] used a screening population of 1208 men to model the effects of an age-specific cut-off versus a standard cut-off value of 4.0 ng/ml. Our large biopsy series proved to be a predictive model for establishing likely cancer yield. Our group determined that age-specific PSA cut-off levels offered a positive predictive value of 38% (50 cancers detected out of 132 biopsies) while a standard PSA cut-off of 4.0 ng/ml has a positive predictive value of 35% (64 cancers detected out of 183 biopsies). Use of the age-specific cut-off level would prevent 51 biopsies, but miss 14 cancers (28% of the saved biopsies). This investigation indicated that using a boundary of 4.0 ng/ml is more efficient in identifying men with cancer.

It does not appear advantageous to apply age-specific PSA cut-off levels for older men, in whom the significant sensitivity is sacrificed for a marginal increase in specificity. The true significance of age-specific PSA cut-off values may be in younger men, in whom a mildly elevated PSA should be looked at more critically than a similar value in an older individual. However, the American Cancer Society[49] and the

Table 8.8 Age-specific normal PSA level ranges[25]	
Age range (years)	**PSA reference range* (ng/ml)**
40–49	0–2.5
50–59	0–3.5
60–69	0–4.5
70–79	0–6.5

* 95% confidence intervals.

American Urologic Association[50] recommend that the serum PSA level is evaluated on an annual basis in men aged over 50 years. There is currently no general application of age-specific cutoffs in a younger population. Further prospective analysis is essential to determine if age-specific cut-off values merit clinical consideration.

Forms of PSA in circulation – free vs total PSA

Three major molecular forms of PSA are recognized in the bloodstream.[51–53] PSA may be unbound (free PSA), complexed with α_1-antichymotrypsin (PSA–ATC), or bound to α_2-macroglobulin (PSA–AMG). The largest portion of circulating PSA is typically complexed with the serine protease inhibitors. Unbound PSA represents only a small fraction of the total PSA in the blood.

The forms of PSA measured can be partly differentiated immunohistochemically. Immunoreactive assays for serum PSA recognize five distinct epitopes on the free PSA molecule. These epitopes are partly masked when a complex is formed (Figure 8.2). For the PSA–ACT complex, three of the epitopes are covered, leaving two available for antibody detection. With the PSA–AMG complex, all the epitopes are covered, and thus this form is not detected by current commercial assays.

Analysis of PSA form has the potential to differentiate between elevated PSA values due to prostate cancer from those due to BPH. Various studies have demonstrated improved PSA predictive value of PSA level when analysis of PSA form was included. In 1991, both Stenman et al[53] and Lilja et al[52] reported that PSA–ACT is the predominant form of PSA in prostate cancer. These findings indicated that measuring the PSA–ACT level may increase the sensitivity of cancer detection over measuring the PSA level alone. A subsequent investigation by the latter group confirmed these initial findings.[5] In this study, free PSA, PSA–ACT, and total PSA were measured in the sera from 121 patients with prostate cancer and 144 patients with BPH. Using a total PSA cut-off of 5.0 ng/ml, the clinical sensitivity was 90% and the specificity was 50%. Combining a minimum total PSA cut-off of 10 ng/ml with a maximum free/total PSA cut-off of 0.18 increased the specificity to 73% while still achieving a sensitivity of 90%.

More recently, Luderer et al[54] investigated

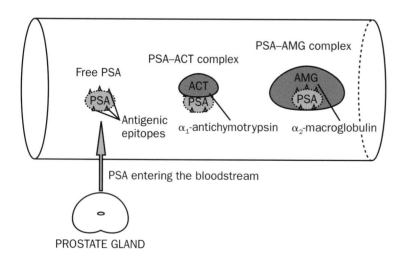

Figure 8.2 Major molecular forms of PSA.

using free/total PSA ratio (F/T PSA) to differentiate between PSA elevations due to BPH and those indicating prostatic carcinoma. Their findings indicated that free/total PSA ratios offered improved diagnostic performance over a total PSA cut-off of 4 ng/ml only in men with PSA values in the range 4.0–10.0 ng/ml. A group of 25 men with cancer was compared with 32 men with BPH; all patients had PSA values between 4.0 and 10.0 ng/ml. The groups were selected such that the total PSA had no predictive value in differentiating between the groups – the mean total PSA for the benign group was 6.2 ng/ml, while the mean total PSA for the cancer group was 6.9 ng/ml. A free/total PSA cut-off of less than 0.2 did significantly differentiate between these groups ($p < 0.001$).

Catalona et al[55] have also studied the utility of free/total PSA ratios in men with total serum PSA values between 4.0 and 10.0 ng/ml. However, they added the additional parameter of prostate volume. Serum was analyzed from 20 patients with prostate cancer and a normal sized gland (<40 cm³), 30 patients with cancer and an enlarged gland (>40 cm³), and 63 patients with BPH. The assumption was that the free PSA value for a prostate cancer patient with concomitant BPH would be deceptively high as a result of the BPH. In this scenario, the free/total PSA ratio would be elevated and could be higher than the free/total PSA cancer threshold. The data support this hypothesis: a cut-off of less than 0.14 was required to maintain a 90% sensitivity in patients with normal sized glands, while a cut-off of less than 0.21 was essential to maintain the same sensitivity for the group with large glands. In these groups, use of the free/total PSA ratio added significant specificity to the predictions made using total PSA alone. A free/total PSA cut-off as high as 0.23 would have prevented 31% of the benign biopsies.

A number of large-scale population-based investigations are in progress with the aim of validating these preliminary findings and determining the appropriate role of the free/total PSA ratio in patient care. These findings should establish normal free/total PSA ratios and the role the ratios can play in multivariate patient assessment. Catalona et al have suggested that the free/total PSA ratio may be of greatest diagnostic power when combined with other parameters such as total PSA and prostate volume.

Our biological variation data indicate that PSA is released by BPH in a fundamentally different manner than it is from cancer.[44] In cancer patients short-term serum PSA variability is less than in patients with only BPH, suggesting a more pulsatile PSA release in BPH. These different release mechanisms may also help explain the variations in the forms of PSA seen in cancer versus those seen in BPH patients. Perhaps a high PSA yield for a BPH patient represents a short-term surge in serum PSA. This periodicity may explain the relatively elevated concentration of free PSA in BPH patients. The free form of PSA is cleared much more rapidly than is the complexed form: the half-life of free PSA is thought to be less than 2 h, while the half-lives of the complexed forms are approximately 3 days. The relative abundance of free PSA found in BPH patients may indicate 'younger' PSA. In cancer patients, where a high concentration of PSA is constantly secreted, it is consistent that the bound form of PSA is seen in a relatively higher concentration.

Interpretation of PSA values may be refined by the addition of a myriad additional parameters. Currently, there is no compelling evidence that any technique provides greater predictive value than the PSA level alone. None the less, PSAD, PSAV, and patient age may all be considered, in addition to PSA alone, to offer an informative follow-up measure in patients with PSA values in the 4–10 ng/ml range – a markedly positive PSA velocity may render a PSA of 5 ng/ml suspect, while a large prostate and a history of BPH may indicate watchful waiting.

Assay variability

Consistent serum PSA measurement is critical in early detection, monitoring, or screening using this analyte. A number of assays measure serum PSA but, as there is no international standard, considerable variations exist between these assays. Inconsistencies may result from assays differing in the ratio of the forms they measure. The Stanford Group has recommended a 90% complexed/10% free approach to PSA standardization.[56]

Our laboratory has compared serum PSA values measured using the IMx assay (Abbott Laboratories, North Chicago, IL), the Tandem-E assay (Hybritech Inc., San Diego, CA), and the restandardized ACS assay (Chiron Diagnostics, Walpole, MA). We found substantial equivalence between the restandardized ACS assay and the Tandem-E assay.[57] However, a significant bias exists between these two assays and the IMx assay, with the IMx assay consistently giving lower values. A comparison between the Tandem-E and IMx assays showed the overall bias to be a 14% lower reading with the IMx assay over the range 2.0–10.0 ng/ml.[58]

Assay variability may have considerable clinical significance. Figure 8.3 demonstrates the number of patients with known malignancy who exceed the thresholds of 2.0–6.0 ng/ml with these three assays. As is particularly evident with cut-off values of 5.0 and 6.0 ng/ml, the Abbott IMx assay identifies substantially fewer men with carcinoma.

This observation mandates standardization. The Stanford group demonstrated that substi-tuting a standard calibrator of 10% free and 90% complexed PSA makes the various PSA assays produced by different manufacturers more comparable.[56] Until such a standard is universal, clinicians must remain cognizant of assay variability and bear in mind the assay used in their laboratory when offering patient-management recommendations.

PSA and clinical stage

The use of PSA to assess clinical stage was originally disappointing. While general trends were observed, there was significant overlap between groups, precluding individual clinical utility. Figure 8.4 demonstrates the results from our radical prostatectomy series, when preoperative serum PSA levels were correlated with pathologic stage. In a subsequent investigation, controls were enacted to insure that PSA serum samples were obtained prior to significant prostate perturbation, including diagnostic biopsy and transurethral resection of the prostate (TURP). Figure 8.4 demonstrates that, in this series, the performance of PSA in detecting advanced disease was enhanced. Thus, all the PSA values above 10 ng/ml indicated non-organ-confined disease. Catalona et al[15] examined a series of 33 men who had undergone

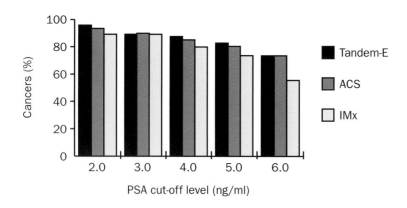

Figure 8.3 Cancers exceeding PSA cut-off levels, as measured using three different assays.

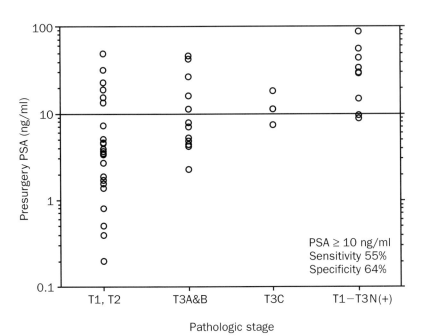

Figure 8.4 Presurgery PSA level and clinical stage of disease.

radical prostatectomy, and observed that 15 out of 16 (94%) of those with a PSA level above 10 ng/ml had non-organ-confined disease. The findings of Catalona et al as well as our own PSA-based screening studies[15,16,19,59] have confirmed that there is significant pathologic upstaging when the serum PSA concentration is greater than 10 ng/ml.

Oesterling et al[60] investigated the relationship between serum PSA values and bone scan results in men with untreated prostate cancer. This group suggested that a serum PSA level above 20 ng/ml is highly indicative of bony metastases. Further investigation is needed to confirm this proposal, which was based on a population of only seven men with positive bone scans.

MONITORING USING PSA

PSA following radical prostatectomy

The serum PSA level is a fundamental measure in monitoring therapy of patients with an established diagnosis of prostate cancer. Following successful surgical excision of the entire gland, the serum PSA should fall below the level of detection. Lange et al[61] found that patients with a PSA level above 4.0 ng/ml following radical prostatectomy always suffered from persistent disease, while men whose PSA values remained below 0.2 ng/ml had no evidence of recurrence. Detection of serum PSA following radical prostatectomy is generally the first indication of progression.

This observation has been corroborated by Stein et al,[62] who followed a series of 230 men with stage D1–D2, N0, M0 disease for

48 months following radical prostatectomy. Detectable serum PSA universally preceded progression. However, a number of men with detectable PSA values did not develop clinical progression during 10 years of follow-up. No patient with a postoperative PSA level below 0.2 ng/ml had a positive biopsy; however, 42% of those with a PSA level above 0.4 ng/ml had clinical evidence of carcinoma. Similar observations have been reported by Abi-Aad et al[63] and Foster et al.[64]

Following a non-curative radical prostatectomy, serum PSA levels tend to drop to an undetectable level, and then proceed to rise gradually. In a series of 542 men, Partin et al[65] demonstrated that the velocity of this rise can differentiate between those patients with clinically localized disease and those with disseminated disease. In the local recurrence group, the median PSA was 5.7 ng/ml and the monthly rate of PSA increase was 0.43 ng/ml; the group with distant metastases exhibited a median PSA

value of 17.0 ng/ml and a PSA increase of 1.8 ng/ml per month.

PSA and radiation therapy

Serum PSA determination may be significant in both identifying successful candidates for radiation therapy and monitoring post-treatment progress. As much of the prostate remains after radiation therapy, it is rare to find PSA levels falling to undetectable levels (Table 8.9). Stamey et al[66] reported that in a series of men treated with radiation therapy, 31% had PSA values that fell to within the normal range, and 11% had measurements that decreased to undetectable levels. Russell et al[67] found that the rapidity of normalization of PSA levels following radiation therapy corresponded with patient prognosis. These observations were confirmed by Zagars et al[68] and Schellhammer et al,[69] who investigated men treated with both

Table 8.9 Nadir in the PSA level following radiation therapy (showing numbers, with percentages in parenthesis)

| Study | Treatment | PSA (ng/ml) | | | | |
		<1.0	<1.5	1.0–2.0	>2.0	<4.0
Zagars and von Eschenbach[68]	External	129 (49)		70 (26)	67 (25)	
Crook et al[89]	External	139 (67)		33 (16)	37 (18)	
Hanks et al[90]	External		31 (40)			55 (71)
	Conformal		138 (66)			188 (90)
Blasko et al[91]	Brachytherapy		113 (82)*			
			134 (97)†			
Stock et al[92]	Brachytherapy		92 (95)			
			74 (76)			

PSA, prostate-specific antigen.
*2 years; †4 years.

external beam therapy and brachytherapy. These groups classified a normal PSA range as less than 4.0 ng/ml.

Pretreatment PSA values are useful in anticipating the response of a neoplasm to external beam therapy. Russell et al[67] demonstrated an 82% complete response rate in patients with pretreatment PSA values of less than 16.0 ng/ml. In contrast, those patients with an initial PSA greater than this cut-off level only had a 30% likelihood of complete response.

PSA after androgen deprivation therapy

An increase in serum PSA following androgen ablation therapy has also been reported to anticipate disease progression.[70–72] Stamey et al[73] first noted a significant decrease in serum PSA in a series of patients receiving androgen-depletion therapy: the serum PSA decreased to normal levels in 31% of patients and below detection in 9%. Subsequently, Miller et al[70] noted a correlation between duration of remission and a nadir of PSA of less than 4.0 ng/ml in a series of patients with skeletal metastases. This finding is supported by observations by Gillat et al[71] and Smith et al.[72]

The 5α-reductase inhibitor finasteride has gained popularity as a treatment for BPH. Finasteride reduces dihydrotestosterone concentrations by more than 90%,[74] resulting in significant atrophy of the epithelial component of the prostate. During the first weeks of treatment, PSA values decrease rapidly to levels below half of baseline. However, finasteride-treated patients with prostate cancer showed only a 26% reduction in serum PSA.[75] This observation suggests that a decrease in serum PSA of less than 50% following finasteride treatment should indicate the possibility of undetected prostatic carcinoma.

CONCLUSION

Significant controversy surrounds the subjects of screening for and early detection of prostatic carcinoma. PSA, the revolutionary keystone of screening, is central to this debate. The marked sensitivity of this analyte deserves the enthusiasm it raises, but the issue of specificity gives pause for thought. The concern is two-fold. First, the lack of specificity of the PSA test results in a considerable number of men without carcinoma undergoing biopsy. The associated cost, measured in financial as well as emotional terms, is significant. Secondly, at present there are no conclusive data to demonstrate a reduction in prostate cancer mortality resulting from early detection.

The discord between our august bodies indicates the intensity of the PSA screening debate. The Canadian Task Force on Periodic Health Examination recommends against the use of PSA for population-based screening.[76] However, the American Cancer Association[49] and the American Urological Association[50] recommend serum PSA determination, in conjunction with a carefully performed DRE, in men seeking evaluation for the possibility of prostatic carcinoma.

Novel diagnostic tools and improved analysis will enhance the diagnostic specificity of PSA measurement, and perhaps simplify this debate. These advances will help us to refine our use of this critical tumor marker.

REFERENCES

1. Wang MC, Kuriyama M, Papsidero LD et al, Prostate antigen of human cancer patients. In: *Methods in Cancer Research* (Busch H, Yeoman LC, eds). Academic Press: New York, 1982: 179–97.

2. Ercole CJ, Lange PH, Mathisen M, Chiou RV, Reddy PK, Vessela RL, Prostate-specific antigen and prostatic acid phosphatase in the monitoring and staging of patients with prostatic cancer. *J Urol* 1987; **138**: 1181–4.

3. Ferro MA, Barnes I, Roberts JBM, Smith PJB, Tumor markers in prostatic carcinoma: a comparison of prostate-specific antigen with acid phosphatase. *Br J Urol* 1987; **60:** 69–73.

4. Hudson MA, Bahnson RB, Catalona WJ, Clinical use of prostate-specific antigen in patients with prostate cancer. *J Urol* 1989; **142:** 1011–17.

5. Stamey TA, Yang N, Hay AR, McNeal JE, Freiha FS, Redwine E, Prostate-specific antigen as a serum marker for adenocarcinoma of the prostate. *N Engl J Med* 1987; **317:** 909–16.

6. Brawer MK, Bostwick DM, Peehl DM, Stamey TA, Keratin immunoreactivity in the benign and neoplastic human prostate. *Cancer Res* 1985; **45:** 3663–7.

7. Brawer MK, Rennels MA, Nagle RB, Schifman RA, Gaines J, Serum PSA and prostate pathology in men having simple prostatectomy. *Am J Clin Pathol* 1989; **92:** 760–4.

8. Ronnett BM, Carmichael MJ, Carter HB, Epstein JI, Does high grade PIN result in elevated serum PSA levels? *J Urol* 1993; **150:** 386–9.

9. Brawer MK, Nagle RB, Bigler SA, Lange PH, Sohlberg OE, Significance of PIN on prostate needle biopsy. *Urology* 1991; **38:** 103–7.

10. Neal DE, Clejan S, Sarma D, Moon TD, PSA and prostatitis: effect of prostatitis on serum PSA in the human and non-human primate. *Prostate* 1992; **20:** 105–11.

11. Dalton DL, Elevated serum PSA due to acute bacterial prostatitis. *Urology* 1989; **33:** 465.

12. Yuan JJ, Catalona WJ, Effect of digital rectal examination, prostate massage, transrectal ultrasonography and needle biopsy of the prostate on serum prostate specific antigen levels. *J Urol* 1991; **145:** 213A.

13. Brawer MK, Schifman RB, Ahmann FR, Ahmann ME, Coulis K, The effect of digital rectal examination on serum PSA and acid phosphatase. *J Urol* 1987; **137**(4/2): 356A.

14. Tchetgen MB, Song JT, Strawderman M, Jacobsen SJ, Oesterling JE, Ejaculation increases the serum prostate-specific antigen concentration. *Urology* 1996; **47:** 511–16.

15. Catalona WJ, Smith DS, Ratliff TL et al, Measurement of PSA in serum as a screening test for prostate cancer. *N Engl J Med* 1991; **324:** 1156–61.

16. Brawer MK, Chetner MP, Beatie J, Buchner DM, Vessella RL, Lange PH, Screening for prostatic carcinoma with PSA. *J Urol* 1992; **147:** 841–5.

17. Cooner WH, Mosley RB, Rutherford CL et al, Prostate cancer detection in a clinical urological practice by ultrasonography, digital rectal examination and prostate-specific antigen. *J Urol* 1990; **143:** 1146–52.

18. Babaian RJ, Camps JL, The role of PSA as part of the diagnostic triad and as a guide when to perform a biopsy. *Cancer* 1991; **68:** 2060–3.

19. Catalona WJ, Smith DS, Ratliff TL, Basler JW, Detection of organ-confined prostate cancer is increased through PSA-based screening. *J Am Med Assoc* 1993; **270:** 948–54.

20. Jacobsen SJ, Katusic SK, Bergstralh EJ et al, Incidence of prostate cancer diagnosis in the eras before and after serum prostate-specific antigen testing. *J Am Med Assoc* 1995; **274:** 1445–9.

21. Mettlin C, Littrup PJ, Kane RA et al, Relative sensitivity and specificity of serum PSA level compared with age-referenced PSA, PSA density and PSA change. *Cancer* 1994; **74:** 1615–20.

22. Gann PH, Hennekens CH, Stampfer MJ, A prospective evaluation of plasma PSA for detection of prostatic cancer. *J Am Med Assoc* 1995; **273:** 289–94.

23. Catalona WJ, Richie JP, Ahmann FR et al, A multicenter evaluation of PSA and digital rectal examination (DRE) for early detection of prostate cancer in 6374 volunteers. *J Urol* 1993; **149:** 798A.

24. Myrtle JF, Klimley PG, Ivor LP, Bruni JF, *Clinical Utility of Prostate Specific Antigen (PSA) in the Management of Prostate Cancer.* Hybritech Inc: San Diego, CA, 1986: 1–4.

25. Oesterling JE, Jacobsen SJ, Chute CG et al, Serum PSA in a community-based population of healthy men: establishment of age-specific reference ranges. *J Am Med Assoc* 1993; **270:** 860–4.

26. Benson MC, Ring KS, Olsson CA, The determination of stage D0 carcinoma of the prostate using PSA density. *Urol Corres Club* 1989; **13:** 7–9.

27. Veneziano S, Pavlica P, Querze R, Lalanne MG, Vecchi F, Correlation between PSA and prostate volume, evaluated by transrectal ultrasonography: usefulness in diagnosis of prostate cancer. *Eur Urol* 1990; **18:** 112–16.

28. Benson MC, Whang IS, Pantuck A et al, Prostate-specific antigen density: a means of distinguishing benign prostatic hypertrophy and prostate cancer. *J Urol* 1992; **147:** 815–16.

29. Benson MC, Whang IS, Olsson CA, McMahon DJ, Cooner WH, The use of PSA density to enhance the predictive value of intermediate levels of serum PSA. *J Urol* 1992; **147:** 817–21.

30. Bangma CH, Kranse R, Blijenberg BG, Schroder FH, The value of screening tests in the detection

of prostate cancer. Part I: Results of a retrospective evaluation of 1726 men. *Urology* 1995; **46:** 773–8.

31. Seaman E, Whang M, Olsson CA, Katz A, Cooner WH, Benson MC, PSA density (PSAD): role in patient evaluation and management. *Urol Clin N Am* 1993; **20:** 653–63.

32. Rommel FM, Augusta VE, Breslin JA et al, The use of PSA and PSAD in the diagnosis of prostate cancer in a community based urology practice. *J Urol* 1994; **151:** 88–93.

33. Bazinet M, Meshref AW, Trudel C et al, Prospective evaluation of prostate-specific antigen density and systematic biopsies for early detection of prostatic carcinoma. *Urology* 1994; **43:** 44–51.

34. Brawer MK, Aramburu EAG, Chen GL, Preston SD, Ellis WJ, The inability of PSA index to enhance the predictive value of PSA in the diagnosis of prostatic carcinoma. *J Urol* 1993; **150:** 369–73.

35. Brawer MK, How to use PSA in the early detection or screening for prostatic carcinoma. *CA* 1995; **45:** 148–64.

36. Ohori M, Dunn JK, Scardino PT, Is prostate-specific antigen density more useful than prostate-specific antigen levels in the diagnosis of prostate cancer? *Urology* 1995; **46:** 666–71.

37. Weber JP, Oesterling JE, Peters CA et al, The influence of reversible androgen deprivation on serum prostate specific antigen levels in men with benign prostatic hyperplasia. *J Urol* 1989; **141:** 987–92.

38. Stamey TA, Making the most out of six systematic sextant biopsies. *Urology* 1995; **45:** 2–11.

39. Carter HB, Pearson JD, Metter EJ et al, Longitudinal evaluation of prostate-specific antigen levels in men with and without prostate disease. *J Am Med Assoc* 1992; **267:** 2215–20.

40. Smith DS, Catalona WJ, Rate of change in serum prostate specific-antigen levels as a method for prostate cancer detection. *J Urol* 1994; **152:** 1168–9.

41. Littrup PJ, Kane RA, Mettlin CJ et al, Cost-effective prostate cancer detection: reduction of low-yield biopsies. *Cancer* 1994; **74:** 3146–58.

42. Porter JR, Hayward R, Brawer MK, The significance of short-term PSA change in men undergoing ultrasound guided prostate biopsy. *J Urol* 1994; **151**(suppl): 293A.

43. Carter HB, Pearson JD, Chan DW, Guess HA, Walsh PC, Prostate-specific antigen variability in men without prostate cancer: effect of sampling interval on prostate-specific antigen velocity. *Urology* 1995; **45:** 591–6.

44. Nixon RG, Wener MH, Smith KM, Parson RE, Strobel SA, Brawer MK, Biological variation of prostate-specific antigen levels in serum: an evaluation of day-to-day physiological fluctuations in a well-defined cohort of 24 patients. *J Urol* 1997; **157:** 2183–90.

45. Dalkin BL, Ahmann FR, Kopp JB, PSA levels in men older than 50 years without clinical evidence of prostatic carcinoma. *J Urol* 1993; **150:** 1837–9.

46. Mettlin C, Murphy GP, Lee F et al, Characteristics of prostate cancer detected in the American Cancer Society – National Prostate Cancer Detection Project. *J Urol* 1994; **152:** 1737–40.

47. el-Galley RES, Petros JA, Sanders WH et al, Normal range prostate-specific antigen versus age-specific prostate-specific antigen in screening prostate adenocarcinoma. *Urology* 1995; **46:** 200–4.

48. Etzioni R, Shen Y, Petteway JC, Brawer MK, Age-specific PSA: a reassessment. *Prostate* 1996; **7:** 70–7.

49. Mettlin C, Jones G, Averette H, Gusberg SB, Murphy GP, Defining and updating the ACS guidelines for the cancer related check-up: prostate and endometrial cancer. *CA* 1993; **43:** 42–6.

50. AUA, *American Urological Association Policy Statement: Early Detection of Prostate Cancer and Use of Transrectal Ultrasound.* AUA: Baltimore, MA, 1992.

51. Christensson A, Laurell CB, Lilja H, Enzymatic activity of prostate-specific antigen and its reaction with extracellular serine proteinase inhibitors. *Eur J Biochem* 1990; **194:** 755–63.

52. Lilja H, Christensson A, Dahlen U et al, PSA in human serum occurs predominantly in complex with alpha-1-antichymotrypsin. *Clin Chem* 1991; **37:** 1618–25.

53. Stenman U, Leinonen J, Alfthan H, Rannikko S, Tuhkanen K, Althan O, A complex between PSA and α1-antichymotrypsin is the major form of PSA in serum of patients with prostatic cancer: assay of the complex improves clinical sensitivity for cancer. *Cancer Res* 1991; **51:** 222–6.

54. Luderer AA, Chen Y, Thiel R et al, Measurement of the proportion of free to total PSA improves diagnostic performance of PSA in the diagnostic gray zone of total PSA. *Urology* 1995; **46:** 187–94.

55. Catalona WJ, Smith DS, Wolfert RL et al, Evaluation of percentage of free serum PSA to

improve specificity of prostate cancer screening. *J Am Med Assoc* 1995; **274:** 1214–20.

56. Stamey TA, Second Stanford Conference on International Standardization of PSA immunoassays: September 1 and 2, 1994. *Urology* 1995; **45:** 173–84.

57. Brawer MK, *Restandardization of the Ciba Corning PSA Assay (PSA2): Clinical Observations and Implications for Cancer Detection.* Chiron Diagnostics Corp: East Walpole, MA, 1996: 1–5.

58. Wener MH, Daum PR, Brawer MK, Variation in measurement of PSA: the importance of method and lot variability. *Clin Chem* 1995; **41:** 1730–7.

59. Brawer MK, Beattie J, Wener MH, Vessella RL, Preston SD, Lange PH, Screening for prostatic carcinoma with PSA: results of the second year. *J Urol* 1993; **150:** 106–9.

60. Oesterling JE, Martin SK, Bergstraih EJ, Lowe FC, The use of PSA in staging patients with newly diagnosed prostate cancer. *J Am Med Assoc* 1993; **269:** 57–60.

61. Lange PH, Lightner DJ, Medini E, Reddy PK, Vessella RL, The effects of radiation therapy after radical prostatectomy in patients with elevated PSA levels. *J Urol* 1990; **144:** 927–33.

62. Stein A, deKernion JB, Smith RB, Dorey F, Patel H, PSA levels after radical prostatectomy in patients with organ confined and locally extensive prostate cancer. *J Urol* 1992; **147:** 942–6.

63. Abi-Aad AS, Macfarlane MT, Stein A, deKernion JB, Detection of local recurrence after radical prostatectomy by PSA and TRUS. *J Urol* 1992; **147:** 952–5.

64. Foster LS, Jajodia P, Fournier G Jr, Shinohara K, Carol P, Narayan P, The value of PSA and transrectal ultrasound-guided biopsy in accurately detecting prostatic fossa recurrences following radical prostatectomy. *J Urol* 1993; **149:** 1024–8.

65. Partin AW, Pearson JD, Pound CR et al, Evaluation of serum prostate-specific antigen velocity after radical prostatectomy distinguish local recurrence from distant metastases. *Urology* 1994; **43:** 649–59.

66. Stamey TA, Kabalin JN, McNeal JE et al, Prostate specific antigen in the diagnosis and treatment of adenocarcinoma of the prostate: II. Radical prostatectomy treated patients. *J Urol* 1989; **141:** 1076–83.

67. Russell KJ, Dunatov C, Hafermann JT, Griffeth L, Pollisssar L, Prostate-specific antigen in the management of patients with localized adenocarcinoma of the prostate treated with primary radiation therapy. *J Urol* 1991; **146:** 1046–52.

68. Zagars GK, von Eschenbach AC, Prostate-specific antigen: an important marker for prostate cancer treated by external beam radiotherapy. *Cancer* 1993; **72:** 538–48.

69. Schellhammer PF, Kuban DA el-Mahdi AM, Treatment of clinical local failure after radiation therapy for prostate carcinoma. *J Urol* 1993; **150:** 1865–6.

70. Miller JI Ahman FR, Drach GW, Emerson SS, Bottaccini MR, The clinical usefulness of serum PSA after hormonal therapy of metastatic prostate cancer. *J Urol* 1992; **147:** 956–61.

71. Gillatt D, Gingell C, Smith PJB, Serum PSA for the assessment of response to hormonal therapy. *J Urol* 1990; **143:** 207A.

72. Smith JA, Crawford ED, Lange PH et al, PSA correlation with response and survival in advanced carcinoma of the prostate. *J Urol* 1993; **149:** 430–6.

73. Stamey TA, Kabalin JN, Ferrari M, Yang N, Prostate specific antigen in the diagnosis and treatment of adenocarcinoma of the prostate: IV. Anti-androgen treated patients. *J Urol* 1989; **141:** 1088–90.

74. Geller J, Effect of Finasteride, a 5-alpha reductase inhibitor, on prostate tissue androgens and prostate-specific antigen. *J Clin Endocrinol Metab* 1990; **71:** 1552–5.

75. Guess HA, Heyse JF, Gormley GJ, The effect of finasteride on prostate-specific antigen in men with benign prostatic hyperplasia. *Prostate* 1993; **22:** 31–7.

76. Feightner JW, The early detection and treatment of prostate cancer: the perspective of the Canadian Task Force on the periodic health examination. *J Urol* 1994; **152:** 1682–4.

77. Brawer MK, PIN and PSA. *Urology* 1989; **34:** 62–5.

78. Brawer MK, Beatie J, Wener MH, PSA as the initial test in prostate carcinoma screening: results of the third year. *J Urol* 1993; **149**(suppl): 299A.

79. Catalona WJ, Richie JP, Ahmann FR et al, A multicenter evaluation of PSA and DRE for early detection of prostate cancer in 630 volunteers. *J Urol* 1994; **151:** 1308–9.

80. Cooner WH, Mosley BR, Rutherford CL Jr, Clinical application of transrectal ultrasonography and prostate specific antigen in the search for prostate cancer. *J Urol* 1988; **139:** 758–61.

81. Lee F, Littrup PJ, Torp-Pederson ST, Mettlin C, McHugh TA, Gray JM, Prostate cancer: comparison of TRUS and DRE for screening. *Radiology* 1988; **168:** 389–94.

82. Mettlin C, Lee F, Drago J, Murphy GP, The American Cancer Society National Prostate Cancer Detection Project. Findings on the detection of early prostate cancer in 2425 men. *Cancer* 1991; **67:** 2949–58.

83. Ellis WJ, Brawer MK, Repeat prostate needle biopsy: who needs it? *J Urol* 1995; **153:** 1496–8.

84. Brawer MK, Lange PH, PSA: its role in early detection, staging and monitoring of prostatic carcinoma. *J Endourol* 1989; **3:** 227–36.

85. Brawer MK, Chetner MP, Ultrasonography of the prostate and biopsy. In: *Campbell's Urology,* Vol 3 (Walsh PC, ed). WB Saunders: Philadelphia, PA, 1997: 2506–17.

86. Catalona WJ, Hudson MA, Scardino PT et al, Selection of optimal PSA cutoffs for early detection of prostate cancer: receiver operating characteristic curves. *J Urol* 1994; **151**(suppl): 449A.

87. Labrie F, DuPont A, Suburu R et al, Serum PSA as pre-screening test for prostate cancer. *J Urol* 1992; **147:** 846–52.

88. Lee FR, Gray JM, McLeary RD et al, Prostatic evaluation by transrectal sonography: criteria for diagnosis of early carcinoma. *Radiology* 1986; **158:** 91–5.

89. Crook JM, Bahadur YA, Bociek RG, Perry GA, Robertson SJ, Esche BA, Radiotherapy for localized prostate cancer: correlation of pre-treatment PSA and nadir PSA with outcome as assessed by systematic biopsy and serum PSA. *Cancer* 1997; **79:** 328–36.

90. Hanks GE, Corn BW, Lee WR, Hunt M, Hanlon A, Schultheiss TE, External beam irradiation of prostate cancer. *Cancer* 1995; **75:** 1972–7.

91. Blasko JC, Wallner K, Grimm PD, Ragde H, Prostate-specific antigen based disease control following ultrasound guided iodine implantation for stage T1/T2 prostatic carcinoma. *J Urol* 1995; **154:** 1096–9.

92. Stock RG, Stone NN, DeWyngaert JK, Lavagnini P, Unger PD, Prostate-specific antigen findings and biopsy results following interactive ultrasound-guided transperineal brachytherapy for early stage prostate carcinoma. *Cancer* 1996; **77:** 2386–92.

9

The role of transrectal ultrasound in prostate cancer and its use in biopsy

Hiroki Watanabe, Munekado Kojima

CONTENTS • Method • Diagnostic ultrasound • Interventional ultrasound • Conclusion

Transrectal ultrasound (TRUS) was the first technique that could be used to visualize the internal architecture and the entire contour of the prostate. It was readily applied to the investigation of prostate disease.[1-4] Currently, TRUS occupies a central position among the diagnostic modalities for diseases of the prostate.[5,6] Along with accumulating evidence indicating the clinical usefulness of TRUS in the diagnosis of prostate cancer, recent developments in interventional ultrasound have confirmed it to be an indispensable technique in the daily practice of urology clinics.[7] This chapter reviews the development and current status of TRUS in the diagnosis and treatment of prostate cancer. The discussion is based mainly on the authors' experience.

METHOD

In 1967, in our laboratory, the first clinical sonogram of the rectal cavity was obtained in a patient in the lithotomy position following the ordinary procedure for urological examinations.[1,2] However, in 1974 we started to carry out the examination with the patient in the sitting position, in order to improve efficacy.[3] With the patient in the lithotomy position, the examiner had to hold the transducer throughout the entire examination, which caused instability in the depth and angle of insertion of the transducer. With this technique, each examination took 10–20 min. In contrast, with the patient in the sitting position the scanning axis is stable, reproducibility is good and the examination takes only 3–4 min per patient.[8]

For these reasons, transverse views obtained with the patient in the sitting position are considered useful for routine work. Using the results from over 10 000 examinations using TRUS, we found the success rate of the method to be 99.4%.[9] Human factors accounted for most of the failures. However, with the patient in the sitting position, it is not possible to obtain images in the sagittal plane, which may be needed for urodynamic examinations or for puncture monitoring. Various electronic linear scanners and biplane scanners have been developed for clinical use for this purpose.[6,10] Therefore, if possible, both chair-type equipment (Figure 9.1) for daily routine work and a biplane transducer for special uses should be available in a urology clinic.

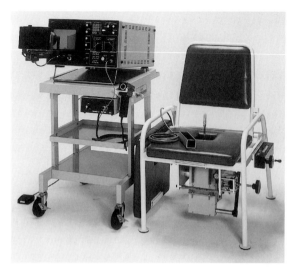

Figure 9.1 A chair with a transducer (5 MHz) for transrectal sonography.

DIAGNOSTIC ULTRASOUND

Size measurement

Ultrasound scanning can be used to obtain accurate measurements of the sizes of organs in the body. In 1974, we published the first measurement of the size of the prostate obtained using TRUS.[11] To obtain the measurement we employed a step-section planimetric method at 5-mm intervals, because this yielded stable and accurate measurements. Many researchers have used a prolate ellipse formula (height × width × length × $\pi/6$) when measuring the size of the prostate, but it should be noted that the elliptical volume involves considerable interobserver variation over repeated measurements.[12]

Research work involving measurement of the size of the prostate is most usually done using TRUS, as only with this technique can prostate size be estimated non-invasively and with an accuracy that is within acceptable measuring limits. Traditional digital rectal examination (DRE) has some limitations in the accurate

estimation of prostate size. We compared size measurements made using DRE and TRUS, and found that DRE was only statistically effective in differentiating between two sizes ('hen's egg' size and smaller) and had little clinical value for making more stratified size classification.[13]

TRUS measurement of the prostate has yielded much important information about the physiology and pathology of this gland. For example, the volume of the prostate in normal subjects increases rapidly between the ages of 10 and 20 years, and then decreases.[14] The diurnal change in prostate volume is nearly 20%.[15] In addition, TRUS has contributed much to the investigation of benign prostatic hyperplasia (BPH).[16–18]

As TRUS is a non-invasive technique, prostate size can be measured frequently in the same patient. The sizes of the prostates of four patients with prostate cancer were measured sequentially over a period of time, during which they received no treatment, and the cancer doubling time was calculated as 180–780 (average 405) days.[19] This possibility of making sequential measurements also means that the effect of therapy on the progress of prostate cancer can be evaluated (see the section on monitoring later in this chapter).

TRUS is an important tool in the screening for and early detection of prostate cancer, not only in terms of diagnosing prostate cancer but also in discriminating between BPH and cancer, particularly in patients with an abnormally high prostate-specific antigen (PSA) level.[20–22] With the aim of diminishing the unfavourable influence of BPH on the serum PSA value, Benson et al[23] proposed the use of a PSA density, which was obtained by dividing the PSA value by the prostate volume. Similarly, Babaian et al[24] defined a prostate volume-referenced PSA range. They reported that both the PSA density and the prostate volume-referenced PSA were superior to the PSA level and the age-referenced PSA level[25] based on receiver operating characteristic curve analysis. Thus, TRUS measurement of the prostate provides important information for volume-based PSA indexes, which could improve the efficacy of detecting prostate cancer.

Diagnosis

In 1974 we proposed diagnostic criteria for prostate diseases, including prostate cancer and BPH (Table 9.1).[4,26] In 1984 these criteria were revised by a research group supported by the Japanese Ministry of Education, and were made the official standard criteria by the Japanese Society of Ultrasonics in Medicine[27] and the Japanese Urological Association.[28] These criteria were based on three categories of findings (the shape, capsular echoes and internal echoes of the prostate) and distinguish between the normal prostate, BPH, prostate cancer and prostatitis.

Originally, in the diagnosis of prostate cancer attention was directed towards the change in the shape of the prostate. At the same time, changes in internal echoes were also evaluated when reading prostate sonograms, and internal echoes in patients with prostate cancer were described in the diagnostic criteria as 'occasionally partially disappeared' (see Table 9.1). This sign was later emphasized by Lee et al[29] as the typical sonographic feature of prostate cancer, the so-called 'hypoechoic lesions' (Figure 9.2). With the prevalent use of high-frequency probes and grey scale displays,[30] too much interest has been directed towards the relationship between prostate cancer and the occurrence of hypoechoic lesions, and this has undoubtedly resulted in the mistaken belief that any 'black' area in the prostate indicates a malignancy. Although this is true in small cancer foci, it is also true that advanced large cancer foci can display a mixed pattern of both hyperechoic and hypoechoic regions.[31]

The overemphasis on the relationship between hypoechoic lesions and prostate cancer has promoted the clinical application of TRUS

Table 9.1 Diagnostic criteria for TRUS of the prostate[4]			
	Prostate normal	**BPH**	**Prostate cancer**
Section:			
Area	Small	Enlarged	Enlarged in most cases
Shape	Triangular or semilunar	Semilunar or circular	Deformed
Symmetry	Positive	Positive	Negative
Anteroposterior diameter	Short	Elongated, keeping balance with lateral diameter	Occasionally highly elongated
Capsular echoes:			
Thickness	Thin	Thick	Irregular
Continuity	Positive	Positive	Negative
Evenness	Positive	Positive	Negative
Internal echoes:			
Quality	Regular	Regular	Irregular
Density	Moderate	Increased	Occasionally partially disappeared

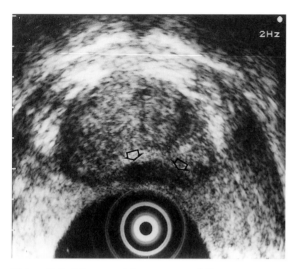

Figure 9.2 A transrectal sonogram of the prostate. The hypoechoic lesion (arrow) indicated a cancer focus.

The advantage of TRUS over DRE in detecting prostate cancer has been cited in several studies.[36–38] Lee et al[36] examined 784 self-referred men over 60 years of age in order to compare the clinical usefulness of TRUS and DRE in detecting prostate cancer. Twenty cases of cancer were detected by TRUS, and 10 by DRE. The sensitivity of TRUS was twice that of DRE. Importantly, all tumours with a favourable prognosis were revealed by TRUS, compared with only 41% by DRE. These authors advocated broader implementation and evaluation of TRUS for the early detection of cancer. More recently, the National Prostate Cancer Detection Project (sponsored by the American Cancer Society) demonstrated that the sensitivity (65.5%) of TRUS was significantly greater than that of DRE (38.7%; $p < 0.0001$) and equivalent to that of the PSA level (69.2%).[22]

Comparative studies of the in vitro sonographic appearance of prostate cancer and histopathological findings have shown that TRUS is not sufficiently sensitive to detect cases of low-volume cancer.[39]

in the early detection of cancer of the prostate. It should be noted that hypoechoic lesions do not always indicate cancer foci; the positive rate of hypoechoic lesions for prostate cancer is reported to be about 35%.[32] This is the basis of the argument doubting the reliability of TRUS in detecting prostate cancer. In sonography, a hypoechoic lesion (region) means only that there is no difference in acoustic impedance in that lesion (region).

A great deal of work has been published on the diagnostic efficacy of TRUS for prostate cancer. In our research, the sensitivity in 102 outpatients was 97.1%.[5] In our mass screening programme the sensitivity and specificity in 3479 cases were 86.3% and 91.4%, respectively,[33] and in an official blind test supported by the Ministry of Health and Welfare, Japan, performed by 21 urologists, the corresponding values were 64.2% and 76.2%, respectively.[34] Carter et al[35] reported that the sensitivity for unpalpable cancer foci was 52% and the specificity was 68%.

Screening

Until the clinical application of TRUS, DRE was the only method available for the detection of prostate cancer. The clinical importance of DRE in this respect remains because of its ease of application and low cost. Despite its prevalent application in urology clinics, however, DRE lacks sensitivity. In spite of the development of computed tomography and, more recently, magnetic resonance imaging, TRUS is the only imaging modality available for screening for prostate cancer.

As early as 1975, we started a mass screening programme using TRUS and DRE of men aged over 55 years,[40] and the first special mobile unit for prostate screening (the Dolphin) was introduced in 1980.[41] The results obtained between 1975 and 1989 showed TRUS to be superior to DRE in both sensitivity and specificity.[7] The mass screening programme revealed prostate cancer in 0.6% (48/7235) of examinees. This result was extraordinarily high compared with the results of mass screening programmes for uterine cervical (0.15%), stomach (0.1%) and breast (0.06%) cancer in Japan. More importantly, 52.1% of the cases of prostate cancer detected in the screening were in their early stages, a much higher rate of detection than that in general outpatient clinics (10–15%). Due to this experience, mass screening programmes for prostate cancer have been performed in many areas in Japan.[42]

In contrast to the situation in Japan, the status of TRUS screening for prostate cancer in the USA, where prostate cancer is the most prevalent cancer in the male population, is varied. The official opinion of the American Urological Association was negative towards the value of TRUS.[43] Despite this, the screening for and early detection of prostate cancer using TRUS is becoming more common at the general clinic level.[36–38] Cooner et al[44] have supported the superiority of TRUS as a screening modality in special age groups.

In this field, the most significant change in the diagnostic approach to prostate cancer must be the introduction of PSA level measurement. Due to its simplicity and low cost, PSA measurement is now an essential test for prostate cancer. As a result of the prevalence of PSA testing in recent years, the number of prostate cancer patients is increasing considerably.[45] The screening for an early detection of this cancer will become more widespread year by year.

Staging

It is firmly believed that correct staging of disease results in the proper selection of treatment. Although DRE is the basic means of evaluating tumour distension, its lack of sensitivity for extracapsular tumour invasion is well known. DRE can only be used to evaluate the status of the prostate margin on the side facing the rectum. In contrast, TRUS can offer information concerning possible extraprostatic extension all around the prostate. The possible use of TRUS in the staging of prostate cancer has been evaluated.

In 1984 the research group supported by the

Ministry of Education, Japan, proposed standard criteria for the staging of prostate cancer using TRUS (Table 9.2).[27,46] The criteria were called the 'UT classification', after the 'T' in TNM classification. In TRUS, the irregularity of capsular echoes is occasionally caused by artefacts. Prostatic calculi generate acoustic shadows, which cause discontinuities in capsular echoes. In addition, the resolution of TRUS is worse at the posterolateral corner of the prostate, because the ultrasound beam is projected in a direction parallel to the capsule. These drawbacks can be compensated for by skill in the reading of sonograms, provided that attention is paid to the overall section of the prostate.

The sensitivity of TRUS to extracapsular invasion confirmed on pathology specimens was 89% in our blind test of 31 cases.[47] The assignment of the same stage using TRUS and pathology occurred in 63% of 27 cases treated with radical prostatectomy in our department,[48] and in 65.2% of cases in the official blind test, by nine senior readers, supported by the Ministry of Health and Welfare, Japan.[49]

The preferred use of TRUS for predicting extracapsular invasion has been reported by several authors. Hamper et al[50] compared TRUS findings with the results of pathological examinations of radical prostatectomy specimens in patients with clinical stage A or B cancers. In their study, local contour deformity and irregularity or an interruption of periprostatic fat echoes were considered to suggest the extracapsular invasion by the cancer. TRUS enabled correct identification of extracapsular invasion in 59 of the 86 hemispheres of the prostates examined. A positive TRUS diagnosis of pericapsular tumour spread correlated moderately well with the depth of penetration demonstrated pathologically. These authors concluded that TRUS is an effective non-invasive procedure for predicting extracapsular invasion by prostate cancer.

TRUS is also useful in predicting invasion into the seminal vesicles. In 1980, Resnick et al[51] reported that TRUS was helpful in assessing tumour invasion around the seminal vesicles. Pontes et al[47,52] noted the poor correlation between asymmetry or dilatation of the seminal

Table 9.2 The UT staging system for prostate cancer[46]*

Stage	Deformity	Capsular interruption	Invasion	TNM	NPCP
UT0	DF0	CA0	NI0	T0	A1–2
UT1	DF0a	CA0	NI0	T1	B1
UT2	DF1	CA0	NI0	T2	B2
UT3a	DF2	CA1	NI0	T2	B2–C1
UT3b	DF2	CA2	NI1	T3	C2
UT4	DF2	CA3	NI4	T4	D1

Deformity

DF0	Deformity (−)
DF0a	Hypoechoic lesion
DF1	Asymmetry only
DF2	Deformity (+)

Capsular interruption

CA0	Interruption (−)
CA1	One portion $< \frac{1}{4}$ circumference
CA2	Two or more portions or $> \frac{1}{4}$ circumference
CA3	Two or more portions or $\frac{1}{4}$ circumference + invasion to pelvic bone

Invasion

NI0	Invasion (−)
NI1	Invasion to seminal vesicle
NI2	Invasion to other organ

NPCP, National Prostatic Cancer Project; TNM, tumour, node, metastasis classification of malignant tumours.
*Each item is first determined independently according to the table. The highest step among the determinations for each item is indicated as the final stage of prostate cancer (UT0 to UT4) for the patient.

vesicles and seminal vesicle invasion, but found that an increase in the internal echoes of the organ provided the best clue of possible seminal vesicle invasion by prostate cancer. A similar result was reported by Terris et al,[53] and this confirmed the importance of hyperechogenicity in the prediction of seminal vesicle invasion. They found invasion to be correlated with a combination of two or more sonographic abnormalities such as cystic dilatation, asymmetry, enlargement and anterior displacement. Further improvement in the detection of seminal vesicle invasion by prostate cancer has been obtained with the use of TRUS-guided seminal vesicle

biopsy[54,55] (see the section on staging using interventional ultrasound later in this chapter).

In addition, TRUS may have the ability to predict pelvic lymph-node metastasia. Scardino et al[56] found that 4 of 40 patients (10%) with ultrasonographically confirmed organ-confined tumours had no lymph-node metastasis, compared with 22 of 60 patients (37%) who had ultrasonographically confirmed extraprostatic invasion ($p < 0.005$).

The determination of the serum PSA level has also been used in staging prostate cancer. Despite its significant correlation with pathological stage, the serum PSA level is considered to be unreliable in individual cases.[57,58] However, when combined with the PSA test, the validity of TRUS in staging prostate cancer is improved. Wolf et al[59] calculated an 'expected PSA value' from the volume of the hypoechoic lesion, the prostate volume and the biopsy Gleason score. Using this value, they found a diagnostic accuracy as high as 83%. The sensitivity and specificity were 84% and 82%, respectively. Thus, the clinical usefulness of TRUS in staging prostate cancer is enhanced by combination with PSA testing.

Monitoring

As the prostate is an androgen-dependent organ, a reduction in its size is expected when the androgen supply is cut off. We have confirmed this expectation by using TRUS measurement of prostate size in healthy adult dogs.[60] Furthermore, we have shown that the prostate volume in patients with prostate cancer diminishes exponentially after castration, before reaching a constant level[61–63] (Figure 9.3). Furthermore, in patients treated with a luteinizing hormone-releasing hormone (LHRH) analogue the reduction in prostate volume was almost parallel to the reduction in the serum testosterone level.[64] The volume of the

hypoechoic lesion also decreased in a similar way after castration.[65]

Based on this kinetic analysis of the change in prostate volume when treating prostate cancer, we have proposed an exponential formula, consisting of three factors (see Figure 9.3):

$$V = a \times 10^{-t/\tau} + b,$$

where V is the total volume of the prostate, a is the volume of the effective portion, b is the volume of the ineffective portion, t is time and τ is the reduction time. The primary factor regulating the activity of the cancer is the reduction time τ. Our results in 42 patients with stage D cancer demonstrated that for survivors the value of τ was low, while for those who died the value was high. All patients having a τ value less than 30 days were still alive 5 years after castration ($p < 0.01$), even those with stage D cancer. With just two exceptions, patients with a τ value greater than 60 days died within 3 years. All patients, except one, with a τ value greater than 32 days died within 5 years ($p < 0.01$).[63]

Similar results were obtained in patients treated with LHRH analogues.[66] All patients having a τ value of less than 41 days neither showed clinical progression within 15 months nor died as a result of prostate cancer during the 5-year follow-up, while the disease-specific 5-year survival rate in patients having a τ value greater than 42 days was as low as 17%. Interestingly, no conventional prognostic parameters significantly predicted the prognosis.

More recently, a further use of the kinetic analysis of prostate volume has been reported by Okihara,[67] who evaluated τ with regard to the manner of prostate cancer progression in patients in whom the disease recurred after castration. According to the change in prostate volume, patients were classified into two types: the local progression type and the metastatic progression type. In the former group, the prostate volume reduced exponentially after castration, and then increased exponentially after a short period. In the latter group, the prostate volume did not change with the progression of the disease, but the degree of bone metastasis increased greatly.

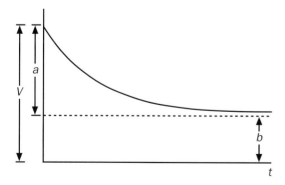

Figure 9.3 A sketch of a typical curve showing the reduction in prostate volume in patients with prostate cancer treated by castration.

The value of τ was significantly larger in the metastatic progression type than in the local progression type. More interestingly, there was an inverse relationship between τ and the doubling time, which was calculated during the relapse period in patients of the local progression type.[67] Thus, TRUS is a promising tool for investigating the pathophysiology of prostate cancer through size measurement.

Colour Doppler flow mapping

A recent topic in investigations using TRUS is colour Doppler flow mapping.[68,69] As early as 1987, we obtained colour Doppler images of the prostate using a transrectal probe, which had been primarily designed for colour Doppler imaging of the renal artery through the gastric cavity.[70,71] Doppler signals from the vessels inside or along the prostate were first visualized successfully using this apparatus. A special transrectal probe for the purpose was subsequently developed.[72]

Blood flows were visualized more frequently in patients with prostate cancer than in normals or those with BPH (Figure 9.4).[73] Following castration, blood flows decreased.[74] These findings suggest that colour Doppler flow mapping is a promising tool for the diagnosis and monitoring of prostate cancer. More recent developments such as the use of an echo contrast agent[75] and the power Doppler method will contribute much to this area. Further experience is needed to confirm the clinical usefulness of colour Doppler flow mapping in investigations of the prostate.

INTERVENTIONAL ULTRASOUND

In 1981, Saitoh et al[54] developed a special unit for interventional ultrasound consisting of a transrectal electronic real-time linear scanner and an attachment for needle guidance for puncture to the prostate or the seminal vesicles. Holm and Gammelgaard[76] also developed a system for precise needle placement, but used

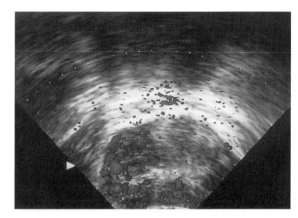

Figure 9.4 A sonogram of transrectal power Doppler colour flow mapping in a patient with prostate cancer. Images of rapid pulsatile blood flows were observed predominantly at hypoechoic lesions.

transaxial ultrasound monitoring. Ultrasound-guided biopsy has many advantages compared with 'blind' (finger-guided) biopsy, not only in targeting but also in decreasing side-effects such as bleeding. There are two routes through which a needle can be inserted under ultrasonic guidance: transperineal and transrectal. When using the latter route, the chance of urinary tract infection must particularly be considered.[77]

Sagittal scanning is more effective than transverse imaging during guidance because the whole puncture process can be monitored on one image.[78] Biplane transducers can provide still better images for needle placement.[6]

Diagnosis

Ultrasound-guided puncture was first applied to the prostate in 1980 by Saitoh et al[54,79] using a transrectal real-time linear scanner. With this technique, it is easy to obtain biopsy specimens from the targeted region with few side-effects. Because of the widespread link between hypoechic lesions and cancer, this technique in particular has become a routine tool for prostate biopsy. The recent development of the biplane probe allows more accurate targeting of the selected area of the prostate.[6]

Since the introduction of the PSA test into the early detection programme for prostate cancer, the number of patients in whom the prostate showed normal TRUS and normal DRE findings but an abnormally elevated PSA level has increased. To diagnose these so-called 'non-palpable and non-visible' cancers, random biopsy of the prostate is necessary. In general, systematic sextant biopsy is now used in such cases.[80] Although these methods might detect clinically insignificant cancers,[81] their combined use with serum PSA measurement would offer a greater chance of detecting prostate cancer in its early stages, when a satisfactory therapeutic outcome can be anticipated.

Staging

As invasion of prostate cancer into the seminal vesicles is a well-known poor prognostic indicator, its accurate prediction provides important information for selecting a treatment option. Hyperechogenicity, asymmetry, deformity and dilatation of the seminal vesicles are considered to be signs suggesting tumour invasion into the organ.[47,53] Unfortunately, TRUS gives only limited information about seminal vesicle invasion. Abe et al[55] have applied an ultrasound-guided puncture system to the seminal vesicles using a real-time linear scanner. They reported significantly better prediction of seminal vesicle invasion using this method compared with DRE. Terris et al[82] have also supported the value of TRUS-guided seminal vesicle biopsy in predicting invasion preoperatively. In their 73 patients with prostate cancer, seminal vesicle invasion was detected by biopsy with a sensitivity of 67% (8/12) and a specificity of 97% (59/61). Currently, seminal vesicle biopsy is the only tool that can give objective and reliable information about tumour invasion.

Treatment

The accurate placement of a needle in the prostate by ultrasound-guided puncture has been used therapeutically for prostate cancer. Implantation of radioactive seeds such as iodine-125 can be performed safely only with ultrasound guidance.[83] The recent development of cryoablation for prostate cancer is directly due to the possibility of accurately placing the cryoprobe inside the prostate.[84]

Recently, interventional TRUS has been used successfully for prostate nerve blockade, with the aim of minimizing the discomfort associated with systematic needle biopsy of the prostate. Nash et al[85] injected 5 ml of 1% lidocaine into the region of the prostate vascular pedicle at the base of the prostate just lateral to the junction between the prostate and the seminal vesicle, and achieved a more comfortable procedure for the patient.

Monitoring

Due to its ease of use and few side-effects, prostate biopsy guided by ultrasound is useful for monitoring the effects of therapy on prostate cancer. In particular, the histopathological evaluation of prostate biopsy specimens is important after definitive therapy for prostate cancer. TRUS-guided biopsy has been used in the follow-up of prostate cancer patients treated either by radioactive seed implantation[86] or by external beam radiotherapy.[87,88] Babaian et al[88] have reported the usefulness of TRUS and PSA measurement in the detection of residual cancer after definitive external beam radiotherapy. In their patients, the most clinically useful model for predicting histologically identifiable residual cancer was either a serum PSA value greater than 2, or a serum PSA value less than or equal to 2 and abnormal TRUS findings. Consequently, ultrasound-guided biopsy revealed residual cancer after definitive radiotherapy with a diagnostic accuracy of 84%.

CONCLUSION

Since the first successful visualization of a sonogram of the prostate on an oscilloscope in 1967, there have been many developments in the clinical application of ultrasonography as well as many advances in ultrasound technology. These efforts have allowed us to increase our understanding of prostate cancer in terms of the relationship between ultrasonographic appearance and pathophysiological changes. Recent developments in interventional ultrasound and colour Doppler flow mapping are also promising in this field.

The next decade will see many more marvellous results obtained using TRUS that hopefully will enable us to deal far more effectively with prostate cancer than we can at present.

REFERENCES

1. Watanabe H, Kato H, Kato T et al, Diagnostic application of the ultrasonotomography to the prostate. *Jpn J Urol* 1968; **59:** 273–9.
2. Watanabe H, Kaiho H, Tanaka M et al, Diagnostic application of ultrasonotomography to the prostate. *Invest Urol* 1971; **8:** 548–59.
3. Watanabe H, Igari D, Tanahashi Y et al, Development and application of new equipment for transrectal ultrasonography. *J Clin Ultrasound* 1974; **2:** 91–8.
4. Watanabe H, Igari D, Tanahashi Y et al, Transrectal ultrasonotomography of the prostate. *J Urol* 1975; **114:** 734–9.
5. Watanabe H, History and application of transrectal sonography of the prostate. *Urol Clin North Am* 1989; **16:** 617–22.
6. Watanabe H, Instrumentation in prostatic ultrasonography. In: *Prostatic Ultrasonography* (Resnick MI, ed). BC Decker: Philadelphia, 1990: 17–23.
7. Watanabe H, Transrectal sonography. A personal review and recent advances. *Scand J Urol Nephrol* 1991; **137**(suppl): 75–83.
8. Watanabe H, Date S, Ohe H et al, A survey of 3000 examinations by transrectal ultrasonotomography. *Prostate* 1980; **1:** 271–8.
9. Watanabe H, Ohe H, Saitoh M et al, A survey of 10 000 examinations by transrectal ultrasonotomography in our clinic. *Jpn J Med Ultrasonics* 1985; **12**(suppl 1): 921–2.
10. Watanabe H, Tanaka N, Hayami H et al, A handytype transrectal scanner equipped with dual transducer (5 MHz and 7.5 MHz). *Jpn J Med Ultrasonics* 1988; **15**(suppl 2): 239–40.
11. Watanabe H, Igari D, Tanahashi Y et al, Measurement of size and weight of prostate by means of transrectal ultrasonotomography. *Tohoku J Exp Med* 1974; 277–85.
12. Bates TS, Reynard JM, Peter TJ et al, Determination of prostatic volume with transrectal ultrasound: a study of intra-observer and interobserver variation. *J Urol* 1996; **155:** 1299–300.
13. Ohe H, Ohnishi K, Watanabe H et al, Accuracy of digital palpation for size measurement of the prostate evaluated by transrectal sonography. *Tohoku J Exp Med* 1988; **154:** 323–8.
14. Mori Y, Measurement of the normal prostate size by means of transrectal ultrasonotomography. *Jpn J Urol* 1982; **73:** 767–81.
15. Ohe H, Kinetics and urodynamics of the prostate. *Jpn J Urol* 1985; **76:** 1637–9.
16. Watanabe H, Natural history of benign prostatic hypertrophy. *Ultrasound Med Biol* 1986; **12:** 567–71.
17. Watanabe H, Diagnosis of benign prostatic hypertrophy by ultrasound and outcome from surgery. *Akt Urol* 1993; **24:** 127–30.
18. Ukimura O, Kojima M, Inui E et al, A statistical study of the American Urological Association symptom index for benign prostatic hyperplasia in participants of mass screening program for prostatic diseases using transrectal sonography. *J Urol* 1996; **156:** 1673–8.
19. Watanabe H, Estimation of the doubling time of prostatic cancer by means of transrectal sonography. *J Kyoto Pref Univ Med* 1989; **98:** 777–80.
20. Watanabe H, Ohe H, Saitoh M et al, PSA assay of

dried blood samples from the ear lobe on a filter paper with special reference to prostatic mass screening. *Prostate* 1995; **27**: 90–4.

21. Kojima M, Babaian RJ, Algorithms for early detection of prostate cancer: current state of the 'art'. *Cancer* 1995; **75**: 1860–8.

22. Mettlin C, Murphy GP, Babaian RJ et al, The results of a five-year early prostate cancer detection intervention. *Cancer* 1996; **77**: 150–9.

23. Benson MC, Whang IS, Pantuck A et al, Prostate specific antigen density: a means of distinguishing benign prostatic hypertrophy and prostate cancer. *J Urol* 1992; **147**: 815–16.

24. Babaian RJ, Kojima M, Ramirez EI et al, Comparative analysis of prostate specific antigen and its indexes in the detection of prostate cancer. *J Urol* 1996; **156**: 432–7.

25. Oesterling JE, Jacobsen SJ, Chute CG et al, Serum prostate-specific antigen in a community-based population of healthy men. Establishment of age-specific reference ranges. *J Am Med Assoc* 1993; **270**: 860–4.

26. Watanabe H, Development and application of transrectal ultrasonotomography. *Jpn J Urol* 1974; **65**: 613–32.

27. Committee for Diagnostic Criteria, Announcement of standard diagnostic criteria in urology. *Jpn J Med Ultrasonics* 1985; **12**: 178–81.

28. Japanese Urological Association. *General Rule for Clinical and Pathological Studies on Prostatic Cancer*. Kanehara: Tokyo, 1985.

29. Lee F, Gray JM, McLeary RD et al, Transrectal ultrasound in the diagnosis of prostate cancer: Location, echogenecity, histopathology, and staging. *Prostate* 1985; **7**: 117–29.

30. Harada K, Tanahashi Y, Igari D et al, Clinical evaluation of inside echo patterns in gray scale prostatic echography. *J Urol* 1980; **124**: 216–20.

31. Miyashita H, Itakura Y, Ohnishi K et al, Ultrasonotomography of prostatic cancer (11th report). Internal echoes in prostatic cancer. *Jpn J Med Ultrasonics* 1986; **13**(suppl 2): 263–4.

32. Chodak GW, Schoenberg HW, Progress and problems in screening for carcinoma of the prostate. *World J Surg* 1989; **13**: 60–4.

33. Watanabe H, Ohe H, Present status and perspectives in mass screening for prostatic diseases. *KARKINOS* 1989; **2**: 1009–14.

34. Watanabe H, Ohe H, Tanahashi Y et al, Evaluation of clinical efficacy of transrectal sonography and computed tomography for prostatic diseases. *Jpn J Urol* 1988; **79**: 1202–9.

35. Carter HB, Hamper UM, Sheth S et al, Evaluation of transrectal ultrasound in the early detection of prostate cancer. *J Urol* 1989; **142**: 1008–10.

36. Lee F, Littrup PJ, Torp-Pedersen ST et al, Prostate cancer: comparison of transrectal ultrasonography and digital rectal examination for screening. *Radiology* 1988; **168**: 389–94.

37. Nesbit JA, Drago JR, Badalament RA, Transrectal ultrasonography: early experience with use as prostate cancer detection tool. *Urology* 1989; **34**: 120–2.

38. Ragde H, Bagley CM, Aldape HC et al, Screening for prostate cancer with high resolution ultrasound. *J Endourol* 1989; **3**: 115–23.

39. Fornage BD, Babaian RJ, Troncoso P, Diagnosis of early prostatic cancer: correlation of in vitro echography and histopathologic mapping. *Ann Radiol* 1989; **32**: 415–19.

40. Watanabe H, Saitoh M, Mishina T et al, Mass screening program for prostatic diseases with transrectal ultrasonotomography. *J Urol* 1977; **117**: 746–8.

41. Watanabe H, Ohe H, Inaba H et al, A mobile mass screening unit for prostatic disease. *Prostate* 1984; **5**: 559–65.

42. Watanabe H, Screening for prostatic cancer. In: *EORTC Genitourinary Group Monograph 5: Progress and Controversies in Oncological Urology II*. AR Liss: New York, 1988: 99–107.

43. American Urological Association, The AUA's current policy on the role of transrectal ultrasonography in the early diagnosis of cancer of the prostate. *AUA Today* 1989; **2**(2): 5.

44. Cooner WH, Mosley MR, Rutherford CL et al, Prostate cancer detection in a clinical urological practice by ultrasonography, digital rectal examination and prostate specific antigen. *J Urol* 1990; **143**: 1146–54.

45. Potosky AL, Miller BA, Albertsen PC et al, The role of increasing detection in the rising incidence of prostate cancer. *J Am Med Assoc* 1995; **273**: 548–52.

46. Watanabe H, A staging system employed in Japan. In: *Clinical Aspects of Prostate Cancer* (Catalona WJ, Coffey DS, Karr JP, eds). Elsevier: New York: 1989: 93–9.

47. Pontes JE, Eisenkraft S, Watanabe H et al, Preoperative evaluation of localized prostatic carcinoma by transrectal ultrasonography. *J Urol* 1985; **134**: 289–91.

48. Watanabe H, The Japanese staging system. In: *Diagnostic Ultrasound of the Prostate* (Resnick MI,

Watanabe H, Karr JP, eds). Elsevier: New York, 1989: 4–12.

49. Watanabe H, Ohe H, Evaluation of diagnostic efficacy for staging of prostatic cancer by transrectal sonography and computed tomography. *Jpn J Med Ultrasonics* 1989; **16**(suppl 2): 751–2.

50. Hamper UM, Sheth S, Walsh PC et al, Capsular transgression of prostatic carcinoma: evaluation with transrectal US with pathologic correlation. *Radiology* 1991; **178**: 791–5.

51. Resnick MI, Willard JW, Boyce WH, Transrectal ultrasonography in the evaluation of patients with prostatic carcinoma. *J Urol* 1980; **124**: 482–4.

52. Pontes JE, Ohe H, Watanabe H et al, Transrectal ultrasonography of the prostate. *Cancer* 1984; **53**: 1369–72.

53. Terris MK, McNeal JE, Stamey TA, Invasion of the seminal vesicles by prostatic cancer: detection with transrectal sonography. *Am J Radiol* 1990; **155**: 811–15.

54. Saitoh M, Watanabe H, Ohe H, Ultrasonically guided puncture for the prostate and seminal vesicles with transrectal real-time linear scanner. *J Kyoto Pref Univ Med* 1981; **90**: 47–53.

55. Abe M, Watanabe H, Kojima M et al, Puncture of the seminal vesicles guided by a transrectal real-time linear scanner. *J Clin Ultrasound* 1989; **17**: 173–8.

56. Scardino PT, Shinohara K, Wheeler TM et al, Staging of prostate cancer. *Urol Clin North Am* 1989; **16**: 713–34.

57. Oesterling JE, Chan DW, Epstein JI et al, Prostate specific antigen in the preoperative and postoperative evaluation of localized prostatic cancer treated with radical prostatectomy. *J Urol* 1988; **139**: 766–72.

58. Lange PH, Ercole CJ, Lightner DJ et al, The value of serum prostate specific antigen determinations before and after radical prostatectomy. *J Urol* 1989; **141**: 873–9.

59. Wolf JS Jr, Shinohara K, Narayan P, Staging of prostate cancer. Accuracy of transrectal ultrasound enhanced by prostate-specific antigen. *Br J Urol* 1992; **70**: 534–41.

60. Miyashita H, Watanabe H, Ohe H et al, Transrectal ultrasonotomography of the canine prostate. *Prostate* 1984; **5**: 453–7.

61. Ohe H, Watanabe H, Saitoh M et al, Evaluation of effect of treatment for primary lesions of stage D2 prostatic cancer by means of transrectal ultrasonography. *Tohoku J Exp Med* 1986; **149**: 307–16.

62. Watanabe H, Ohe H, Ando K et al, The effect of estramustine phosphate on prostatic cancer esti-

mated by transrectal ultrasonotomography. *Prostate* 1981; **2**: 155–61.

63. Ohe H, Watanabe H, Kinetic analysis of prostatic volume in treating prostatic cancer and its predictability for prognosis. *Cancer* 1988; **62**: 2325–9.

64. Kojima M, Watanabe H, Ohe H et al, Kinetic evaluation of the effect of LHRH analog on prostatic cancer using transrectal ultrasonotomography. *Prostate* 1987; **10**: 11–17.

65. Okihara K, Watanabe M, Saitoh M et al, Kinetic analysis of focal hypoechoic lesion in the prostate treated by castration. *Prostate* 1994; **24**: 252–6.

66. Kojima M, Ohe H, Watanabe H, Kinetic analysis of prostatic volume in patients with stage D prostatic cancer treated with LHRH analogues in relation to prognosis. *Br J Urol* 1995; **75**: 492–7.

67. Okihara K, Kinetic study of local relapse in prostatic cancer. *Jpn J Urol* 1995; **86**: 878–997.

68. Watanabe H, Saitoh T, Saitoh M et al, Color Doppler sonography in urology. *Jpn J Urol Surg* 1994; **7**: 213–18.

69. Saitoh M, An application of color flow imaging for urodynamic study. *Jpn J Urol Surg* 1994; **7**: 329–34.

70. Inaba T, Watanabe H, Ohe H et al, Non-invasive transgastric detection of ultrasonic Doppler signals from canine renal vessels. *Tohoku J Exp Med* 1987; **153**: 75–6.

71. Miyashita H, Watanabe H, Ohe H et al, Application of 2D Doppler color flow mapping to the prostate. *Jpn J Urol* 1988; **79**: 235–8.

72. Watanabe H, Tanaka T, Ohnishi K et al, 2D-Doppler color flow mapping of the prostate using transrectal biplane probe. *Jpn J Med Ultrasonics* 1990; **17**(suppl 2): 169–70.

73. Watanabe M, Hongo F, Inoue W et al, Study on sound spectrogram of the prostatic diseases using color Doppler sonography. *Jpn J Med Ultrasonics* 1992; **19**(suppl 2): 265–6.

74. Watanabe M, Ohnishi K, Hayami H et al, Ultrasonography of prostatic cancer (the 16th report): study of blood flow images in prostatic cancer during therapy by 2D-Doppler flow mapping. *Jpn J Med Ultrasonics* 1990; **17**(suppl 1): 443–4.

75. Watanabe H, Saitoh M, Orikasa S et al, Efficacy of an echo contrast agent, SH/TA-508, in color Doppler sonography of mass lesions in urology. *Urol Oncol* 1995; **1**: 215–22.

76. Holm HH, Gammelgaard J, Ultrasonically guided precise needle placement in the prostate and seminal vesicles. *J Urol* 1981; **125**: 385–7.

77. Keizur JJ, Lavin B, Leidich RB, Iatrogenic urinary

tract infection with *Pseudomonas cepacia* after transrectal ultrasound guided needle biopsy of the prostate. *J Urol* 1993; **149:** 523–6.

78. Watanabe H, Ultrasound in association with endoscopy. *Br Med Bull* 1986; **42:** 318–24.

79. Abe M, Hashimoto T, Matsuda T et al, Prostatic biopsy guided by transrectal ultrasonography using real-time linear scanner. *Urology* 1987; **29:** 567–9.

80. Hodge KH, McNeal JE, Terris MK, Random systematic versus directed ultrasound guided transrectal core biopsies of the prostate. *J Urol* 1989; **142:** 71–5.

81. Epstein JI, Walsh PC, Carmichael M et al, Pathologic and clinical findings to predict tumor extent of nonpalpable (stage T1c) prostate cancer. *J Am Med Assoc* 1994; **271:** 368–74.

82. Terris MK, McNeal JE, Freiha FS et al, Efficacy of transrectal ultrasound-guided seminal vesicle biopsies in the detection of seminal vesicle invasion of prostate cancer. *J Urol* 1993; **149:** 1035–9.

83. Holm HH, Juul N, Pedersen JF et al, Transperineal [125]Iodine seed implantation in prostatic cancer guided by transrectal ultrasonography. *J Urol* 1983; **130:** 283–6.

84. Onik GM, Cohen JK, Reyes GD et al, Transrectal ultrasound-guided percutaneous radical cryosurgical ablation of the prostate. *Cancer* 1993; **72:** 1291–9.

85. Nash PA, Bruce JE, Indudhara R et al, Transrectal ultrasound guided prostatic nerve blockade eases systematic needle biopsy of the prostate. *J Urol* 1996; **155:** 607–9.

86. Lee F, Torp-Pederden S, Meiselman L et al, Transrectal ultrasound in the diagnosis and staging of local disease after ^{125}I seed implantation for prostate cancer. *Int J Radiat Oncol Biol Phys* 1988; **15:** 1453–9.

87. Kabalin JN, Hodge KK, McNeal JE et al, Identification of residual cancer in the prostate following radiation therapy: role of transrectal ultrasound guided biopsy and prostate specific antigen. *J Urol* 1989; **142:** 326–31.

88. Babaian RJ, Kojima M, Saitoh M et al, Detection of residual prostate cancer after external radiotherapy. *Cancer* 1995; **75:** 2153–8.

10 Evaluation of metastases

10.1

Nuclear medicine in prostate cancer

John Buscombe, Andrew Hilson

CONTENTS • Bone scintigraphy • Assessment of soft tissue metastases • Therapy • Conclusions

Nuclear medicine is concerned with the applications of radioisotopic tracers to diagnosis and therapy. If differs from other forms of imaging in being primarily concerned with function and changes in physiology occurring in pathological states. The tracer technique demands that tiny traces of substances (normally less than 10^{-9} g) be given which are specific to a particular physiological event. These have no pharmacological effect and, therefore, do not disturb the function of the organ that they are imaging. By using a radioactive label it is possible to image these tracers. Specific tracers have been designed for particular jobs. For example, methylene diphosphonate (MDP) is taken up into bone depending on the metabolic turn-over of that bone. As bone tries to heal around infection, fracture or metastasis it is metabolically more active and will appear as a focal area of increased uptake (a 'hot spot') on a bone scan.

Radioisotopes have the same chemical characteristics as their stable counterparts, but decay by emitting a characteristic radiation. Radiation comes in three main forms: α, β and γ. The first two types are particulate and can cause significant short-range tissue damage; therefore, these types are used for therapy rather than imaging. γ-rays (like X-rays) with sufficient energy are able to pass through the body with minimal attenuation and can be detected using a specialist machine – the γ-camera. For most imaging, a medium half-life isotope with a suitable energy is required. It must be readily available and cheap. Technetium-99m (^{99m}Tc), an artificial metallic isotope, has ideal physical properties (half-life 6 h) and can be 'manufactured' by a generator at a central pharmacy or within a nuclear medicine department. Thus [^{99m}Tc]MDP is the ideal combination of a radioisotope and a pharmaceutical (a radiopharmaceutical) for bone imaging.[1]

Uptake into the bone normally constitutes

about 20% of the injected dose and occurs within the first 20–30 min; however, it may take 2–3 h for the remaining blood pool to clear. In patients with significant tumour load, more than 20% of the injected activity may be taken up, and in the so-called 'super scan' almost all the injected tracer is taken into the bones with little or none left to be excreted via the kidneys. The clearance of tracer via the kidneys depends on the glomerular filtration rate (GFR). This can be impaired in some patients with prostate cancer, with effective outflow obstruction leading to loss of renal function. In these patients images may appear fuzzy due to high background activity. To ensure good-quality imaging, it is important that the patient is kept well hydrated and a longer delay between injection and scanning should be considered in patients with known renal impairment. [^{99m}Tc]hydroxy-ethylidene diphosphonate (HEDP) has a faster clearance rate and imagining can be performed 2–2.5 h after injection. However, the difference in time does not often justify change to the more expensive [^{99m}Tc]HEDP, and [^{99m}Tc]MDP remains the most commonly used agent for bone scintigraphy world-wide.

BONE SCINTIGRAPHY

Bone scintigraphy in carcinoma of the prostate is concerned almost exclusively with identifying the presence and site of bone metastases. Bone metastases from carcinoma of the prostate almost all arise via haematological spread of cancer cells, not to the bone but to the bone marrow. As the tumour in the bone marrow grows, lysis of bone occurs. This does not in itself excite an increased uptake of [^{99m}Tc]MDP. However, the resulting attempt of the bone to heal and remodel leads to increased osteoblastic activity, which leads to increased uptake of tracer. As this can only really occur at sites of red marrow, the bone scan can be confined to the axial skeleton and proximal humeri and femora. Painless single distal bone metastases are extremely rare and need not be considered in the normal scanning protocol. Images are obtained of part of the skeleton, individual

images being required to cover the whole axial skeleton (Figure 10.1.1). Anterior chest images should be recorded at a 30° oblique angle so that activity in the sternum does not overlay the spine. An alternative is to use a system with a fixed couch and one or two γ-cameras (one viewing the anterior, one the posterior), so that a whole-body image can be obtained (Figure 10.1.2). Essentially the same information can be gained using each imaging system, although imaging may be faster with a whole-body scanner and with two heads imaging can be completed in 15–20 min as against 45 min using multiple spot views.

Additional imaging may be needed in those patients for whom the standard bone scan is not clear. In the spine it may be possible to characterize any spinal lesion better by using three-dimensional imaging (single photon emission tomography (SPECT)). It is not uncommon for patients referred for a bone scan for carcinoma of the prostate to be elderly and have an increased probability of spinal degenerative disease. This can look similar to early metastases on the bone scan, but by performing SPECT the true nature of such a lesion can be elucidated (Figure 10.1.3).

As the [^{99m}Tc]MDP is excreted in the urine, patients with bladder-emptying problems may have difficulty voiding radioactive urine from the bladder. This may lead to a large amount of urinary activity obscuring the surrounding pelvic bones and sacrum, both of which are common sites of bone metastases. Urinary catheterization may be possible, but most nuclear medicine departments are not ideally located and do not have the staff to perform urinary catheterization using a sterile method while ensuring there is no contamination of the surrounding environment by radioactive urine. In this case, a 'squat' view can be taken by sitting the patient on the camera face. This separates the activity in the bladder from that of the surrounding bones (Figure 10.1.4). Alternatively, a late image at 24 h can be performed when some activity remains within the bone but hopefully all the bladder activity has washed out. As the radiation is injected at the start of the study all these extra images can be

nt
it

RAO

AIP

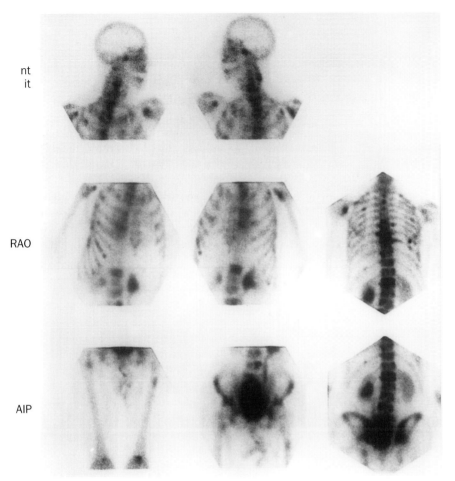

Figure 10.1.1 Multiple spot views of bone scintigraphy showing 'hot spots' due to metastases in the spine and ribs. Note, however, that despite the image being taken after micturition, bladder activity obscures the pelvic bones.

obtained without the need for any extra radiation burden to the patient.

The classic pattern of bone metastases seen in patients with prostate cancer is of multiple, small, occasionally congruent, metastases involving almost all the axial skeleton. However, this is often a late change and is unlikely to occur without there being a markedly raised blood level of prostate-specific antigen (PSA). A further classically described pattern is that of diffusely increased uptake throughout the axial skeleton, proximal femora and proximal humeri, with suppression of activity in the nor-

mal bone and no or minimal renal or urinary uptake (Figure 10.1.5). This is often described as a 'super scan'; it is a very rare occurrence. More common, however, is non-homogeneous uptake with no urinary tract activity.

These more spectacular patterns are not those seen in most clinical practice, especially in patients with only a slightly elevated PSA level. While a single bone metastasis in carcinoma of the prostate is unusual, it can occur and is often found in the pelvis and lumbar spine. Single rib lesions are less likely to be metastatic than benign, and are often associated with minor rib

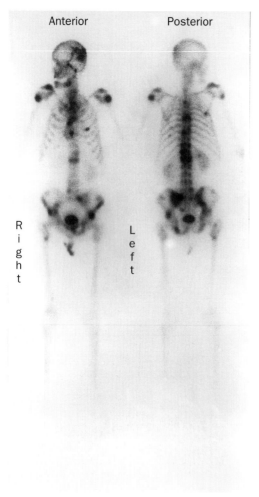

Anterior   Posterior

R
i
g
h
t

L
e
f
t

Figure 10.1.2 Whole-body anterior and posterior images showing bone metastases in the skull, ribs, sternum, and proximal femora and humeri.

trauma. Within the spine sites of predilection for metastases include the vertebral body and the pedicles. When these lesions are multiple, a diagnosis of metastatic carcinoma is not difficult. However, in the spine the results of bone scintigraphy may be less clear, with some confusion between degenerative disease and metastases.

The pattern of uptake of the [^{99m}Tc]MDP within the spine may suggest that a particular lesion is benign or malignant. For example, uptake in the lumbar facet joints (best seen on SPECT or oblique views) is certain to be benign. Likewise, linear uptake across the body of the vertebra is classically seen in osteoporotic collapse, but may be seen in vertebral collapse secondary to tumour. More common, however, is diffuse slightly increased uptake throughout the lumbar and cervical spine. This is normally attributed to degenerative disease, but it may be difficult to exclude coexisting bone metastases. Attempts to use more tumour-specific methods such as fluorine-18-labelled fluorodeoxyglucose ([^{18}F]FDG) have proved to be both insensitive and non-specific. Radiological techniques, such as coned views and computed tomography (CT) to look for bone destruction, or magnetic resonance imaging (MRI) to assess marrow involvement, may need to be employed. It may also be necessary to use serial scans at 4–6 month intervals. Metastatic lesions tend to progress, degenerative lesions do not progress. However, even this may not be true if small spinal metastases are being controlled by hormone therapy. It may also be difficult to differentiate between Paget's disease, particularly if mono-ostotic, and metastatic carcinoma of the prostate, especially if the uptake is in the pelvis (Figure 10.1.6). The presence of other lesions make carcinoma of the prostate more likely. However, it may be necessary to perform extra radiology and sometimes bone biopsy to differentiate between the two. Despite these difficulties, bone scintigraphy remains the most cost-effective and least time-consuming method for localizing bone metastases.

Bone scintigraphy has proven to be valuable in the diagnosis of bone metastases, and attempts have been made to use this method to predict the outcome of the disease on the assumption that the appearance of metastases on the initial bone scintigram is a crude but effective estimate of disease load. It also reflects the biological behaviour of the tumour. Whilst counting the number of lesions on the initial bone scintigram has been used, this is a very complex procedure. An association between the

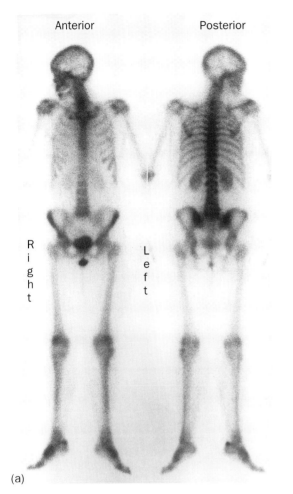

Anterior   Posterior

Right   Left

(a)

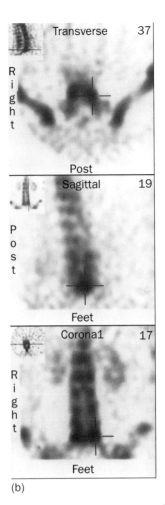

Transverse   37

Right

Post

Sagittal   19

Post

Feet

Coronal   17

Right

Feet

(b)

Figure 10.1.3 A patient with what appears to be a normal bone scan in the planar image (a) except for some mildly increased uptake in the lower lumbar spine. Tomographic images (b) displayed as transverse, sagittal and coronal slices show focal uptake in the left-hand side of L5 due to a single bone metastasis.

number of lesions seen and poor survival has been noted, but was no better indicator than the initial serum prostatic acid phosphatase level.[2] It was noted, however, that bone metastases outside the spine and pelvis held a poorer prognosis for the patient than did limited disease. Simple comparisons with serum PSA seem to show that a normal PSA level means that bone

scintigraphy is not indicated.[3] However, in the same study, 30% of patients with a normal PSA level had bone metastases. We would recommend that at initial diagnosis bone scintigraphy should be done in all patients, regardless of the serum PSA level. There is an added advantage in that a bone scintigram recorded at initial diagnosis provides a baseline

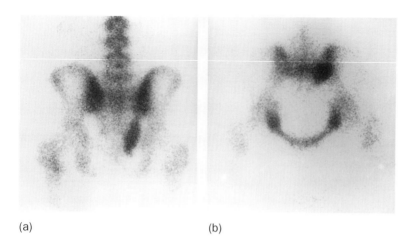

(a) (b)

Figure 10.1.4 The posterior planar view of the pelvis (a) suggests that uptake could be in bone or could be a urinary artefact. The 'squat' view (b) shows that uptake is due to metastases in the right-hand side of the sacrum.

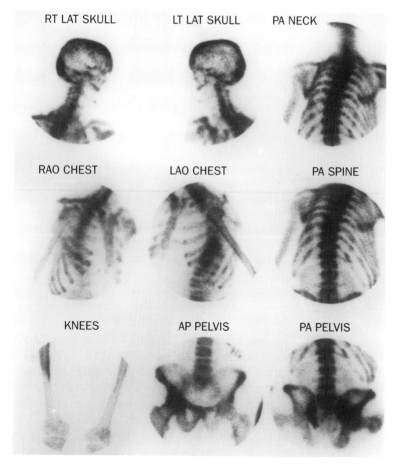

Figure 10.1.5 A 'super scan' with increased uptake of tracer seen through the axial skeleton. Note the lack of renal or bladder activity.

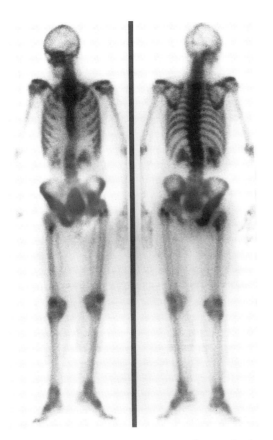

Figure 10.1.6 The increased uptake of tracer in the right hemi-pelvis could represent metastatic disease or pagetic changes. However, the abnormal uptake in the proximal femora is more characteristic of metastases, and the probability is that the pelvic uptake is metastatic and not pagetic.

Table 10.1.1 Semiquantitative grading of the extent of bone metastases on initial bone scintigraphy (after Soloway et al[4]) *

Grade	Appearance of bone scintigram
0	No lesions compatible with bone metastases
1	1–5 lesions compatible with bone metastases
2	6–20 lesions compatible with bone metastases
3	> 20 lesions compatible with bone metastases, but not a 'super scan'
4	A 'super scan' (> 75% of axial skeleton, proximal humeri and femora involved)

* In the spine each half-vertebra counts as a single site for metastases. Therefore, if a lesion is limited to or is less than half a vertebra in size it is counted as one lesion, but if it involves more than half a vertebra it counts as two lesions.

from which any subsequent changes can be measured. A systematic method is to use a semiquantitative approach using a five-step grading system to assess tumour load such that grade 0 is normal and grade 4 a 'super scan', as described by Soloway et al[4] (Table 10.1.1). Using such a system and comparing the Soloway grade with the PSA level, the histological grade of the tumour and the extent of disease locally, it was found that the best predictor of survival was the Soloway grade and the local extent of disease (Figure 10.1.7). The initial PSA level was not as good a predictor of survival.[5] This use of the bone scan to predict survival is another reason why all patients should have a bone scintigram at initial diagnosis.

Whilst in prostate cancer bone scintigraphy is generally used as a diagnostic and staging tool, effective regimens of therapy using endocrine manipulation and chemotherapy have resulted in patients showing a regression of bone metastases. Therefore, these patients should undergo serial bone scintigraphy in order to assess the effect of treatment on the bone metastases. The normally recommended interval between scans is 4–6 months. It is unlikely that more frequent imaging, unless pain arises at a new site, will yield any useful

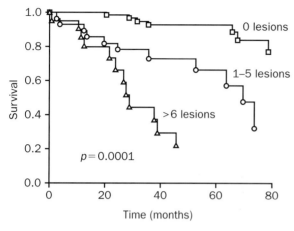

Figure 10.1.7 Differential survival of patients with carcinoma of the prostate according to the number of metastatic lesions seen on the bone scan at diagnosis. There is significantly poorer survival for patients presenting with six or more lesions.

standard nuclear medicine techniques are its higher sensitivity of the system and its better resolution (lesions of 6–7 mm can be resolved, compared with the resolution of standard γ-camera systems of >10 mm). The most commonly used tracer is [18F]FDG, a false glucose substrate that is taken into metabolically active cells preferentially, phosphorylated and then remains unaltered within the cell. The half-life of this tracer is only 110 min, and so the PET camera must be close to the cyclotron producing the fluorine-18 and specialist staff are needed. This has meant that the cost of a PET scan has tended to be 2–3 times that of MRI, although the cost is falling with newer technology. PET has been shown to have a high sensitivity in the detection of cancer, and is particularly good in finding nodal disease.[6] However, the results in prostate cancer, in both nodal disease and skeletal metastases, have been disappointing, with reported sensitivities of 50%, particularly in bone metastases.[7,8]

clinical information. Also, as the uptake on the bone scan reflects attempts at healing rather than bone destruction, it is possible to see a transient increased uptake in the 2–6 weeks following hormone manipulation. This is often described as a 'flare' reaction, but is not often accompanied by an increase in bone pain as occurs in a clinical flare, and the term should not be used. If such a phenomenon is suspected a repeat study 2–3 months later will normally differentiate between progression of the bone disease and a generalized increase in uptake of tracer secondary to hormone manipulation.

ASSESSMENT OF SOFT TISSUE METASTASES

Positron emission tomography

Positron emission tomography (PET) is a new imaging method that uses short-lived positron-emitting isotopes and a special type of radiation detector (a PET camera). Its advantages over

Immunoscintigraphy

The ideal method of imaging would be the direct visualization of prostate cancer using some unique physiological properties of the tumour cell compared to normal prostate or normal surrounding tissue. Unfortunately, as seen with [18F]FDG imaging, there are few properties in the prostate cancer cell that can be exploited directly to perform this type of imaging. However, the cell does express certain unique antigens on its surface, the most common being prostatic acid phosphatase and PSA. While it is common to use blood levels of these antigens to measure disease activity, it is also possible to raise antibodies that have specific bonding to these antigens. These can then be radiolabelled and used for imaging. The technique is known as immunoscintigraphy. The aim of immunoscintigraphy is to combine a highly specific antibody with a suitable isotope for imaging. Initial studies using an antiprostatic acid phosphatase antibody labelled with iodine-131 produced some promising results in a small group of patients with widespread metastases. However, the antibody is not specific to prostatic cancer, the iodine-131 does not give ideal imaging and a high radiation dose is delivered.[9] Better results have been obtained using an indium-111-labelled antibody, with which localization is seen in soft tissue and bone metastases.[10]

Another strategy has been to use a general tumour marker such as carcinoembryonic antigen (CEA). There is evidence that carcinoma of the prostate can be imaged with anti-CEA antibodies. Sensitivities of 55% for bone metastases and 86% for nodal metastases were obtained in a group of 40 patients with disseminated disease. This antibody (designated CYT-356) is now entering phase III clinical trials, and may become the first commercially available agent for immunoscintigraphic imaging of lymph-node metastases with a sensitivity higher than CT or MRI.[11] Logically, antibodies directed at PSA should have more specific action. An indium-111-labelled product has been used in a group of 11 patients with encouraging results.[12] Radioimmunoscintigraphy has not, however, proved to be sufficiently reliable to become a standard imaging technique. The trials that have been reported so far have contained too few patients, with too advanced disease, for the results to be considered reliable, although this situation may change in the next year or two.

Molecular methods

Prostate cancer, in common with breast cancer, is one of the few human cancers that is susceptible to hormone manipulation. This suggests that these cancers may have specific hormone receptors that could be used for imaging. Radiolabelled progestins have high binding affinities for cancer cells in vitro, but to date no clinical studies involving these agents have been applied to prostate cancer.[13] Such a method may be of use not only in the diagnosis of metastases, but also in the in vivo characterization of the hormone status of the tumour, which might be of use in tailoring treatment.

THERAPY

Nuclear medicine does not involve only the diagnostic use of unsealed radioisotopes, but also includes therapy. Unlike external radiotherapy, which depends on the anatomical localization of the tumour, targeted radiotherapy depends on the differential uptake of tracer in or close to the tumour. Ideally pure α- or β-radiation emitters should be used, as these deposit the highest amounts of energy in tissue. Phosphorus-32, a β-emitter, has been used in the form of sodium phosphate to treat widespread bone metastases. Response rates, in terms of reduction in bone pain, have been recorded in 80% of patients,[14] but the compound has significant toxicity. Strontium-89, a calcium analogue, is less toxic and has a shorter half-life. It is given as a standard 150 MBq (4 mCi) dose. It has been shown that 67% of patients have some response to this compound, in terms of pain relief lasting up to 6 months, at which time the treatment can be repeated. Mild toxicity with transient reduction in platelets has been recorded, and about 1% of patients may require supportive therapy.[15] In a cost–benefit study done in Canada, strontium-89 was found to be as effective as hemibody irradiation and more effective than local radiotherapy, with similar overall costs.[16]

It is also possible to combine a therapeutic isotope similar to technetium-99m, such as samarium-153 or rhenium-186, with diphosphonates in order to localize the isotope at the site of bone metastases. The advantage of these agents is that they have a shorter half-life and the myelotoxicity is less. A similar number of patients (about 67%) have relief of pain, but this tends to last for only 3 months, at which time a repeat dose has to be given. Both agents are given with an activity of 37 MBq (1 mCi) per kilogram body weight.[17]

All these treatments can be given as outpatient procedures, and all are only palliative. They are ideally used in patients with bone metastases in more than four sites spread around the body that have escaped hormonal control. These treatments should not be given to patients with platelet counts of less than

Table 10.1.2 Comparison of unsealed therapy used as palliation for bone metastases

Radiopharmaceutical	Efficacy	Bone marrow toxicity	Cost	Repeat
Phosphorus-32	++++	+++++	$	6 monthly
Strontium-89	++++	+	$$$$$	6 monthly
[^{153}Sm]EDTMP	+++	+	$$$	3 monthly
[^{186}Re]HEDP	+++	+	$$$	3 monthly

EDTMP, ethyldiaminetetramethylene diphosphonate; HEDP, hydroxyethylidene diphosphonate.

80 000/ml or total leukocytes of less than 2000/ml, or in whom survival is likely to be less than 2 months. Pain relief occurs at about 1–2 weeks after treatment, but can be preceded by a transient increase in pain. This can be covered by the use of steroids, anti-inflammatory drugs and/or increasing pain relief for the first 2 weeks after treatment. Generally, however, the treatments offer a good method of pain relief and are underused (Table 10.1.2).

CONCLUSIONS

Despite many attempts, there are no proven methods of imaging soft tissue metastases with nuclear medicine. Immunoscintigraphy may be able to do this better than CT or MRI, but more data are needed. [^{18}F]FDG PET has been disap-pointing. The imaging of bone metastases remains the main use of nuclear medicine in prostate cancer and probably offers the best method by which bone metastases can be identified.

An initial bone scintigram is indicated in all patients, even in patients with a normal PSA level. Bone scintigraphy should be repeated in all patients undergoing active treatment for bone metastases, those with a sudden rise in PSA and those with new onset of localized bone pain. In elderly men it may be difficult to differ-entiate between degenerative and metastatic disease in the spine. Repeat bone scintigraphy at 4–6 months may be the best method. Metastases tend to progress, while degenerative lesions do not.

Nuclear medicine can offer effective palli-ation for those patients who do not experience pain relief from hormone manipulation.

REFERENCES

1. Shearer RJ, Constable AR, Girling M, Hendry WF, Fergusson JD, Radioactive bone scintigra-phy with the gamma camera in the investigation of prostatic cancer. *Br Med J* 1974; **ii:** 362–5.

2. Merrick MV, Ding CL, Chilsolm GD, Elton RA, Prognostic significance of alkaline and acid phosphatase and skeletal scintigraphy in carci-noma of the prostate. *Br J Urol* 1996; **20:** 715–20.

3. Oomen R, Geethanjali FS, Gopalakrishnan Chacko N, John S, Kanangabapathy AS, Roul RK, Correlation of serum prostate specific antigen levels and bone scintigraphy in carcinoma of the prostate. *Br J Radiol* 1994; **67:** 469–71.

4. Soloway MS, Hardiman SW, Hickey D, Stratification of patients with metastatic prostate cancer based on extent of disease on initial bone scan. *Cancer* 1988; **61:** 195–202.

5. Buscombe JR, Richmond PJM, Kaisary AV, Hilson AJW, Bone scintigraphy as a predictor of outcome in carcinoma of the prostate. *J Nucl Med* 1995; **36:** 196P.

6. Strauss LG, Conti PS, The application of PET in clinical oncology. *J Nucl Med* 1991; **32:** 623–48.

7. Laubenbacher C, Hofer C, Avril N et al, Can 18-FDG PET differentiate local recurrent prostatic cancer and scar? *Eur J Nucl Med* 1995; **22:** 803.

8. Shreeve P, Grossman HB, Wahl RL, Initial assessment of FDG/PET detection of skeletal metastatic prostate cancer and scar? *J Nucl Med* 1993; **34:** 223P.

9. Goldenburg DM, DeLand FH, Bennett SJ et al, Radioimmunodetection of prostatic cancer. *J Am Med Assoc* 1983; **250:** 630–5.

10. Babaian RJ, Lamki LM, Radioimmunoscintigraphy of prostate cancer. *Semin Nucl Med* 1989; **19:** 309–21.

11. Abdel-Nabi H, Wright GL, Gulfo JV et al, Monoclonal antibodies and immunoconjugates in the diagnosis and treatment of prostate cancer. *Semin Urol* 1992; **10:** 45–55.

12. Dillman RO, Beauregard J, Ryan KP et al, Radioimmunodetection of cancer with the use of indium-111 labeled monoclonal antibodies. *Natl Cancer Inst Monogr* 1987; **3:** 33–6.

13. Katzenellenbogen JA, Designing steroid receptor-based radiotracers to image breast and prostate tumours. *J Nucl Med* 1995; **36:** 8S–13S.

14. Montebello JF, Hartson-Easton M, The palliation of osseous metastasis with ^{32}P or ^{89}Sr compared with external beam and hemibody irradiation: a historical perspective. *Cancer Invest* 1989; **7:** 139–60.

15. Silberstein EB, Williams C, Strontium-89 therapy for the pain of osseous metastases. *J Nucl Med* 1985; **26:** 345–8.

16. McEwan AJB, Amoyotte GA, McGowan DG, MacGillvary JA, Porter AT, Retrospective analysis of the cost effectiveness of treatment with Metastron (strontium-89) and conventional radiotherapy in patients with prostate metastases to bone. *Nucl Med Commun* 1994; **15:** 499–504.

17. Turner JH, Claringbold PG, A phase II study of treatment of painful multifocal skeletal metastases with single and repeated dose samarium-153 ethylenediaminetetramethylene phosphonate. *Eur J Cancer* 1991; **27:** 1084–6.

10.2

Computed tomography and magnetic resonance imaging in the management of prostate cancer

Janak Saada, Sarbjinder S Sandhu, Anthony F Watkinson

CONTENTS • **Essential problems with the interpretation of imaging studies** • **Computed tomography** • **Magnetic resonance imaging** • **Comparative imaging** • **Value of imaging in clinically localized prostate cancer** • **Detection of metastasis** • **Monitoring therapy** • **Future imaging developments** • **Conclusion**

Almost every imaging modality has been applied to the evaluation of prostate cancer. The principal role of imaging in patients with prostate cancer is staging and the evaluation of therapy. Imaging can help in answering three main questions: what is the volume of the primary tumour, is the lesion locally invasive, and how far has it spread? The answers to these questions have important prognostic and therapeutic implications. The role of imaging in diagnosis is currently limited to the guidance of biopsies. Biopsies may be taken from the prostate, lymph nodes or a metastasis.

The imaging modalities in current use are transrectal ultrasonography (TRUS), computed tomography (CT) and magnetic resonance imaging (MRI). The role of TRUS has been discussed elsewhere (see Chapter 9), therefore in the main only the application and efficacy of CT and MRI in staging prostate cancer are reviewed here.

ESSENTIAL PROBLEMS WITH THE INTERPRETATION OF IMAGING STUDIES

A number of problems with imaging-based studies need to be appreciated before evaluating their efficacy. Comparative data on competing prostatic imaging methods are difficult to obtain because few institutions have sufficient patient numbers to produce rigorous, statistically meaningful evaluations. Many of the available studies have been retrospective, performed on selected populations with different prevalences of prostatic cancer. This makes comparisons unreliable.

Poor study design without 'blinding' readers to non-imaging-based factors results in bias. Improved levels of accuracy may be obtained when clinical data (prostate-specific antigen or PSA, locations of positive biopsies) are known. Assessing the extent to which imaging has influenced patient management is often difficult (verification bias), for example, carrying out a prostatic biopsy on the basis of a suspicious lesion detected on imaging. Increased detection rates are also in part related to the increasing use of sextant biopsies. A selection bias exists in most studies; patients with only clinically localized disease are included and not patients with advanced disease. The study population has therefore been biased towards cases of minimal disease.

The introduction of a new imaging technique is associated with a number of problems. First, the 'learning curve' phenomenon is a potent source of error and an important contributor to interobserver variation.[1] The initial enthusiasm and expectation may result in biased interpretation. There is often considerable delay in reporting the potential pitfalls and limitations of the new test.

The criteria for abnormality based on imaging (for example, definition of capsular penetration) are frequently subjective, often based on non-standardized parameters, making a meta-analysis difficult. The penetration of the capsule by cancer is initially a microscopic event. No current imaging modality has the resolution to define this. The quality of pathological correlation is also variable and frequently the methodology is not reported. Adoption of rigorous pathological methods may result in the increased documentation of more advanced disease. Only a few studies have attempted to correlate imaging with histopathological maps of the entire specimen, on a lesion-by-lesion basis. Even with histopathological mapping of the entire specimen, correlating the position of the detected lesion with the map is still difficult.[2] This is particularly important with a multifocal disease such as carcinoma of the prostate.

Advances in imaging technology have resulted in studies being done on equipment of different generations which are not comparable. This is particularly important with MRI-generated images. Most imaging variables can critically influence the image quality and make comparisons between different studies invalid.

COMPUTED TOMOGRAPHY

CT diagnosis of prostatic cancer

The CT attenuation of tissue is principally determined by the physical density of its components. Similarities in the CT density of prostatic carcinoma, benign prostatic hyperplasia (BPH) and the normal prostate make detection and early diagnosis of intracapsular cancers, even with intravenous contrast agents, impractical.[3]

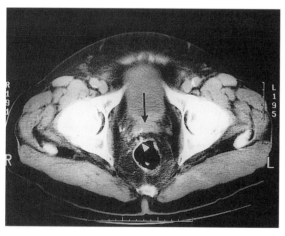

(a)

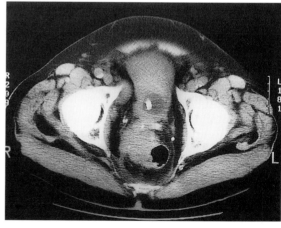

(b)

Figure 10.2.1 (a) CT scan showing non-organ-confined carcinoma of the prostate with seminal vesicle and early perirectal invasion; (b) the same patient a year later. Despite hormonal ablation there has been marked growth of tumour resulting in symptoms of rectal obstruction.

Occasionally, rare mucinous carcinoma and focal tumour necrosis can be identified as a hypodense area. Although asymmetry or nodularity of the glandular contour, with or without enlargement, may suggest a cancer,[3] differentiation from benign prostatic hypertrophy is imprecise.

The role of CT in the detection of extracapsular spread (Figure 10.2.1) has been extensively investigated. Irregularity of the prostatic margin is suspicious and an increase in the density of the periprostatic and perirectal fat, in a patient without a history of pelvic surgery or irradiation, may indicate tumour invasion. Distinguishing between the artefactual changes secondary to intervention and relapse may be possible only with serial follow-up examinations. The mean sensitivity, specificity and accuracy of CT detection of transcapsular exten-

sion are 53%, 72% and 56%, respectively (Table 10.2.1).

Attention has also been focused on specifically identifying seminal vesicle involvement (Figure 10.2.2), because this portends a much worse prognosis than capsular penetration alone and often coexists with microscopic nodal metastases.[9] Seminal vesicle size, symmetry of enlargement and obliteration of the seminal vesicle angle have all been employed as criteria to judge seminal vesicle involvement. Obliteration of the seminal vesicle angle is reported as the most accurate sign.[10] The mean sensitivity, specificity and accuracy of CT detection of a seminal vesicle invasion is 35%, 78% and 67%, respectively (see Table 10.2.1).

Invasion of the urinary bladder (see Figure 10.2.1b) can be suspected in cases of localized thickening associated with contour irregularities

Table 10.2.1 Pooled data from six studies evaluating the usefulness of computed tomography

		Flanigan et al[4] 1985	Platt et al[5] 1987	Salo et al[6] 1987	Hricak et al[7] 1987	Hammerer et al[8] 1992	Konety et al[9] 1996	Mean value
Detection of	Sn		75				30	53
extracapsular	Sp		60				83	72
spread (%)	Acc		64				48	56
Detection of	Sn		33	36				35
seminal vesicle	Sp		60	96				78
invasion (%)	Acc		58	76				67
Detection of	Sn	50	0		22	6	8	17
lymph node	Sp	100	96		100	96	97	98
metastasis (%)	Acc	91	81		–	–	89	87
Distinguishing	Sn		50	25	55		30	40
T2 and T3 (%)	Sp		75	89	73		79	79
	Acc		57	60	65		51	58

Sn, sensitivity; Sp, specificity; Acc, accuracy.

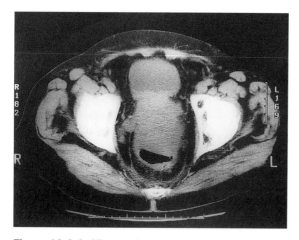

Figure 10.2.2 CT scan demonstrating gross seminal vesicle, bladder and rectal invasion by prostate cancer.

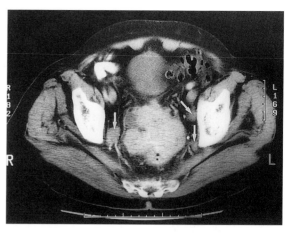

Figure 10.2.3 T4 carcinoma of the prostate involving the rectum and pelvic lymph nodes.

in a distended bladder. Thickening of the bladder secondary to outlet obstruction and detrusor hypertrophy can make the assessment difficult. An obstructed ureter is, however, a reliable indicator of invasion of the bladder with involvement of the ureterovesical junction. Infiltration of the bladder base or rectum cannot be accurately detected because of the limitations of the transaxial plane of imaging. Invasion of the internal obturator and levator ani muscles or the rectum leads to difficulties in identifying these structures as distinct entities. However, in some patients the levator ani muscle and the anterior rectal wall are difficult to distinguish from the prostate as a result of the lack of interposed fat and so the interpretation is made more difficult.

CT detection of pelvic lymph node involvement (Figure 10.2.3) with prostate carcinoma has been extensively studied with a reported mean sensitivity, specificity and accuracy of 17%, 98% and 87%, respectively (see Table 10.2.1). Despite the low sensitivity, the accuracy is high as a result of the relatively high specificity. There is a diagnosis of lymph node metastases if the nodes are enlarged, asymmetrical or increased in number (Figure 10.2.4). The

internal structure of normal-sized nodes cannot be evaluated, making differentiation between metastatic and reactive nodes impossible on imaging alone. Lymph nodes larger than 15 mm are considered suspicious for metastases, but this is an arbitrary value; Oyen et al[11] performed CT-guided aspiration cytology on asymmetrical nodes as small as 6 mm with a significant yield of tumour. Their sensitivity, specificity and accuracy rates were 78%, 100% and 97%, respectively. This compares favourably with surgical or laparoscopic lymphadenectomy.

Unfortunately, early stage disease is more likely to be associated with microscopic metastatic disease than bulky nodal disease which is seen in the later stages.[5] This accounts for the poor sensitivity of lymph node staging based on size criteria. The yield from CT imaging of the para-aortic region is very low and unnecessary in the absence of enlarged pelvic nodes.[12] Differentiation between metastatic involvement and non-specific enlargement of lymph nodes is impossible without cytological evaluation. Evaluation of the regional lymph nodes is difficult because of the lack of fat planes. Lymph nodes that are only marginally

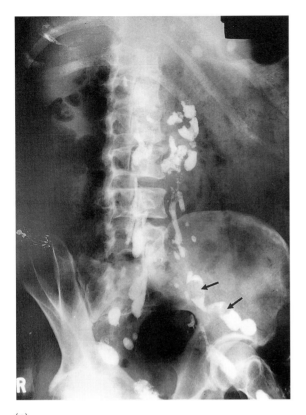

(a)

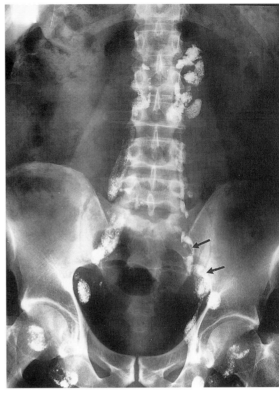

(b)

Figure 10.2.4 Lymphangiogram demonstrating iliac and aortic node involvement (a) pre- and (b) post-oestrogen treatment. (Courtesy of Dr R Dick, Consultant Radiologist, The Royal Free Hospital, London.)

enlarged are occasionally indistinguishable from neighbouring blood vessels, nerves or small bowel loops. Intravenous contrast administration can improve nodal demonstration in these situations.

Skeletal metastases may be visualized if the involved parts of the skeleton are imaged on the CT studies. Local recurrences of tumour after radical prostatectomy present as a soft tissue mass within the prostatic bed; this may be confused with postoperative scar formation. Follow-up examinations are therefore important to differentiate between scar tissue and tumour recurrences. A baseline examination 6–8 weeks after a radical prostatectomy may be of value because at this time the postoperative reactive changes are completed.

CT staging

T1 tumours cannot be identified by CT. T2 tumours are detected only if they lead to a nodular contour irregularity accompanied by a lack of evidence of extension beyond the prostatic capsule. Evidence of invasion into periprostatic fat tissue or seminal vesicles classifies the tumour as T3. Extensive invasion of the urinary bladder, rectum and pelvic floor muscles is classified as T4. The N category is assigned on the basis of the identification of enlarged or multiple lymph nodes within the regional or juxtaregional lymph node. The mean sensitivity, specificity and accuracy for T2 versus T3 staging is 40%, 79% and 58%, respectively (see Table 10.2.1). This has led some authors to conclude that CT has minimal utility in detecting extraprostatic extension of disease in patients with clinically local disease and should not be used to influence decisions concerning management.[5,9] In summary CT is of limited use in the staging and detection of localized disease but it may be helpful in detecting unsuspected nodal involvement.

MAGNETIC RESONANCE IMAGING

MRI is a rapidly evolving, versatile technique offering multiplanar imaging, with excellent contrast and spatial resolution of tissues. Early attempts at pelvic imaging were hampered by excess motion artefact and so associated with poor image resolution. The quality of MRI of the prostate has improved with the development of improved coil technology and faster imaging sequences, resulting in a reduced motion artefact and improved resolution.

Before the development of endorectal coils,[13] imaging was performed with body coils. Body coils had the advantage of providing a large field of view encompassing the entire pelvis and so allowing evaluation of adenopathy and bones, but the limited signal-to-noise ratio resulted in relatively poor quality images of the prostate. Introduction of fast sequences (for example, multiplanar fast spin echo), for use with both body and surface coils, has resulted in reduction of the motion artefact and use of higher resolution matrix, and allowed time to produce more T2 weighting for pathological evaluation compared with images obtained with conventional spin echo sequences.[14] Fat-suppression techniques have also contributed to improving image quality.[14]

MRI techniques

Technical aspects of MRI are constantly evolving. To date three basic techniques have been adopted. Earlier studies used only body coil imaging (BCMR) and resulted in poor prostatic resolution. This was followed by the development of endorectal coil MRI (ERMR), which provided high-resolution images of the structures around the rectum, particularly the mid and posterior aspects of the prostate, but poor evaluation of the anterior margin; the ERMR examination is performed in conjunction with body coil imaging. This allows simultaneous pelvic imaging and so the position of the endorectal coil can be optimized.

The third technical modification is the use of an additional, phased-array, pelvic-surface coil combined with the endorectal coil to produce high-resolution images of the entire prostate and pelvis. This coil configuration produces a more homogeneous signal through the prostate, and a higher signal-to-noise ratio, with a decreased reliance upon filtering. The body coil is also used to image the kidneys and the retroperitoneum for lymphadenopathy. The use of surface coils (including the endorectal coil) is technically challenging and associated with important artefacts (for example, near field effect, ghosting) which should be appreciated before image interpretation.[14]

In general, T1-weighted, sagittal localizer and axial images are obtained from the renal hilum to symphysis pubis, using the body coil. This can be followed by T2-weighted multiplanar images using the endorectal coil alone or the endorectal–surface coil combination. The use of fast imaging sequences, with or without fat saturation sequences, is used to improve visualization of the periprostatic structures, particularly the neurovascular bundles.

The MRI contrast agent, gadolinium chelate, has been used in the preoperative imaging of prostatic cancer. It has been found to be of marginal benefit and is not for routine use.[14] However, early reports with fast sequence, for example, subtracted Turbo FLASH, has shown potential for improved tumour localization and staging.[15]

Appearance of the prostate gland

On T1-weighted images the entire prostate has a low-intensity signal, surrounded by high-signal periprostatic fat. With T2 weighting the zonal anatomy can be appreciated; the

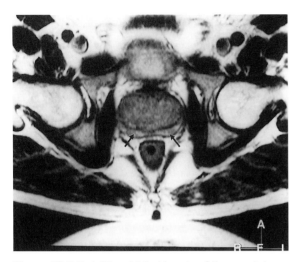

Figure 10.2.5 A T2-weighted image of the prostate obtained with a body coil. The peripheral zone appears brighter than the central gland as a result of its increased water content.

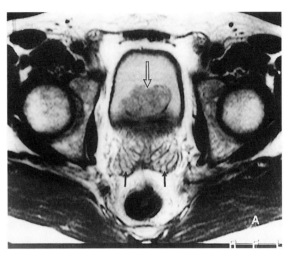

Figure 10.2.6 This body coil MRI demonstrates normal seminal vesicles and hyperplasia of the central zone resulting in invagination of the bladder.

increased water content of the peripheral zone allows T2 weighting to return a high signal intensity relative to the central gland (Figure 10.2.5). The prostate gland–periprostatic fat interphase is seen as a hypointense line incorporating the prostatic capsule.

The central gland consists of the central and transition zones which return a similar low-intensity signal.[16] The central zone may contain nodules of BPH which can have a variable signal intensity with a higher signal representing the glandular element.[17] The anterior fibromuscular stroma, the prostatic capsule and its associated ligamentous attachments are imaged as low-signal structures on T2-weighted images. The bilateral neurovascular bundles appear as low- and high-signal regions on T1- and T2-weighted images respectively.

Seminal vesicles are easily visualized with MRI as a result of the fluid within their lumina. On T1 weighting they appear as symmetrical, low-signal structures; the tubular walls have a higher signal than the luminal contents. The signal intensity of the tubular walls and contents is reversed with T2 weighting, and they appear as a low and high signal respectively

(Figure 10.2.6). The confluence of the vas deferens and seminal vesicles can usually be seen as they form the ejaculatory ducts on coronal imaging.

In the normal prostate the central zone enhances more than the peripheral zone after the administration of contrast agent. Both zones enhance in a homogeneous fashion. In the presence of BPH the enhancement pattern is heterogeneous.[18,19] BPH may occasionally arise in the peripheral zone and so result in inhomogeneous enhancement.

Appearance of prostate cancer

The typical appearance of a cancer in the peripheral zone is a low-signal lesion on T2-weighted images (Figure 10.2.7).[17] The very rare mucin-producing cancers will appear as high-signal lesions on T2 weighting. Central gland cancers (accounting for about 30% of prostate cancers) have intermediate signal. These are often inconspicuous compared with the background of mixed signal arising from benign hyperplastic nodules (Figure 10.2.8).

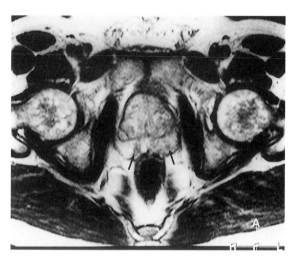

Figure 10.2.7 T2-weighted fat-suppression body coil MRI of the prostate demonstrating hypointense foci within the right and the left peripheral zone, with no evidence of extracapsular spread. There are also changes consistent with BPH within the central gland.

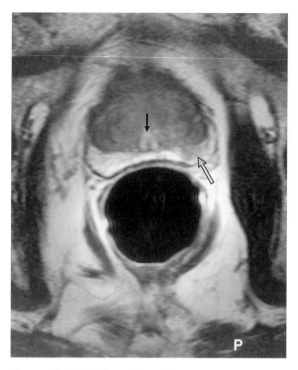

Figure 10.2.8 A T2-weighted ERMR study of the prostate, taken at the level of the veru montanum, distinguishes the hyperintense peripheral zone from the hypointense central gland. The left peripheral zone nodule was confirmed as tumour on pathological mapping.

The transition and central zones are therefore potential 'blind spots' for cancer detection using MRI.[14]

The histopathological basis of the signal intensity is highly complex. Schiebler et al,[17] in their excellent review on endorectal coil imaging, described 27 variations of signal intensity attributed to physiological and pathological intraprostatic conditions. Apart from carcinoma, there are many other causes of a hypointense image in the peripheral zone, including inflammatory, fibrotic and hyperplastic lesions; infarction, radiotherapy and a previous biopsy will also return a low signal. Jager et al[2] reported a false-positive rate of 22% on ERMR using hypointense signal lesions as indicators of carcinoma (Figure 10.2.9). This suggests that histology will continue to be essential for diagnosis of carcinoma of the prostate.

Imaging the primary lesion using MRI is currently unsatisfactory. The abnormal MRI signal results principally from changes in the water content, caused by distortion of prostatic glandular tissue and a possible local tissue reaction to cancer. There are very few studies that have specifically addressed detection of early prostate cancer with detailed pathological correlation using histological mapping of the whole surgical specimen. Two groups[20,21] using BCMR have reported sensitivity for cancer detection within the prostate of 60% and 62%, respectively (Table 10.2.2); both these studies considered only lesions sized 5 mm or more. The reported sensitivity for ERMR from two other groups[2,22] was 48% and 65%, respectively (Table 10.2.3); the minimum size for detected cancers in these studies was not reported. All these studies used different methodologies for histological correlation. This variation limits the value of direct comparison. Nevertheless these studies indicate that 35–52% of pathologically proven cancers are undetected by ERMR imaging

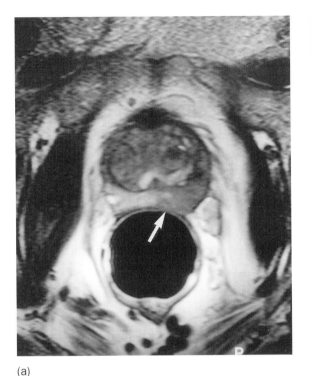

(a)

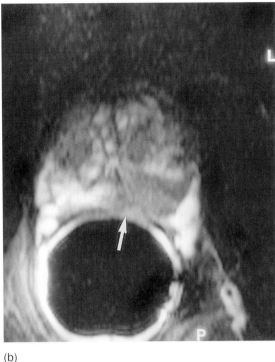

(b)

Figure 10.2.9 (a) T2-weighted and (b) short-tau inversion recovery (STIR) sequences show a hypointense region involving the left peripheral zone with focal disruption of the prostatic capsule, indicating capsular invasion by tumour. The STIR sequence (b), which is fluid sensitive and suppresses signal from fat, demonstrates capsular invasion with greater clarity in this case.

(Figure 10.2.10). As with ultrasonography, detection of tumour in the central gland is more difficult than in the peripheral zone.[15]

Tumour volume is of prognostic importance. If the volume is less than 4 cm³, metastatic disease is unlikely, whereas volumes in excess of 12 cm³ are strongly associated with metastatic disease.[34] The high frequency of cancers undetected by MRI also explains the poor correlation between tumour volume estimations by ERMR and pathological evaluation.[35] Jager et al[2] found that only 21% of imaged lesions had volumes within a 25% range of their histologically matched counterparts.

Use of gadolinium chelate to increase MRI diagnostic information is well described.[18,35,36] These studies suggest that contrast administration generally does not provide additional information; however, it may help in the detection of seminal vesicle invasion in equivocal cases.[18,35]

A critical role of staging is to separate patients with organ-confined disease from those with extracapsular spread (that is, stage T2 from T3) (Figure 10.2.11). A number of MR diagnostic criteria have been described for capsular penetration. Outwater et al[29] studied six of these criteria: extracapsular tumour spread, capsular thickening, stranding, capsular retraction, length of focal bulge and capsular bulging. Of these the highest positive predictive value was obtained with extracapsular tumour spread; all of the diagnostic criteria had moderate-to-poor accuracy. Failure to locate the site and extent of the tumour correctly was a major impediment to correct interpretation, as

Table 10.2.2 Pooled data from nine studies evaluating the usefulness of body coil MRI

		Hricak et al[9] 1987	Biondetti et al[22] 1987	Bezzi et al[23] 1988	Rifkin et al[21] 1990	Scheibler et al[24] 1991	McSherry et al[25] 1991	Schnall et al[26] 1991	Tempany et al[27] 1994	Ellis et al[20] 1994	Mean values
Detection of prostate cancer (%)	Sn				60					62	61
	Sp										
	Acc										
Detection of extracapsular spread (%)	Sn		57								57
	Sp		86								86
	Acc		80						61		71
Detection of seminal vesicle invasion (%)	Sn				28				21		25
	Sp				88				85		87
	Acc										
Detection of lymph node metastasis (%)	Sn	44	100	69	4		0				43
	Sp	100	100	95	96		100				98
	Acc										
Distinguishing T2 and T3 (%)	Sn	75		72		47			61		69
	Sp	88		84		63			62		78
	Acc	83		78		52		66	62		72

Sn, sensitivity; Sp, specificity; Acc, accuracy.

Table 10.2.3 Pooled data from nine studies evaluating the usefulness of endorectal coil MRI

		Schnall et al[26] 1991	Chelsky et al[28] 1993	Tempany et al[27] 1994	Outwater et al[29] 1994	Huch Boni et al[30] 1995	Jager et al[2] 1996	Bates et al[31] 1996	Presti et al[32] 1996	Perroti et al[33] 1996	Mean values
Detection of prostate cancer (%)	Sn				48		65				57
Detection of extracapsular spread (%)	Sn		38		68		42	50	91	22	52
	Sp		96		72		87	100	49	84	81
	Acc		66	45	71		75			64	64
Detection of seminal vesicle invasion (%)	Sn		63	21			36	100	50	23	49
	Sp		97	85			89	94	94	93	92
	Acc		91				79			77	82
Detection of lymph node metastasis (%)	Sn									0	0
	Sp									91	91
	Acc							77		76	76
Distinguishing T2 and T3 (%)	Sn	93	58	60		89	67			73	73
	Sp	84	78	42		87	68			72	72
	Acc	91	68	67		88	68			77	77

Sn, sensitivity; Sp, specificity; Acc, accuracy.

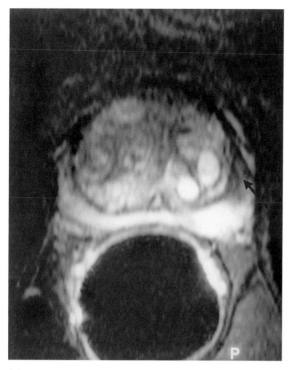

(a)

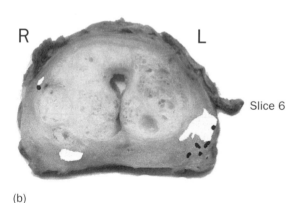

R　　　　　　L

Slice 6

(b)

Figure 10.2.10 (a) An ERMR study using a STIR sequence of a patient with localized carcinoma. A hypointense region is seen adjacent to the pseudocapsule within the left peripheral zone. (b) Pathological map obtained post-radical prostatectomy confirms this as being tumour and the central zone cysts as being BPH (white areas = tumour, black areas = PIN). Note the only one of three foci of tumour was detected on the imaging study. (Pathology courtesy of Dr M Jarmulowicz, Consultant Pathologist, The Royal Free Hospital, London.)

was microscopic invasion. The mean sensitivity, specificity and accuracy of pooled studies evaluating capsular penetration are 52%, 81% and 64%, respectively, for ERMR (see Table 10.2.3). Assessing the usefulness of the periprostatic venous plexus signal in detecting extracapsular tumour extension signal, Biondetti et al[22] reported their preliminary results in 1987 using the BCMR, claiming sensitivity, specificity and accuracy of 57%, 86% and 80%, respectively. The extent of capsular transgression and the size of the primary lesion were not reported; these results have not been reproduced recently and comparison with more recent endorectal coil studies is probably not justified. Yu et al[1] demonstrated that obliteration of the rectoprostatic angles and asymmetry of the neurovascular bundles were the most reliable ERMR features of extracapsular extension.

Seminal vesicle invasion has been more extensively studied with ERMR than with BCMR (see Figure 10.2.11). On T2-weighted images the main conditions that will cause a reduced signal intensity of the seminal vesicles are tumour infiltration, radiation, hormonal therapy and postbiopsy sequelae.[14] The mean sensitivity, specificity and accuracy of pooled studies evaluating seminal vesicle invasion are 49%, 92% and 82%, respectively, with ERMR (see Table 10.2.3). The corresponding values with BCMR are sensitivity 21–28% and specificity 85–88% (see Table 10.2.2).

As with CT there is a tremendous variation in the detection rates of lymphadenopathy with MRI. The criteria for lymph node involvement are size dependent and similar to CT. Multiplanar MRI can evaluate nodal size with greater accuracy than CT, but is still limited by its inability to detect metastasis in normal size-nodes. The mean sensitivity and specificity of the pooled studies evaluating lymph node involvement are 17% (range 0–50%) and 98%, respectively (see Table 10.2.1). Rifkin et al[21] reported results from a large study comprising 185 patients with a sensitivity of only 4%, although the specificity was 96%. Using a size limit of 8 mm, Jager et al[37] reported a sensitivity of 60%, a specificity of 98%, and an accuracy of 89% in patients with localized carcinoma of the prostate.

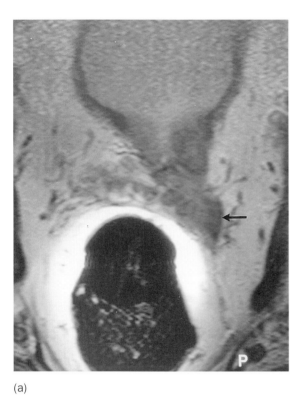

(a)

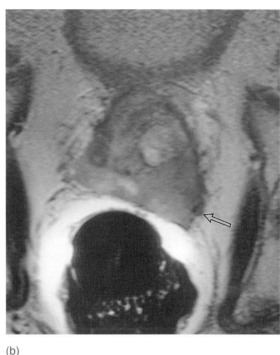

(b)

Figure 10.2.11 A T2-weighted endorectal MRI of a patient with advanced prostate cancer detected at transurethral resection of the prostate demonstrating: (a) bladder base and left seminal vesicle invasion and (b) left neurovascular invasion.

The routine use of imaging to evaluate lymph node metastases is probably not justified as a result of low diagnostic yield – particularly in patients with early prostate cancer. Analysis of cost by Wolf et al[38] demonstrated that imaging should be restricted to patients with a high probability of lymph node disease. Jager et al[37] recommend MRI staging only for patients who are candidates for radical total prostatectomy, with a Gleason score of more than 7 and PSA of more than 10 ng/ml.

Staging of prostate cancer

The staging efficacy of ERMR and BCMR is of great interest. Schiebler et al[14] performed an extensive meta-analysis of both techniques.

They reported sensitivity, specificity and accuracy of pooled data as 65%, 69% and 66% for BCMR. The corresponding values for ERMR were 87%, 81% and 83%, respectively. These authors concluded that the staging superiority of ERMR was most probably the result of superior image resolution. None of the studies incorporated protocols including both BCMR and ERMR. The conclusions therefore lack the power of a truly comparative study.

COMPARATIVE IMAGING

Comparative studies evaluate competing imaging modalities, so patients undergo imaging by all the modalities being evaluated. The superiority of imaging-based evaluation over clinical

Table 10.2.4 Pooled data from eight comparative studies

Study	Year	CT (%)			TRUS (%)			BCMR (%)			ERMR (%)		
		Sn	Sp	Acc	Sn	Sp	Acc	Sn	Sp	Acc	Sn	Sp	Acc
Salo et al[8]	1987	25	89	60	86	94	90						
Hricak et al[9]	1987	55	73	65				75	88	83			
Rifkin et al[21]	1990				58			62					
Schnanal et al[26]	1991									66	93	94	91
Ellis et al[20]	1994				64			60					
Tempany et al[27]	1994							61	62	62	60	42	67
Huch Boni et al[30]	1995				42	100	70	68	87	76	89	87	88
Presti et al[32]	1996				48	71							
Mean value		40	81	63	60	88	80	65	79	72	83	66	82

Sn, sensitivity; Sp, specificity; Acc, accuracy.

staging by digital rectal examination (DRE) which often understages the local extent of the disease,[39] is generally accepted. Some imaging modalities are better than others. CT and BCMR lack the resolution to detect subtle extracapsular or seminal vesicle invasion and offer little advantage for the purpose of local staging. The results of some of the major comparative studies performed to date are summarized in Table 10.2.4. No study has evaluated CT, TRUS, BCMR and ERMR simultaneously. Huch Boni et al[30] performed a small (33 patients), prospective, comparative study to evaluate the diagnostic value of ERMR, BCMR, TRUS, DRE and PSA levels. They found that ERMR was the most sensitive, specific and accurate test. The staging accuracy of ERMR was 88%, BCMR 76%, TRUS 70% and DRE 57%, with further improvement in accuracy when imaging was combined with PSA levels.

Currently both MRI and TRUS are used to stage patients with clinically localized disease. Rifkin et al,[21] in a multicentre study of 219 patients, found BCMR to be more sensitive than TRUS for staging prostatic cancer (77% vs 66%, respectively). Ellis et al[20] have performed the largest study involving over 340 patients, but failed to demonstrate a significant difference in sensitivity between BCMR and TRUS.

The comparison between ERMR and TRUS is less controversial. Huch Boni et al[30] demonstrated a 22% advantage when comparing ERMR with TRUS in terms of staging accuracy. Presti et al,[35] using fast spin echo sequences and phased array pelvic coils, also showed that ERMR was more sensitive than TRUS in detecting extracapsular spread. However, the patients included in these studies had localized disease defined by TRUS and so a selection bias may have influenced these results.

The choice of the optimal MRI technique is not well established. Tempany et al[27] performed a multicentre evaluation of three techniques in 213 patients, comparing BCMR (conventional spin echo) without fat suppression, with BCMR (conventional spin echo) with fat suppression and ERMR (conventional spin echo). The pooled staging accuracy varied from 60% for ERMR to 64% for BCMR with fat suppression. A marked variation in the performance of individual radiologists was also noted, with sensitivities varying between 33% and 83%. These results illustrate the importance of experience when interpreting MRI scans. Huch Boni et al[30] demonstrated a 12% improvement in staging accuracy with ERMR when compared with BCMR. The excellent staging accuracies reported from such small studies have not been reproduced in larger studies. To our knowledge there are no large studies comparing ERMR (using fast spin echo sequences and pelvic phased-array coils) with conventional ERMR or BCMR. Early results with ERMR using fast spin echo sequences and pelvic phased-array coils are promising.[32]

VALUE OF IMAGING IN CLINICALLY LOCALIZED PROSTATE CANCER

The value of imaging is controversial and is determined by its impact on therapeutic decision-making. In the setting of prostatic cancer, new developments result in new demands from imaging. As with all imaging modalities the urological surgeon wants to know which patients have resectable disease. Radiologists can usually detect patients with irresectable disease, but find it difficult to rule out localized microscopic or low-volume macroscopic disease because these processes are beyond the resolution of current imaging modalities. The potential value of imaging modalities is dependent on many factors (availability of equipment, experience of radiologist, cost, patient selection, etc). It is therefore difficult to predict the value of imaging at a local centre based on studies performed at other institutions. Each centre must therefore audit its own results and determine the impact of imaging on local clinical management.

Perroti et al[33] evaluated ERMR (using conventional spin echo). Patients with localized disease detected and staged conventionally underwent ERMR before radical retropubic total prostatectomy. ERMR images were compared with the pathological findings. Using this technique the authors found that 21% of patients were overstaged, so these patients could have been denied potentially curative surgery. These authors concluded that ERMR in their institutions, using local patient selection criteria, was not sufficiently accurate to influence the treatment of patients with clinically localized disease. It is possible that the clinical impact of their imaging could be improved using fast spin echo sequences and phased-array pelvic coils; however, this is only one of many factors with a potential clinical impact. The 'best' published series should serve only as an indicator of best practice in a specified centre. One should not assume that these results are directly translatable into local practice.

DETECTION OF METASTASIS

MRI and CT are comparable in their ability to detect lymph node metastases. Introduction of newer techniques, such as fine needle aspiration biopsy of nodes, under CT guidance (and MRI more recently), has further enhanced the accuracy of imaging.[11] These cross-sectional modalities have largely replaced lymphography (see Figure 10.2.4) for the evaluation of nodal disease.

The routine skeletal survey has no role in imaging advanced disease. Plain radiographs should be used to evaluate equivocal lesions on bone scintigraphy or to evaluate complications of metastatic bone disease. Bone scintigraphy remains the method of choice for routine evaluation of bone metastases. MRI has been shown to be a valuable tool for skeletal imaging, particularly with early skeletal metastases when bone scintigraphy, CT and plain films are negative.[40] MRI is more sensitive because it can detect bone marrow lesions before the development of any secondary cortical change (Figure 10.2.12). Routine MRI staging of prostate cancer includes images of the lumbar spine, sacrum and pelvis. These areas are commonly involved by metastases. In the current economic climate, the cost of MRI makes the evaluation of the

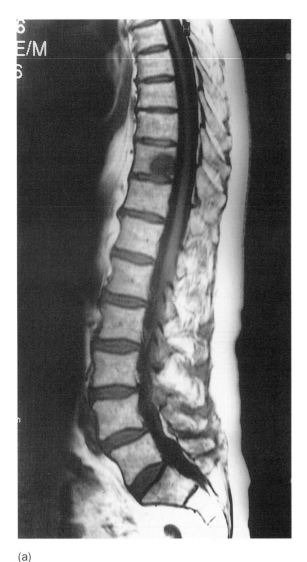

(a)

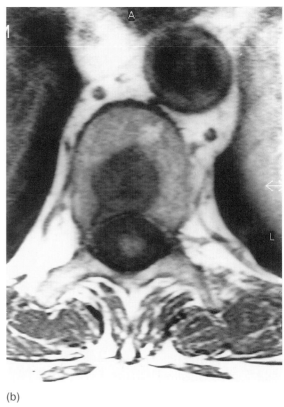

(b)

Figure 10.2.12 A solitary metastasis within the T10 vertebral body demonstrated on (a) sagittal MRI and (b) axial T1-weighted MRI.

appendicular skeleton with MRI an impractical option. Therefore MRI for routine evaluation cannot at present be recommended and should be reserved for patients with equivocal results on bone scintigraphy and plain films.

Intrathoracic metastatic disease is not uncommon in patients with prostate cancer. At presentation, 6% of patients will have intrathoracic metastases.[41] The manifestations of intrathoracic malignancy are varied and include pleural effusions, pulmonary nodules, medi-

astinal adenopathy and lymphangitis carcinomatosis. The chest radiograph remains the first imaging investigation; coexisting pathology (for example, cardiac insufficiency, pneumonia and pulmonary infarction) can complicate radiographic appearances. Thoracic CT is useful in situations where there is uncertainty.

Postmortem studies show a high incidence of intra-abdominal metastatic disease. A study of 1885 patients[42] showed a high incidence of liver (35%) and adrenal (17%) metastases. A significant number of patients also had renal, peritoneal, splenic and pancreatic deposits. These intra-abdominal lesions can be detected using ultrasonography, CT or MRI. The choice of imaging is determined by local availability, cost and potential impact on the clinical management.

MRI is the method of choice for the detection of spinal disease, particularly when associated with clinical features of spinal cord or nerve root compression. Myelography is almost exclusively performed in centres with limited access to MRI. Intracranial metastatic disease is readily imaged with MRI or contrast-enhanced CT.

MONITORING THERAPY

A number of prostate ablative therapies (cryosurgery, laser photocoagulation and hormonal treatments) can be evaluated using MRI.[43–45] ERMR has also been reported to be highly successful in the evaluation of postsurgical recurrence.[46]

FUTURE IMAGING DEVELOPMENTS

The value of current imaging modalities can be enhanced by patient selection using nonimaging parameters, that is, PSA, Gleason scores and age. Seltzer et al[47] further refined this integrated approach using a radiologist–computer system which substantially improved staging accuracy.

Developments in technology, particularly in faster imaging sequences (echo planar sequences), improved coil design and dynamically enhanced MRI, are likely to make a significant impact. The dynamic subtracted Turbo FLASH sequence has the potential to discriminate between high- and low-grade cancers. Jager et al[15] demonstrated more rapid enhancement and washout in the more poorly differentiated lesions. These findings are promising even though they did not impact directly upon staging in prostate cancer. These techniques may be useful in differentiating between postbiopsy residual tumour, oedema, scar and granulation tissue.[48]

MR spectroscopy is currently attracting considerable attention. Spectroscopic evaluation of the prostate can give valuable chemical information. Estimation of the choline and citrate proton spectra can aid in distinguishing benign from malignant prostate tissue.[49]

CONCLUSION

Histology remains the gold standard for diagnosis. Staging based upon imaging is more accurate than clinical evaluation alone. CT has no role in the routine evaluation of localized prostatic cancer, although CT-guided fine needle biopsy of suspicious nodes seen on CT or MRI may be useful. ERMR is probably superior to TRUS in the staging of clinically localized disease, but there is doubt as to whether either modality is sufficiently accurate to influence the management of patients with clinically localized disease. Therefore the results of imaging should be combined with other parameters of disease activity in determining optimal patient management. The wider availability of fast imaging sequences and spectroscopy are likely to make a significant impact.

Each centre treating patients with prostate cancer must develop and continually evaluate imaging protocols based on local expertise and resources. This process will be aided by well-designed, prospective, comparative studies with pathological correlation.

REFERENCES

1. Yu KK, Hricak H, Alagappan R, Chernoff DM, Bacchetti P, Zaloudek CJ, Detection of extracapsular extension of prostate carcinoma with endorectal and phased-array coil MR imaging: multivariate feature analysis. *Radiology* 1997; **202:** 697–702.

2. Jager GJ, Ruijter ET, Van de Kaa CA et al, Local staging of prostate cancer with endorectal MR imaging: correlation with histopathology. *AJR* 1996; **166:** 845–52.

3. Price JM, Davidson AJ, Computed tomography in the evaluation of the suspected carcinomatous prostate. *Urol Radiol* 1979; **1:** 39.

4. Flanigan RC, Mohler JL, King CT et al, Preoperative lymphnode evaluation in prostatic cancer patients who are surgical candidates; the role of lymphangiography and CT scanning with directed fine needle aspiration. *J Urol* 1985; **134:** 84.

5. Platt JF, Bree RL, Schwab RE, The accuracy of CT in the staging of carcinoma of the prostate. *AJR* 1987; **149:** 315–18.

6. Salo J, Kivisari L, Rannokko S et al, Computerised tomography and transrectal ultrasound in the assessment of local extension of prostatic cancer before radical retropubic prostatectomy. *J Urol* 1987; **137:** 435–8.

7. Hricak H, Dooms GC, Jeffrey RB et al, Prostatic carcinoma: Staging by clinical assessment, CT and MR imaging. *Radiology* 1987; **162:** 331–6.

8. Hammerer P, Huland H, Sparenberg A, Digital rectal examination, imaging, and systematic sextant biopsy in identifying operable lymphnode negative prostatic carcinoma. *Eur Urol* 1992; **22:** 281.

9. Konety BR, Naraghi R, Gooding W et al, Evaluation of computerised tomography for staging of clinically localised adenocarcinoma of the prostate. *Urol Oncol* 1996; **2:** 14–19.

10. Larner J, Gay S, Grizos W et al, Significance of CT scan detected seminal vesicle enlargement in prostate cancer. A pilot study. *Urology* 1993; **41:** 259–61.

11. Oyen RH, Van Poppel HP, Ameye FE et al, Lymph node staging of localised prostatic carcinoma with CT and CT guided fine needle aspiration biopsy: Prospective study of 285 patients. *Radiology* 1994; **190:** 315–22.

12. Pilepich MV, Perez CA, Prasas S, Computed tomography in definitive radiotherapy of prostatic carcinoma. *Int J Radiat Oncol Biol Phys* 1980; **6:** 923–7.

13. Schnall MD, Lenkinski RE, Gatsonis CA et al, MR imaging with an endorectal surface coil. *Radiology* 1989; **172:** 570–4.

14. Schiebler ML, Schnall MD, Pollack HM et al, Current role of MR imaging in the staging of adenocarcinoma of the prostate. *Radiology* 1993; **189:** 339–52.

15. Jager GJ, Ruijter ETG, Van de Kaa CA et al, Dynamic Turbo FLASH subtraction technique for contrast enhanced MR imaging of the prostate. *Radiology* 1997; **203:** 645–52.

16. Hricak H, Dooms GC, McNeal JE et al, MR imaging of the prostate gland: Normal anatomy. *AJR* 1987; **148:** 51–7.

17. Schiebler ML, Tomaszewski JE, Bezzi M et al, Prostatic carcinoma and benign prostatic hyperplasia: Correlation of high resolution MR and histopathological findings. *Radiology* 1989; **172:** 131–7.

18. Mirrorwitz SA, Brown JJ, Heiken JP, Evaluation of the prostate and prostatic carcinoma with gadolinium-enhanced endorectal coil MR imaging. *Radiology* 1993; **186:** 153–7.

19. Brown G, MacVicar DA, Ayton V, Husband JE, The role of intravenous contrast enhancement in magnetic resonance imaging of prostatic carcinoma. *Clin Radiol* 1995; **50:** 601–6.

20. Ellis JH, Tempany C, Sarin MS et al, MR imaging and sonography of early prostatic cancer: pathologic and imaging features that influence identification and diagnosis. *AJR* 1994; **162:** 865–72.

21. Rifkin MD, Zehourni EA, Gatsonis CA et al, Comparison of magnetic resonance imaging and ultrasonography in staging early prostate cancer. *N Engl J Med* 1990; **323:** 621–6.

22. Biondetti PR, Lee JK, Ling D et al, Clinical stage B prostate carcinoma: Staging with MR imaging. *Radiology* 1987; **162:** 325–9.

23. Bezzi M, Kressel HY, Allen KS et al, Prostatic carcinoma: Staging with MR imaging at 1.5T. *Radiology* 1988; **169:** 339–46.

24. Scheibler ML, McSherry S, Keefe B et al, Comparison of the digital rectal examination, endorectal ultrasound and body coil magnetic resonance imaging in the staging of adenocarcinoma of the prostate. *Urol Radiol* 1991; **13:** 110–18.

25. McSherry SA, Levy F, Schiebler ML et al, Preoperative prediction of pathological tumour volume and stage in clinically localised prostate cancer: Comparison of digital rectal examina-

tion, transrectal ultrasonography and magnetic resonance imaging. *J Urol* 1991; **146:** 85.

26. Schnall MD, Imai Y, Tomaszewski J et al, Prostate cancer: Local staging with endorectal surface coil MR imaging. *Radiology* 1991; **178:** 797–802.

27. Tempany CM, Zhou X, Zerhouni EA et al, Staging of prostate cancer: Results of Radiology Diagnostic Oncology Group Project comparison of three MRI techniques. *Radiology* 1994; **192:** 47–54.

28. Chelsky MJ, Schnall MD, Seidmon EJ et al, Use of endorectal surface coil magnetic resonance imaging for local staging of prostate cancer. *J Urol* 1993; **150:** 391–5.

29. Outwater EK, Petersen RO, Siegelman ES et al, Prostate carcinoma: Assessment of diagnostic criteria for capsular penetration on endorectal MR images. *Radiology* 1994; **193:** 333–9.

30. Huch Boni RA, Boner JA, Dbatin JF et al, Optimisation of prostate carcinoma staging: Comparison of imaging and clinical methods. *Clin Radiol* 1995; **50:** 593–600.

31. Bates TS, Cavanagh PM, Speakman M et al, Endorectal MRI using a 0.5T mid field system in the staging of localised prostate cancer. *Clin Radiol* 1996; **51:** 550–3.

32. Presti JC, Hricak H, Narayan PA et al, Local staging of prostatic carcinoma: comparison of transrectal sonography and endorectal MR imaging. *AJR* 1996; **166:** 103–8.

33. Perrotti M, Kaufman RP, Jennings TA et al, Endorectal coil magnetic resonance imaging in clinically localised prostate cancer: Is it accurate? *J Urol* 1996; **156:** 106–9.

34. McNeal JE, Cancer volume and site of origin of adenocarcinoma of the prostate: relationship to local and distant spread. *Human Pathol* 1992; **23:** 258–66.

35. Huch Boni RA, Boner JA, Lutolf UM et al, Contrast enhanced endorectal coil MRI in local staging of prostate carcinoma. *J Comput Assist Tomogr* 1995; **19:** 232–7.

36. Sommer FG, Nghiem HV, Herfkens R et al, Gadolinium-enhanced MRI of the abnormal prostate. *Magn Reson Imaging* 1993; **11:** 941–8.

37. Jager GJ, Barentsz JO, Oosterhof GO, Witjes JA, Ruijs SJ, Pelvic adenopathy in prostatic and urinary bladder carcinoma: MR imaging with a 3D

T1 weighted MP RAGE sequence. *AJR* 1996; **167:** 1503–7.

38. Wolf JS, Cher M, Dalla'Era M et al, The use and accuracy of cross-sectional imaging and fine needle aspiration cytology for the detection of pelvic lymph node metastases before radical prostatectomy. *J Urol* 1995; **153:** 993–9.

39. Mukamel E, Hannah J, DeKernion JB, Pitfalls in preoperative staging in prostate cancer. *Urology* 1987; **30:** 318–21.

40. Avrahami E, Tadmore R, Dally O et al, Early MR demonstration of spinal metastases in patients with normal radiographs, and CT and radionuclide bone scans. *J Comput Assist Tomogr* 1989; **13:** 598–602.

41. Lindell MM, Doubleday LC, Von Eschenbach AC et al, Mediastinal metastases from prostatic carcinoma. *J Urol* 1982; **128:** 331–4.

42. Saitoh H, Hida M, Shimbo T et al, Metastatic patterns of prostate cancer: Correlation between the sites and number of organs involved. *Cancer* 1984; **54:** 3078–84.

43. Kalbhen CL, Hricak H, Shinohara K et al, Prostate carcinoma: MRI findings after cryosurgery. *Radiology* 1996; **198:** 807–11.

44. Chen M, Hricak H, Kalbhen CL et al, Hormonal ablation of prostatic cancer: effects on prostate morphology, tumour detection, and staging by endorectal coil MRI. *AJR* 1996; **166:** 1157–63.

45. Kurhanewwicz J, Vigneron DB, Hricak H et al, Prostate cancer: metabolic response to cryosurgery as detected with 3D H-1 MR spectroscopic imaging. *Radiology* 1996; **200:** 489–96.

46. Silverman JM, Krebs TL, MR imaging evaluation with a transrectal surface coil of local recurrence of prostatic cancer in men who have undergone radical prostatectomy. *AJR* 1997; **168:** 379–85.

47. Seltzer SE, Getty DJ, Tempany CM et al, Staging prostate cancer with MR imaging: a combined radiologist-computer system. *Radiology* 1997; **202:** 219–26.

48. Barentsz JO, Jager GJ, van Vierzen PBJ et al, Staging urinary bladder cancer after transurethral biopsy: Value of fast dynamic contrast-enhanced MR imaging. *Radiology* 1996; **201:** 185–93.

49. Kurhanewwicz J, Vigneron DB, Hricak H et al, 3D H-1 MR spectroscopic imaging of the in situ human prostate with high (0.24–0.77 cm^3) spatial resolution. *Radiology* 1996; **198:** 795–805.

11 Surgery

11.1 RADICAL RETROPUBIC PROSTATECTOMY • 11.2 RADICAL PERINEAL PROSTATECTOMY • 11.3 LAPAROSCOPIC PELVIC LYMPHADENECTOMY

11.1

Radical retropubic prostatectomy for localized prostate cancer

Apoorva R Vashi, Joseph E Oesterling

CONTENTS • Anatomy pertinent to radical prostatectomy • Indications • Patient preparation • Technique • Postoperative care • Efficacy • Complications • Summary

The diagnosis of prostate cancer has been revolutionized in recent years by the discovery of prostate-specific antigen (PSA) and the application of transrectal ultrasound (TRUS) with biopsy. PSA has been shown to diagnose significantly more cancers than digital rectal examination (DRE) as well as a greater proportion of organ-confined cancers.[1-3] TRUS-guided prostate biopsy and the development of the sextant biopsy have further enhanced our diagnostic ability.[4] These advances in cancer detection have been paralleled by significant advances in prostate cancer therapy, namely the development of the anatomical radical retropubic prostatectomy. The anatomical radical prostatectomy has allowed us to apply surgical therapy to an increasingly younger population, with minimal morbidity and excellent cancer control.

The origins of radical surgery for prostate cancer date to work done at the Johns Hopkins Hospital. In 1904, Hugh Young, with the assistance of his chief William Halstead (pioneer of the radical mastectomy), utilized a perineal approach to perform the first radical prostatectomy for prostate cancer.[4,5] Hugh Jewett, Elmer Belt, GG Smith and others further popularized this approach. In 1945, Terrence Millin[6] introduced a retropubic operation for benign prostatic hyperplasia (BPH) and later modified it for radical prostatectomy. For numerous reasons, this is now the most popular form of radical prostatectomy.

However, until approximately 15 years ago this procedure had unacceptable morbidity, including urinary incontinence, erectile dysfunction and major blood loss. As efforts at early detection were reaching new heights, it became increasingly necessary to develop a more effective form of therapy. Much of the credit belongs to Patrick C Walsh, whose meticulous work redefined the anatomical radical prostatectomy. Walsh and Reiner outlined the penile venous drainage in the area of the prostate gland, and then developed a method to control the dorsal venous complex and eliminate significant hemorrhage.[7] Walsh also delineated the autonomic innervation to the corpora cavernosa, and developed and popularized the nerve-sparing radical prostatectomy.[8] Similarly, Myers and others[9] enhanced our understanding of the male urethral sphincteric mechanism and the importance of apical dissection, which decreases the incidence of urinary incontinence.

This knowledge has given the retropubic approach further advantages over the perineal approach. The approach provides easy access to the pelvic lymph nodes and allows for preservation of sexual function. In the most experienced hands,[10] the perineal approach preserves sexual function in only 25–30% of patients, which is significantly less than the retropubic approach (see below). Since the anatomy has been carefully outlined, the approach is easier to teach and learn. In addition, the approach leads to fewer rectal injuries.

In this chapter we describe the anatomical radical retropubic prostatectomy as it is performed at the University of Michigan. This technique provides excellent vascular control and exposure, allowing for preservation of the autonomic innervation to the corpora cavernosa. In addition, it allows for preservation of the urethra (when indicated) to maximize the chance of urinary continence.

ANATOMY PERTINENT TO RADICAL PROSTATECTOMY

A general overview of pelvic anatomy is illustrated in Figure 11.1.1.

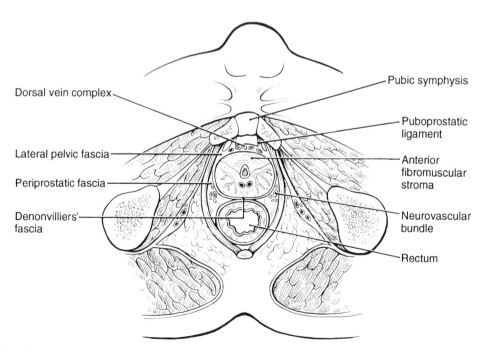

Figure 11.1.1 General anatomical relationships of the prostate gland.

Fascial relations

The endopelvic (pelvic) fascia is a thin layer of connective tissue that sweeps down from the lateral pelvic side wall and covers the bladder and prostate. The parietal pelvic fascia covers the levator ani musculature, and the visceral pelvic fascia covers the bladder and prostate. The convergence of these two leaves forms a white line (the tendinous arch) and superiorly forms the puboprostatic ligaments.[11] During radical prostatectomy, the endopelvic fascia is incised just lateral to this white line. After incision, a remnant levator fascia remains attached to the prostate, and this is termed the 'lateral pelvic fascia'. The lateral pelvic fascia covers the neurovascular bundle, which lies posterolateral to the prostate. Posteriorly, a thin layer of connective tissue facilitates mobilization between the prostate and rectum. This structure is termed 'Denonvilliers' fascia', and must be included in the specimen as it has been shown to be invaded in approximately 19% of radical prostatectomy specimens.[12]

Arterial and venous anatomy

The arterial supply of the prostate originates from the inferior vesical artery (Figure 11.1.2). This artery terminates in two groups of prostatic vessels: the urethral and capsular branches.[13] The capsular vessels travel in the lateral pelvic fascia, along with the cavernous nerves, to form the neurovascular bundle.[8]

The venous drainage of the prostate is highly variable and is known as Santorini's plexus (Figure 11.1.3). The multitude of penile sinuses coalesce to form the deep dorsal vein, which exits the penile hilum anterior to the membra-

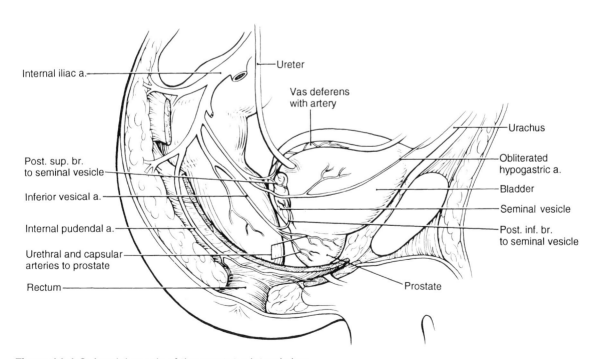

Figure 11.1.2 Arterial supply of the prostate: lateral view.

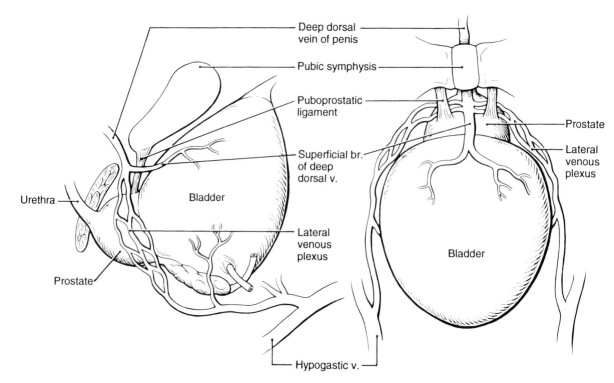

Figure 11.1.3 Venous drainage of the prostate gland: lateral and anterior views. Note the relationship of the dorsal venous complex to the urethra and puboprostatic ligaments.

nous urethra and the apex of the prostate. At this level it divides into a superficial branch, which travels between the puboprostatic ligaments, and the right and left tributaries that course posterolaterally, eventually emptying into the internal iliac vein.[7,13] Proper control of these veins is essential in obtaining exposure and a bloodless field, which are necessary to preserve urinary continence and normal erectile function.

Cavernous nerves

Sympathetic nerve fibers from T11 to L2 give rise to the sympathetic nerve chain, which forms the hypogastric nerve. Parasympathetic fibers from S2 to S4 form the pelvic nerve, and together with the hypogastric and pelvic nerve enter the pelvic plexus. The cavernous nerves arise from the pelvic plexus cephalad and posterior to the tips of each seminal vesicle. They course posterolaterally (at the 5 and 7 o'clock positions) to the prostate contained in the neurovascular bundle covered by the lateral pelvic fascia.[8,11]

Anatomy of the urethral sphincter and membranous urethra

Knowledge of the anatomy of the urethral sphincter is necessary to preserve urinary continence (Figure 11.1.4). Turner-Warwick[14,15]

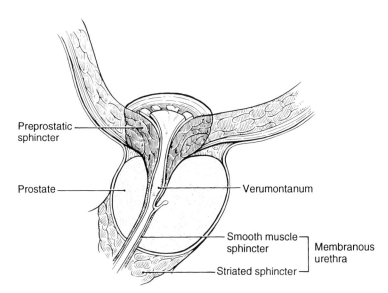

Figure 11.1.4 Anatomy of the genitourinary sphincters. Note the preprostatic sphincter centered at the bladder neck and extending to the verumontanum. The membranous urethra, consisting of the striated and smooth muscle sphincter, also extends to the level of the verumontanum.

Preprostatic sphincter

Prostate

Verumontanum

Smooth muscle sphincter

Striated sphincter

Membranous urethra

divided the posterior urethra into two continence zones. The proximal zone consists of smooth muscle fibers centered at the bladder neck and extending periurethrally to the level of the verumontanum. This is known as the preprostatic sphincter. The distal zone is the membranous urethra, which extends from the verumontanum to the perineal membrane. It is not a flat structure which the prostatic apex rests upon. Together, these two 'continence zones' make up the functional urethral length.[14,15]

The striated sphincter is an array of muscle fibers which extend for a variable distance from the prostate apex to the perineal membrane.[14] During development, the striated sphincter extends to the bladder neck, but as the prostate grows the upper parts of the sphincter are lost.[16] The membranous urethra is composed of four key elements: (1) mucosa and infolding of the urethral crest; (2) longitudinal smooth muscle of the urethral wall (smooth muscle sphincter); (3) striated muscle sphincter; and (4) levator ani musculature. The exact contribution of the striated sphincter to continence is not clear. Although it appears that the smooth mus-

cle sphincter is primarily responsible for continence, both should be considered as sharing in the continence mechanism. Therefore, every attempt should be made to preserve the entire membranous urethra.[14]

Myers and others[9,14] have documented the importance of the apical dissection and transecting the urethra as close to the apex as possible in order to preserve the entire distal continence mechanism. Despite these efforts, some patients are still incontinent postoperatively. In these patients, a greater functional length of urethra needs to be preserved.

Using this knowledge, we have been performing a urethral-sparing radical prostatectomy at the University of Michigan in selected men with small well-differentiated tumors. By preserving the bladder neck, the proximal urethra, and membranous urethra, both continence zones can be preserved and cause the functional length of the urethra to increase. The importance of this length was demonstrated by Hutch and Fischer.[17] On cystogram, they demonstrated a length of 0.7–1.6 cm in five incontinent patients and of 2.6–3.4 cm in seven continent patients. Since the bladder neck and prostatic urethra are distinct structures from the prostatic parenchyma, they can be preserved both proximally and distally, without the concern of leaving positive margins.[18] We feel that this development adds further to the development of postprostatectomy continence.

INDICATIONS

Radical prostatectomy is indicated for a patient with clinically localized prostate cancer (stage T1 or T2) and a life expectancy of 10–15 years or more. No absolute values of Gleason score or serum PSA should preclude surgical therapy, as long as the tumor is felt to be clinically localized. In recent years, specific indications for eliminating lymphadenectomy, cavernous nerve preservation, and urethral preservation have been evolved.

Pelvic lymphadenectomy can be safely eliminated in select patients with prostate cancer, thus decreasing cost and morbidity. The probability of positive pelvic lymph nodes can be predicted from the serum PSA level, primary Gleason grade, and clinical stage from the DRE. Bluestein et al[19] reviewed 1632 consecutive patients and found positive lymph nodes in only 0.7% (predicted false-negative rate 3%)

when the criteria listed in Table 11.1.1 were applied. Using these criteria, up to 60% of patients can be spared the potential cost and morbidity of lymphadenectomy.

Preserving normal erectile function is also possible in select patients by unilateral or bilateral preservation of the neurovascular bundles. Criteria for preservation include: preoperative erectile function, tumor confined to the prostate, lack of induration or nodularity at the apex or posterolateral borders of the prostate, and a serum PSA concentration of less than 10.0 ng/ml. Contraindications include: absent or marginal preoperative erectile function, tumor extension into the neurovascular bundle, induration of the lateral sulcus on preoperative examination, induration of lateral pelvic fascia intraoperatively, or fixation of the bundle to the capsule of the prostate.[20]

Urethral preservation is indicated in men with early stage, well-differentiated tumors that do not involve the transition zone. Contraindications to urethral preservation include: (1) transition-zone tumor; (2) tumor involving the base of the prostate; (3) previous surgery involving the bladder neck; and (4) a large median lobe. In these selected men, pathological evaluation of the specimen has not demonstrated positive margins, including

Table 11.1.1 Criteria for eliminating pelvic lymphadenectomy

Clinical stage	Primary Gleason grade	Serum PSA (ng/ml)
T1 or T2a,b	1–2	<17
	3	<8
	4–5	<4
T2c	1–2	<4
	3	<2
	4–5	<1

where the bladder neck and urethra are dissected from the prostate gland.[21] A well-defined plane exists between the prostate parenchyma and the bladder neck and urethra. If the dissection is difficult, then preservation of the urethra should be abandoned. In these men, cancer control is not compromised and early return of urinary continence is realized.

PATIENT PREPARATION

Preoperative teaching

The patient undergoing an anatomical radical retropubic prostatectomy requires a complete medical evaluation and referral to a subspecialist if indicated. Once clearance has been obtained, preoperative teaching is instituted. This includes incentive spirometer teaching, exercises to prevent deep venous thrombosis, and perineal exercises to strengthen the urinary sphincter.

Autologous blood donation

One of the most important concerns for patients undergoing radical prostatectomy is the need for blood transfusions and autologous blood donation. The literature is highly variable on this topic. Toy et al[22] studied 163 patients from seven hospitals, reporting an average blood loss of 1631 ml and allogeneic blood transfusions in 66% of patients who did not pre-donate and in 20% of those who did. Catalona et al[23] showed similar results with 70% of patients without autologous units requiring allogeneic transfusions compared to 16% of those patients with autologous units. With these data, many authorities have routinely recommended autologous pre-donation of 3–4 units.[22,24]

In contrast, the Mayo Clinic series[25] has shown a dramatic decrease in the rate of transfusion. They reported a decrease in mean blood loss from 1030 ml (before 1988) to 600 ml (after 1988). In addition, the risk of any transfusion decreased from 76% (before 1988) to a current rate of <5% (since 1991).

Goh et al[26] recently reviewed the experience with blood transfusion using the anatomical radical retropubic prostatectomy at the University of Michigan. Overall, 95% of patients did not require an allogeneic blood transfusion; this includes a 0% allogeneic transfusion rate for pre-donors and a 8% rate for non-donors. Of those transfused, 4.4% required one or two units, and only 0.6% required three or more units. Autologous donors were found to have a significantly lower preoperative hematocrit than did non-donors, and only 27% of donors received any of their units back. Pre-donors had an increased rate of blood transfusion (autologous blood only), which was a reflection of their lower preoperative hematocrit, as well as increased physician willingness to transfuse autologous blood. In addition, the average cost of each autologous unit was US$745. Therefore, due to significant cost and a demonstrated lack of necessity, we generally discourage autologous blood donation.

Preoperative preparation and anesthesia

On the night prior to surgery, the patient abstains from oral intake. On the day of surgery, the patient self-administers an enema early in the morning. A formal bowel preparation is not necessary. The authors prefer epidural anesthesia, unless the patient has a strong preference for general anesthesia or there is a contraindication to placing an epidural catheter. Using this approach, the patient can avoid postoperative drowsiness, the postoperative discomfort from the endotracheal tube, and the nausea and vomiting associated with general anesthesia.

TECHNIQUE

Incision and lymphadenectomy

The patient is placed in the supine position with the umbilicus over the break in the table. The table is flexed maximally, and the patient is placed in 20° of Trendelenburg position. The skin is prepared and draped in the standard sterile fashion for radical prostatectomy. An 18-French Foley catheter is placed in the bladder and inflated with 50 ml of saline solution.

A lower midline incision is made from 2 cm below the umbilicus to the pubic symphysis. The linea alba is incised, the rectus muscles separated, and the transversalis fascia incised sharply to enter the space of Retzius. The peritoneum is swept cephalad and mobilized from the external iliac vessels to the bifurcation of the common iliac artery. A self-retaining Balfour retractor is placed.

If clinically indicated, a staging bilateral pelvic lymphadenectomy is performed. This is considered a staging and not a therapeutic procedure. The lymphadenectomy begins with dissection of the lymphatic tissue overlying the external iliac vein. It proceeds superiorly to the bifurcation of the common iliac artery. Lymphatic vessels are ligated with clips as needed. The tissue in the obturator fossa is separated from the pelvic side wall and removed. Care must be taken to avoid injury to the obturator nerve. The obturator vessels usually are not injured, but can be ligated if excessive bleeding occurs. The dissection continues inferiorly to the level of the circumflex iliac vein or node of Cloquet. The lymph-node packet is removed en bloc and evaluated for metastatic disease (Figure 11.1.5).

Incision of endopelvic fascia and division of puboprostatic ligaments

The malleable blade of the Balfour retractor is repositioned in the midline, with the Foley catheter balloon retracted cephalad to provide exposure to the anterior surface of the prostate. The preprostatic adipose tissue is carefully dissected off the prostate to fully expose the endopelvic fascia (Figure 11.1.6). The endopelvic fascia is carefully incised lateral to the tendinous arc (white line), and all the fibers of the levator ani are separated cleanly away from the prostate. Santorini's plexus (formed from the dorsal venous complex) lies medially to this white line in the visceral pelvic fascia and can be visualized after the incision has been made. Therefore, incising the endopelvic fascia too medially risks injury to the venous complex, with potential for significant hemorrhage. The incision in the endopelvic fascia is extended toward the puboprostatic ligaments.

The superficial branch of the dorsal vein lies immediately posterior to the puboprostatic ligaments. Therefore, adequate visualization of these ligaments must be obtained prior to transection. Using Metzenbaum scissors, the fibrous fatty tissue covering the ligaments is teased away, and the scissors are used to separate the venous complex off the posterior edge of the

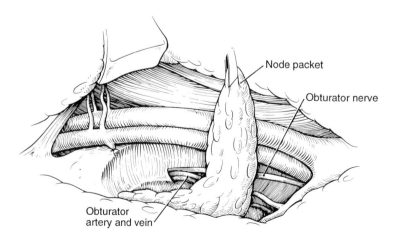

Node packet

Obturator nerve

Obturator artery and vein

Figure 11.1.5 Completion of the lymphadenectomy and removal of the nodal packet. The external iliac vein and obturator nerve are fully exposed. The obturator artery, which contributes to the blood supply of the corpora cavernosa, can be preserved as shown.

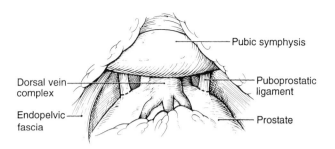

Figure 11.1.6 The periprostatic adipose tissue is removed to expose the endopelvic fascia and puboprostatic ligaments.

ligament. The puboprostatic ligaments are transected sharply under direct vision to enhance the mobility of the apex of the prostate gland. To avoid injury to the underlying vein, only the major portion of the ligament is divided sharply. The residual fragments are fractured bluntly by finger compression.

Control of the dorsal vein complex

As developed by Myers,[27] a special curved Babcock clamp is used to bring all the tissue anterolateral to the prostate together in the midline anterior to the prostate (Figure 11.1.7). Two 0-Chromic sutures are placed through this tissue to prevent back-bleeding when the dorsal venous complex is transected subsequently. A McDougal right-angle clamp is placed in the avascular plane between the anterior aspect of the urethra and the posterior aspect of the dorsal venous complex. A 0-Vicryl suture is passed to this clamp to ligate the dorsal venous complex just distal to the anterior apex of the prostate (Figure 11.1.7, inset). To further secure the complex distally, a sponge stick is used to

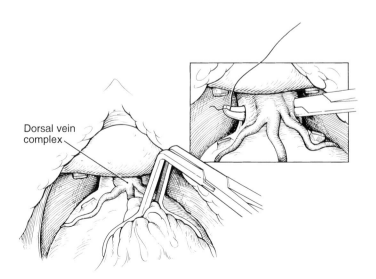

Figure 11.1.7 Control of the dorsal venous complex. A modified Babcock clamp is used to grasp the cut edges of the endopelvic fascia and a 0-Chromic suture is placed to prevent back-bleeding. (Inset) A MacDougal clamp is placed in the avascular plane between the dorsal venous complex anteriorly and the urethra posteriorly and used to grasp a 0-Vicryl tie to secure the complex distally.

expose the lateral aspects of the prostate gland and a 0-Chromic suture is precisely placed on the dorsal vein complex in a figure-of-eight fashion. Care is taken to make sure the stitch is distal to the apex of the prostate, but that it does not incorporate any of the pelvic floor musculature.

With the dorsal venous complex ligated proximally and distally, it can be transected sharply with no bleeding. The absence of hemorrhage at this point allows the surgeon to be precise in his or her transection, so that it occurs at the level of the prostatic apex. This is most important so that the prostatic parenchyma is not violated and the entire urinary sphincter can be left intact and remain functional.

The apical dissection

After ligation of the dorsal vein, because there is minimal bleeding, the anterior membranous urethra comes into view. The periurethral tissue is separated bilaterally from the urethra, and a narrow right-angle clamp is used to pass a thin polyethylene tube around the urethra. Careful and meticulous dissection is now employed to dissect the urethra from the apex of the prostate gland. It must be remembered that the more distal the transection, the shorter the functional length of urethra. A sponge stick is placed anteriorly on the prostate, thereby displacing it cephalad and posteriorly. In this manner, the urethra can be mobilized for at least 1 cm into the apex of the prostate, without violating any prostate parenchyma. The urethra is transected as far proximal toward the bladder neck as possible (Figure 11.1.8). The catheter comes into view, and it is divided and used to manipulate the prostate gland for the remainder of the operation.

The posterior urethra is now dissected to the same level proximally as the anterior urethra. This can be at the level of the verumontanum. With the polyethylene tubing in place and a bloodless field, the posterior urethra only is transected. Care is taken not to enter the prostatic parenchyma either laterally or posteriorly. In

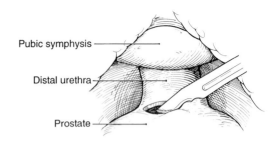

Figure 11.1.8 Transection of the anterior urethra. With a sponge stick providing cephalad–posterior traction, Metzenbaum scissors or a sharp knife are used to incise the anterior urethra.

this manner, the entire distal 'continence mechanism', which extends up to the verumontanum, is preserved.

The dissection continues by maneuvering distally before transecting the 'pillars of the prostate' laterally and the rectourethralis muscle in the midline. This distal maneuver is most important so that there is no violation of the apical prostate posterior to the urethra.

Preservation or excision of the neurovascular bundle

Next, the plane between the prostate and anterior wall of the rectum is developed. At this point, a decision must be made regarding the preservation or excision of the neurovascular bundles. It must be remembered that cancer control is the primary goal, and erectile function a secondary concern. Specific indications/contraindications are detailed above.

If the autonomic innervation to the corpora cavernosa is to be preserved, a delicate right-angle clamp is used to delineate the lateral pelvic fascia located on the posterolateral surface of the prostate gland (Figure 11.1.9, inset). The lateral pelvic fascia is incised from the apex of the prostate to the seminal vesicles at the 4 and 8 o'clock positions. The neurovascular bundles originate from the pelvic plexus cephalad and posterior to the tip of the seminal vesicle

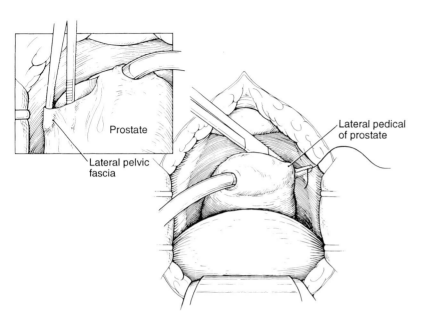

Prostate

Lateral pelvic fascia

Lateral pedical of prostate

Figure 11.1.9 Preservation of the neurovascular bundles. The lateral pelvic fascia is incised to ensure that injury does not occur to the neurovascular bundles. (Inset) A delicate right-angle clamp is used to delineate this fascia located on the posterolateral surface of the prostate gland. The pedicles to the prostate are ligated using a laterally placed tie or clip.

and course posterolaterally at the 5 and 7 o'clock positions beneath the lateral pelvic fascia. This incision thus allows the neurovascular bundles to fall away posterolaterally. With these 'out of harm's way', the pedicles to the prostate can be transected using a laterally placed tie or clip and a small, sharp, right-angle clamp (Figure 11.1.9). The pedicles are taken in small increments, so as not to 'tent up' the neurovascular bundles and inadvertently transect them. Electrocautery should not be used during a nerve-sparing dissection.

Alternatively, it may become necessary to excise one or both neurovascular bundles. If one bundle can be preserved, it is initially separated from the prostate apex. The contralateral bundle is excised as widely as possible and ligated at the tip of the seminal vesicle.

Identification of the vasa deferentia and seminal vesicles

After securing the pedicles to the prostate, Denonvilliers' fascia is visualized and incised to expose the vasa deferentia and seminal vesicles laterally. The vasa deferentia are sharply dissected to the level of the tips of the seminal vesicles. A large hemoclip is applied and the vasa deferentia are transected. The seminal vesicles are then dissected from the surrounding tissues (Figure 11.1.10). Care is taken not to injure the pelvic plexus, which is located in close proximity to the tip of the seminal vesicle. Usually, a blood vessel enters the seminal vesicle at this location. A hemoclip should be applied before transecting the tissue in this area.

Dissection and preservation of the bladder neck

With both vasa deferentia and seminal vesicles dissected free, the plane between the prostate and bladder comes into view (Figure 11.1.11). Using a combination of blunt and sharp dissection, this plane is developed at the level of the seminal vesicles. The dissection continues circumferentially from posterior to anterior until

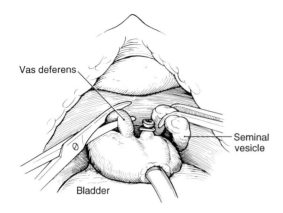

Figure 11.1.10 Dissection of the vasa deferentia and seminal vesicles. Upon transecting Denonvilliers' fascia, the vasa and seminal vesicles are visible. The vasa are dissected to the tip of the seminal vesicles and a large hemoclip is applied. Right-angled scissors are used to transect the vas deferens as shown. The seminal vesicles are then dissected free of the surrounding tissues to free them from the posterior surface of the bladder.

the longitudinal fibers of the bladder neck are identified. At this point, using semiblunt Metzenbaum scissors, the bladder neck and proximal prostatic urethra are dissected from the prostatic parenchyma. The urethra is then transected. Again, the urethra is a separate

structure with its own blood supply, coursing through the prostate gland.[18] The entire remaining urethra inside the prostate can be dissected free and left intact if desired. The balloon of the catheter is deflated, and the prostate gland is removed. The proximal 'continence zone' is preserved.

Reconstruction of the bladder neck

If the contraindications exist or the dissection is difficult, the bladder neck should not be preserved. In these patients, the bladder neck must be reconstructed. Interrupted sutures of 3:0-Chromic incorporate full-thickness muscularis and mucosa to create a 'tennis racket' closure (Figure 11.1.12). The closure starts at the level of the ureteral orifices and continues until the bladder neck is tightened to the size of a 16-French Foley catheter. The bladder mucosa is everted at the bladder neck using interrupted 4:0-Monocryl sutures to create a mucosal bud. The urethrovesical anastomosis is performed as outlined below.

Creation of the urethrourethral anastomosis

After complete hemostasis is achieved at the bladder base, attention is turned to creating the

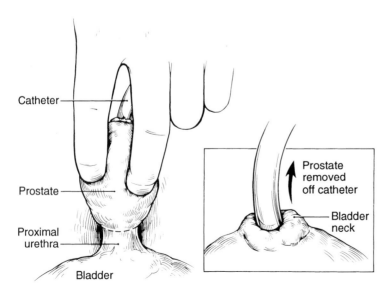

Figure 11.1.11 Preservation of the bladder neck. The bladder neck, as it becomes the prostatic urethra, is defined by utilizing blunt and sharp dissection. The proximal prostatic urethra can be dissected free without violation of the prostate parenchyma. As illustrated, several centimeters of urethra can be preserved. (Inset) The urethra is transected and the prostate removed.

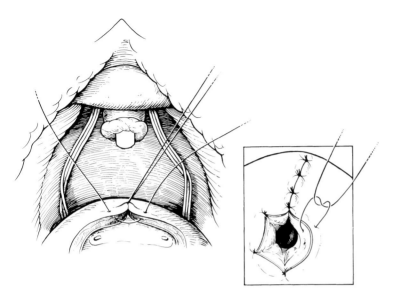

Figure 11.1.12 'Tennis racket' closure of the bladder following non-urethral sparing dissection. (Inset) Creation of mucosal bud using 4:0-Monocryl sutures.

urethrourethral anastomosis (Figure 11.1.13). Using 3:0-Monocryl sutures on a UR6 needle, five sutures are placed into the distal urethral stump at the 1, 4, 6, 8, and 11 o'clock positions. They are placed inside to outside, incorporating only the urethral wall at all but the 6 o'clock position. At this location, the rectourethralis muscle is also included to ensure adequate posterior support to the urethra. Using a French-eye needle, corresponding sutures are placed in the proximal prostatic urethra at the bladder neck. All sutures are placed from inside to outside to ensure that the mucosa will be everted.

A 16-French Foley catheter is placed across the anastomosis into the bladder. The bladder is then brought down into the pelvis and the mucosa-to-mucosa, watertight anastomosis is completed. The sutures are tied in the following order: 4, 1, 6, 8, and 11 o'clock. Water (10 ml) is placed in the balloon, and a closed drainage system is placed in each obturator fossa. The fascia is approximated in the midline using a continuous No. 2 nylon suture. The skin is closed using a running 4:0-Monocryl subcuticular stitch.

POSTOPERATIVE CARE

The postoperative care for the patient undergoing the anatomical radical retropubic prostatectomy is generally uncomplicated. We use a standard protocol, as outlined in Table 11.1.2.

Using this protocol, most patients are discharged on the second postoperative day, with a few being discharged on the third day following surgery. Of the last 100 patients, 85% have been discharged home on the second postoperative day. Patients are discharged home on the stool softener regimen, pain medication (Tylox), and iron if the hematocrit is less than 30%. Patients return 2 weeks after surgery for catheter removal. They are instructed to perform only light activity for 4 weeks. Most men return to work part time by 4 weeks and full time by 6–8 weeks.

EFFICACY

The efficacy of the anatomical radical retropubic prostatectomy can be analyzed in terms of pathology, cancer control, overall survival, and patient satisfaction.

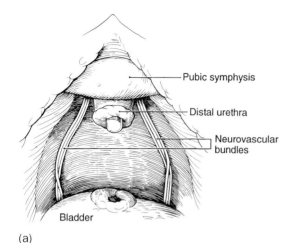

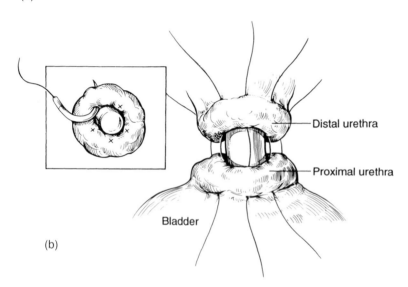

(a)

(b)

Figure 11.1.13 Creation of the urethrourethral anastomosis. (a) View of the pelvis showing the new urethral catheter emerging from the urethral stump. As can be seen, the entire membranous urethra remains intact, and both neurovascular bundles are preserved. (b) The new urethral catheter is brought up out of the pelvis and into the bladder. The bladder is brought down into the pelvis and the sutures are tied. (Inset) Placement of five 3:0-Monocryl sutures on the urethral stump at appropriately marked locations.

Pathological analysis

Walsh et al[28] reviewed their 10-year experience of 955 men with clinically localized prostate cancer who underwent anatomical radical prostatectomy in regard to the pathologic specimen and cancer control. Pathologic stages were as follows: organ confined in 37%, focal capsular penetration in 20.3%, established capsular penetration in 28.3%, seminal vesicle involve-

ment in 7%, and nodal involvement in 4%. In a contemporary series of 3170 patients from the Mayo Clinic,[25] organ-confined disease was noted in 47%, capsular penetration or seminal vesicle involvement in 42%, and nodal involvement in 11%.

With increasing efforts at early detection, one would expect a stage migration to more organ-confined tumors. In a unique comparison of two series separated by 10 years, Beduschi et

Table 11.1.2 University of Michigan radical retropubic prostatectomy protocol

Day of surgery

Discontinue epidural catheter in recovery room

Cefotetan 1 g i.v. every 12 h for 24 h

Pain:

    Toradol 15 mg i.v. every 6 h for 48 h

    Patient-controlled anesthesia (PCA)

Clear liquid diet

Incentive spirometry

Sequential compression devices at all times

Dorsiflexion of feet 100 times each hour while awake

Postoperative day 1

Regular diet

Heplock i.v.

Discontinue PCA at 18:00 h

Tylox 1 tablet every 4 h as necessary

Ambulate 6 times daily

Discontinue sequential compression devices

Begin discharge and leg bag teaching

Postoperative day 2

Remove drain if output < 80 ml per 24 h

Colace 100 mg orally twice daily

$FeSO_4$ 324 mg orally twice daily for 6 weeks if hematocrit < 30

Dulcolax suppository as necessary

Discharge to home

al[29] have confirmed these findings. They compared the first 200 consecutive radical prostatectomies performed at the University of Michigan (by JE Oesterling) with the results reported by Walsh[30] regarding his first 100 consecutive nerve-sparing radical retropubic prostatectomies. The results are summarized in

Table 11.1.3. The data confirm stage migration, with more men having organ-confined disease and less extraprostatic extension and seminal vesicle invasion.

Cancer control

In Walsh's series of 955 men,[28] excellent cancer control was achieved. At 10 years, the likelihood of an undetectable PSA was 70%, isolated elevation of PSA 23%, local recurrence 4%, and distant metastasis 7%. Freedom from biochemical recurrence was 85% in men with organ-confined disease and 82% in those with focal capsular penetration. The majority of patients with progression had an isolated elevation of PSA as their only manifestation of recurrent disease. The significance of this is uncertain.

Ohori et al[31] reported similar rates of non-progression (defined as absence of PSA elevation, local recurrence, or distant metastasis). At 5 years, the non-progression rate was 64% for patients with positive margins (16% of the group) and 83% for those with negative margins. Catalona and Smith[32] also reported promising results in 925 consecutive men who underwent anatomical radical prostatectomy. The overall 5-year probability of non-progression was 78%. For non-palpable tumors, the 5-year non-progression rates were 90% for T1a or T1b tumors and 97% for T1c tumors.

Therefore, while positive margins occur in 24–39% of radical prostatectomy specimens,[31] they do not necessarily portend a poor prognosis. Clearly, excellent cancer control is achieved. Epstein et al[33] have stated that the most likely explanation for the discrepancy between margins and progression is that some of these margins represent artifactually positive margins caused by unique problems with handling radical prostatectomy specimens. Epstein et al have also shown that only approximately 50% of patients with positive margins experience progression, and 61% of these have only an elevated PSA as their sole manifestation of progression.

Epstein et al[33] have conclusively demonstrated that the nerve-sparing modification does

	Incidence (%)	
Pathologic parameter	**Michigan[29]**	**Hopkins[30]**
Organ-confined disease	60	38
Focal extraprostatic extension	14	21
Extensive extraprostatic extension	31	41
Seminal vesicle invasion	9	15
Extensive positive margins	7	7
Focal positive margins	21	20

Table 11.1.3 Stage migration of localized prostate cancer

not compromise cancer control. In a study of 507 men, 4.7% had positive margins only at the site of the neurovascular bundle. However, the majority of these men did not demonstrate progression, and thus only 0.8% of the total population was potentially affected by the nerve-sparing procedure. Similarly, urethral preservation has been shown not to compromise cancer control. Gomez et al[34] demonstrated that there was no increased risk of a positive margin when compared to a more standard dissection. In their series, no patient had a positive bladder neck margin who did not have a positive margin elsewhere. Licht et al[21] have also confirmed these findings.

Overall survival

The efficacy of radical prostatectomy as a treatment option for localized prostate cancer can also be analyzed in terms of overall and cause-specific survival. The Mayo Clinic recently reported their long-term follow-up of 1143 patients. The 10- and 15-year crude survival rates were 75% and 60%, respectively, compared with an expected survival of a control group of 67% and 46%, respectively.[25,35] Cause-specific survival rates were 90% and 83% at 10 and 15 years respectively. It is clear that patients who undergo radical prostatectomy have survival comparable to the general population.

Patient satisfaction

Patients appear to have a favorable view of the procedure. A national sample of Medicaid patients were surveyed by mail, telephone, or interview. Postsurgical patients scored high on quality-of-life measures; the results were similar to those from men who underwent transurethral resection of the prostate (TURP). In addition, 81% reported feeling positive about the results, and 89% would choose to have the anatomical radical prostatectomy again.[36]

COMPLICATIONS

The development of the anatomical radical retropubic prostatectomy has significantly decreased mortality and morbidity. Complications can be divided into intraoperative, and early and late postoperative complications. A

Table 11.1.4 Complications of radical retropubic prostatectomy

Complication	Incidence (%)			
	Washington University[37,38]	Mayo Clinic[25]	Michigan	Hopkins[13]
Pulmonary embolism	2.3	1.1	0.3	1
Deep venous thrombosis	0.8	0.7	0.6	1
Myocardial infarction	0.4	0.4	0	NR
Rectal injury	0.1	0.6	0	1.0
Postoperative bleeding	0.1	NR	0.2	0.5
Anastomotic leak	0.1	NR	0	NR
Death	0	0	0	0.2
Vesical neck contracture	5.0	NR	1.8	NR
Potency	60	NR	NR	68
Total continence	94	95	97	92
Artificial sphincter	NR	0.5	0	0.2

NR, not reported.

comparison of complications from four recent large series is shown in Table 11.1.4.[13,25,37,38]

Intraoperative complications

The major intraoperative complication is hemorrhage. However, proper knowledge of pelvic anatomy and control of the dorsal venous complex can minimize blood loss. Some have advocated temporary occlusion of the hypogastric arteries,[13] but we have not found this to be particularly useful. Instead, adequate exposure and a bloodless field are obtained by control of the dorsal vein complex as outlined above.

Rectal injury occurs in 0–1% (see Table 11.1.4) of cases. The majority of patients do not require diverting colostomy. Intraoperative recognition is the key to management. After the defect has been recognized, the radical prostatectomy should be completed. The anal sphincter is dilated and the defect closed in two layers (an inner layer of 2:0 Chromic and an outer layer of 2:0 silk Lembert sutures). A small pedicle of omentum is mobilized to cover the repair, and the urethral anastomosis is completed. The patient is maintained on broad-spectrum antibiotics. Using this approach, Borland and Walsh[39] noted no wound infections, pelvic abscesses, or urethrorectal fistulas in nine patients. Large defects or those discovered postoperatively are best managed by a diverting colostomy.

Early complications

Postoperative bleeding
Significant postoperative hemorrhage is defined as bleeding that requires acute transfusion of blood to support blood pressure. Fortunately, this scenario is quite rare. Hedican and Walsh[40] reported a 0.5% rate of significant postoperative bleeding. A total of four patients were

re-explored and three were managed conservatively. Patients managed conservatively had an average 1 week longer hospitalization, a 100% rate of vesical neck contracture, and 66% rate of long-term incontinence. In contrast, only one of the four patients re-explored had mild incontinence. Therefore, aggressive re-exploration of postoperative hemorrhage is recommended.

Thromboembolic complications
Pulmonary embolism (PE) and deep venous thrombosis (DVT) are potentially fatal complications of radical prostatectomy. They occur in 0.3–3% of patients (see Table 11.1.4). The most important step is prevention. Use of sequential compression devices, calf exercises, and early ambulation are important preventative measures.

However, a high level of clinical suspicion must be maintained. Any unexplained fever, dyspnea, tachypnea, tachycardia, hypoxia, or leg swelling must be evaluated. A proper evaluation includes: arterial blood gases, chest X-ray, electrocardiogram, duplex Doppler scan of extremities, and a ventilation/perfusion ($\dot{V}/\dot{Q}$) scan of the lungs. Systemic heparinization should be started immediately if suspicion exists.

With the increasing number of patients being discharged home on postoperative day 2, patient instruction regarding signs and symptoms is necessary. Indeed, Cisek and Walsh[41] have recently shown that the average time to presentation of DVT is 11 days or longer.

Anastomotic leak
Anastomotic leak is a relatively rare complication. Persistent fluid drainage through the pelvic drain should prompt a creatinine determination to determine if the fluid is urine or lymph. If the creatinine is high, a urine leak is diagnosed and can be confirmed by cystogram. Most leaks will resolve with prolonged catheter drainage.

Other early complications
Fortunately, with improved anesthetic technique and development of the anatomical radical prostatectomy, the mortality rate approaches zero. Other complications also occur infrequently. These include wound infection (1–2%), prolonged ileus (0–2%), pneumonia (0.4%), and myocardial infarction (0.4%) (see Table 11.1.4).

Late complications

Vesical neck contracture
Vesical neck contracture can be a significant untoward effect associated with radical prostatectomy. The authors have noted a rate of 1.8%, Keetch et al[37] have reported a rate of 5%, while Surya et al[42] have reported a rate of 11.5%. Surya et al[42] noted excess blood loss, urine extravasation, and prior transurethral resection to be contributing factors. Surya et al recommended simple dilatation as primary management, but reported a 50% failure rate. If dilatation failed, cold knife incision was successful in 65% of patients.

In a more recent study, Dalkin[43] utilized a different algorithm and achieved an 88% success rate. He defined mature strictures as those that occurred more than 8 weeks postoperatively and immature strictures as those occurring before 8 weeks. For immature strictures he recommended simple dilatation followed by cold knife incision when the stricture matured. For mature strictures, he recommended cold knife incision as primary treatment.

Continence
Urinary incontinence is probably the most feared complication of radical prostatectomy. However, the development of the anatomical radical retropubic prostatectomy provides for excellent exposure and a precise apical dissection. This has significantly lowered the rate of incontinence. Contemporary series report complete continence rates of 92–97% (see Table 11.1.4). The remaining 3–8% usually have mild stress incontinence, and only 0.2–0.5% require placement of a genitourinary sphincter (see Table 11.1.4).

Return of complete urinary continence following radical prostatectomy usually occurs within 12 months. It usually returns in three stages: (1) the patient is dry when lying at night; (2) the patient is dry when ambulatory; and (3) the patient is dry when straining or rising from a seated position. Unfortunately, for some, incontinence continues to be a major problem. Depending on the degree of incontinence, this can be managed with pads, a Cunningham clamp, transurethral collagen injection, or an artificial urinary sphincter.

Clearly, one can perform an identical prostatectomy on two separate patients, and one will be immediately continent while the other will have persistent incontinence. Although why this occurs is unknown, the fact that a minimal functional urethral length is necessary has been known for many years.[44] Using sound anatomical and urodynamic concepts, we have further modified the radical prostatectomy to include urethral preservation in selected patients. This modification reduces the time to the development of continence and decreases the overall rate of incontinence. This statement is supported by Licht et al,[21] who have found that preservation of the bladder neck alone results in an earlier return of continence.

Using the anatomical radical retropubic prostatectomy at the University of Michigan, we have noted excellent continence rates. As illustrated in Table 11.1.4, a 97% complete continence rate is achieved at 6 months. Of the 416 evaluable patients, 404 reported the use of no pads, eight (2%) required one or two pads/day, and four (1%) required the use of three or more pads daily. No patient on follow-up required placement of an artificial urinary sphincter.

Interestingly, the nerve-sparing radical prostatectomy as first described by Walsh may also aid in the postoperative development of continence. O'Donnell and Finan[45] noted that functional urethral length and resting urethral pressure were significantly higher in patients who had undergone the nerve-sparing technique. Moreover, continence rates were higher in the nerve-spared group. In a recent Johns Hopkins review of 593 patients, a 94% continence rate was realized with bilateral preservation of the neurovascular bundles, compared with 92% for unilateral preservation, and 81% if both bundles were sacrificed.[46]

Erectile function

Potency is defined as the ability to have an erection sufficient for vaginal penetration and orgasm. Until 15 years ago, radical prostatectomy was uniformly associated with impotence. Walsh and Donker's delineation of the autonomic innervation of the corpora cavernosa decreased the incidence of impotence, without compromising cancer control. Using his modification, Walsh[28,47] was able to preserve potency in 68% of 503 patients. Factors that correlated with return of sexual function included (1) age, (2) clinical and pathologic stage, and (3) excision or preservation of one or both neurovascular bundles.[28,47] Clinical stage is the major determinant of surgical technique, and correlates well with preservation or excision of the neurovascular bundles.[47] Advancing age has a detrimental effect on erectile function, as does unilateral excision of the neurovascular bundle, except in patients aged less than 50 years. A summary of the results of Walsh's series is presented in Table 11.1.5.

Catalona and Bigg[48] have confirmed the excellent results of nerve-sparing prostatectomy. In 112 men who had bilateral preservation of the neurovascular bundles, 71 (63%) retained potency postoperatively, as compared with 13 of 33 (39%) who underwent unilateral preservation. In accordance with Walsh's findings, younger men had a much higher rate of potency preservation.

SUMMARY

The anatomical radical retropubic prostatectomy has revolutionized the treatment of clinically localized prostate cancer. Using sound anatomical and pathological concepts, the procedure has been modified and morbidity significantly decreased. At the same time, cancer control has not been compromised and this has translated into excellent overall survival. Combined with increasing efforts and innovations in early detection, the anatomical radical prostatectomy will no doubt translate into decreased mortality from prostate cancer.

Table 11.1.5 Potency following radical prostatectomy[28,47]

Patient age (years)	Potency (%)		
	Overall	BNS	UNS
<50	91	90	91
50–60	75	82	58
60–70	58	69	47
>70	25	22	–

BNS, bilateral nerve sparing; UNS, unilateral nerve sparing.

REFERENCES

1. Brawer MK, Chetner MP, Beatie J, Buchner DM, Vessela RL, Lange PH, Screening for prostatic carcinoma with prostate specific antigen. *J Urol* 1992; **147:** 841–5.
2. Catalona WJ, Richie JP, Ahmann FR et al, Comparison of digital rectal examination and serum prostate specific antigen in the early detection of prostate cancer: results of a multi-center clinical trial of 6630 men. *J Urol* 1994; **151:** 1283–90.
3. Catalona WJ, Smith DS, Ratliff TL, Basler JW, Detection of organ confined cancer is increased through prostate specific antigen based screening. *J Am Med Assoc* 1993; **270:** 948–54.
4. Scott WW, Historical overview of the treatment of prostate cancer. *Prostate* 1983; **4:** 435–43.
5. Young HH, *A Surgeon's Autobiography*. Harcourt Brace: New York, 1940.
6. Millin T, *Retropubic Urinary Surgery*. Williams & Wilkins: Baltimore, MD, 1947.
7. Reiner WG, Walsh PC, An anatomical approach to the surgical management of the dorsal vein and Santorini's plexus during radical retropubic surgery. *J Urol* 1979; **121:** 198–200.
8. Walsh PC, Donker PJ, Impotence following radical prostatectomy: insight into etiology and prevention. *J Urol* 1982; **128:** 492–7.
9. Myers RP, Goellner JR, Cahill DR, Prostate shape, external striated urethral sphincter and radical prostatectomy: the apical dissection. *J Urol* 1987; **138:** 543–50.
10. Gibbons RP, Radical perineal prostatectomy: definitive treatment for patients with localized prostate cancer. *AUA Update Ser* 1994; **XIII:** 34–43.
11. Myers RP, Practical pelvic anatomy pertinent to radical retropubic prostatectomy. *AUA Update Ser* 1994; **XIII:** 26–31.
12. Villers A, McNeal JE, Freitha FS et al, Invasion of Denonvilliers' fascia in radical prostatectomy specimens. *J Urol* 1993; **149:** 793–7.
13. Walsh PC, Radical retropubic prostatectomy. In: *Campbell's Urology*, 6th edn (Walsh PC, Retik AB, Stamey TA, Vaughan ED Jr, eds), Vol 3, Chap 78. WB Saunders: Philadelphia, 1992.
14. Myers RP, Male urethral sphincteric anatomy and radical prostatectomy. *Urol Clin North Am* 1991; **18:** 211–27.
15. Turner-Warwick R, The sphincter mechanisms: their relation to prostate enlargement and its treatment. In: *Benign Prostate Hypertrophy* (Hinman F Jr, ed). Springer-Verlag: New York, 1983.
16. Oelrich TM, The urethral sphincter muscle in the male. *Am J Anat* 1980; **158:** 229–34.

17. Hutch JA, Fisher R, Continence after radical prostatectomy. *Br J Urol* 1968; **40**: 62–7.

18. Oesterling JE, Anatomical radical retropubic prostatectomy. *Profiles in Urology*, Surgical Communications, Inc: New York, 1995.

19. Bluestein DL, Bostwick DG, Bergstralh EJ, Oesterling JE, Eliminating the need for bilateral pelvic lymphadenectomy in select patients with prostate cancer. *J Urol* 1994; **151**: 1315–20.

20. Hatcher PA, Oesterling JE, Nerve sparing procedures in urologic cancer surgery – an overview. *AUA Update Ser* 1993; **XII**: 90–5.

21. Licht MR, Klein EA, Tuason L, Levin H, Impact of bladder neck preservation on continence and cancer control. *Urology* 1994; **44**: 883–7.

22. Toy PT, Menozzi D, Strauss RG, Stehlinng LC, Kruskall M, Ahn DK, Efficacy of preoperative donation of blood for autologous use in radical prostatectomy. *Transfusion* 1993; **33**: 721–4.

23. Goodnough LT, Grishaber JE, Birkmeyer JD, Monk TG, Catalona WJ, Efficacy and cost-effectiveness of autologous blood predeposit in patients undergoing radical prostatectomy procedures. *Urology* 1994; **44**: 226–31.

24. Ness PM, Baldwin ML, Walsh PC, Pre-deposit autologous transfusion in radical retropubic prostatectomy. *Transfusion* 1987; **27**: 518A.

25. Zincke H, Oesterling JE, Blute ML, Bergstralh EJ, Myers RP, Barret DM, Long-term (15 years) results after radical prostatectomy for clinically localized (stage T2c or lower) prostate cancer. *J Urol* 1994; **152**: 1850–7.

26. Goh M, Kleer CG, Kielczewski PA, Wojno KJ, Kim KM, Oesterling JE, Autologous blood donation prior to anatomical radical prostatectomy. Is it really necessary? *Urology* 1997; **49**: 569–74.

27. Myers RP, Improving the exposure of the prostate in radical retropubic prostatectomy: longitudinal bunching of the deep venous plexus. *J Urol* 1989; **129**: 1007–8.

28. Walsh PC, Partin AW, Epstein JI, Cancer control and quality of life following anatomical radical retropubic prostatectomy: results at 10 years. *J Urol* 1994; **152**: 1831–6.

29. Beduschi MC, Wojno KJ, Oesterling JE, Proportion of organ-confined prostate cancer is increasing: findings from two radical prostatectomy series separated by 10 years. Presented at AUA Annual Meeting, New Orleans, LA, 1997.

30. Eggleston JC, Walsh PC, Radical prostatectomy with preservation of sexual function: pathological findings in the first 100 cases. *J Urol* 1985; **134**: 1146–8.

31. Ohori M, Wheeler TM, Kattan MW, Goto Y, Scardino PT, Prognostic significance of positive surgical margins in radical prostatectomy specimens. *J Urol* 1995; **154**: 1818–24.

32. Catalona WJ, Smith DS, Five-year tumor recurrence rates after anatomical radical retropubic prostatectomy for prostate cancer. *J Urol* 1994; **152**: 1837–42.

33. Epstein JI, Pizov G, Walsh PC, Correlation of pathologic findings with progression after radical retropubic prostatectomy. *Cancer* 1993; **71**: 3582–93.

34. Gomez CA, Soloway MS, Civantos F, Bladder neck preservation and its impact on positive surgical margins during radical prostatectomy. *Adult Urol* 1993; **42**: 689–94.

35. Zincke H, Bergstralh EJ, Blute ML et al, Radical prostatectomy for clinically localized prostate cancer: long term results of 1143 patients from a single institution. *J Clin Oncol* 1994; **12**: 2254–63.

36. Fowler FJ, Barry MJ, Lu-Yao G, Wasson J, Roman A, Wennberg J, Effects of radical prostatectomy for prostate cancer on patient quality of life: results from a Medicare survey. *Urology* 1995; **45**: 1007–15.

37. Keetch DW, Andriole GL, Catalona WJ, Complications of radical retropubic prostatectomy. *AUA Update Ser* 1994; **XIII**: 46–51.

38. Andriole GL, Smith DS, Rao G, Goodnough L, Catalona WJ, Early complications of contemporary anatomical radical retropubic prostatectomy. *J Urol* 1994; **152**: 1858–60.

39. Borland RN, Walsh PC, The management of rectal injury during radical retropubic prostatectomy. *J Urol* 1992; **147**: 905–7.

40. Hedican SP, Walsh PC, Postoperative bleeding following radical retropubic prostatectomy. *J Urol* 1994; **152**: 1181–3.

41. Cisek LJ, Walsh PC, Thromboembolic complications following radical retropubic prostatectomy. Influence of external sequential pneumatic compression devices. *Urology* 1993; **42**: 406–8.

42. Surya BV, Provet J, Johanson K-E, Brown J, Anastomotic strictures following radical prostatectomy: risk factors and management. *J Urol* 1990; **43**: 755–9.

43. Dalkin B, Endoscopic evaluation and treatment of anastomotic strictures after radical retropubic prostatectomy. *J Urol* 1996; **155**: 206–8.

44. Lapides J, Ajemian EP, Stewart BH et al, Further observations on the kinetics of the urethrovesical sphincter. *J Urol* 1960; **84**: 86–90.

45. O'Donnell PD, Finan BF, Continence following nerve-sparing radical prostatectomy. *J Urol* 1989; **142:** 1227–30.

46. Steiner MS, Morton RA, Walsh PC, Impact of anatomical radical prostatectomy on urinary continence. *J Urol* 1991; **145:** 512–17.

47. Quinlan DM, Epstein JI, Carter BS, Walsh PC, Sexual function following radical prostatectomy: influence of preservation of neurovascular bundles. *J Urol* 1991; **145:** 998–1002.

48. Catalona WJ, Bigg SW, Nerve-sparing radical prostatectomy: evaluation of results after 250 patients. *J Urol* 1989; **143:** 538–42.

11.2

Radical perineal prostatectomy for clinically localized prostate cancer

Laurent Boccon-Gibod

CONTENTS • **Surgical procedure** • **Intraoperative complications** • **Postoperative care** • **Conclusion**

The perineal approach for radical prostatectomy may be considered when the spread of cancer cells to the lymph nodes has been ruled out by a prior open or endosurgical lymphadenectomy or when the clinical biological and pathological features of the cancer are consistent with a very limited risk of cancer-positive lymph nodes (prostate-specific antigen (PSA) level (< 10, less than three positive biopsies, no cancer in the extraprostatic spaces).[1-3] In this setting, the perineal approach has many advantages: it leads quickly to the prostate gland; the vesicourethral anastomosis can be made watertight under direct vision control; and blood loss is usually extremely limited. These advantages very often outweigh the inconveniences associated with the perineal approach: the relative narrowness of the operative field; difficulty in preserving the neurovascular bundles; and, sometimes, some difficulty in removing the seminal vesicles.[4-6] The urologist should also be aware that the perineal approach should never be used in the following circumstances:

- in a patient with osteoarthritis of the hip or a hip prosthesis, these being incompatible with the exaggerated lithotomy position;
- when the prostate gland is large (>60 g);
- when there is a large median lobe, which will make dissection of the bladder neck from the perineum difficult;
- in a patient with large haemorrhoids, which may make the dissection of the rectal wall perilous.

Once the indication for radical perineal prostatectomy has been confirmed, before surgery the patient must:

- buy a pair of varicose vein stockings, which he will wear from the day of surgery to the day of discharge in order to avoid thrombophlebitis;
- see the anaesthetist, during consultation with whom a programme of autologous blood transfusion can be planned, if necessary;
- see the physiotherapist, who will advise on the muscular exercises that will be necessary during the recovery phase, so as to minimize the duration of the period of incontinence; and
- in the 2 days preceding surgery, follow a

regimen identical to that used prior to colo-rectal surgery.

Instrumentation

Radical perineal prostatectomy does not require any specific instrumentation, but the author finds the following useful:

- a head lamp,
- a cold light sucker,
- right-angle clip applicators,
- right-angle scissors,
- two prostatic tractors – one straight (Young) and one curved (Lowsley),
- autostatic retractors (Bookwalter type) (these are not strictly indispensable to the operation).

Anaesthesia

Usually general anaesthesia with endotracheal intubation is used, as the position of the patient is incompatible with comfortable spinal or peridural anaesthesia.

Positioning the patient

The patient should be positioned in the exag-gerated lithotomy position: the thighs are flexed over the abdomen so that the knees are almost in contact with the shoulders, the legs are verti-cal, and the table is tilted so that the plane of the perineum is parallel to the ceiling of the operating theatre (Figure 11.2.1).

Pads should be used at every site that can be associated with nerve compression (shoulders, knees, etc.).[7] Once the patient has been draped, the surgeon sits between the legs of the patient, the first assistant on his left side, the second assistant on his right side, and the scrub nurse behind the surgeon.

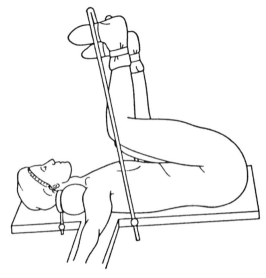

Figure 11.2.1 The exaggerated lithotomy position. (Modified from reference 4, with permission from *Contemporary Urology*, Medical Economics Company.)

SURGICAL PROCEDURE

Introduction of the curved Lowsley tractor

Before introducing the Lowsley tractor, it is wise to pass into the urethra a succession of well-lubricated metallic sounds of increasing calibre, so that the well-lubricated Lowsley trac-tor will pass easily into the bladder once it has been opened. Depressing the tractor towards the lower abdomen will bring the prostate into the perineum, where the gland can be palpated easily. Once it has been checked that the Lowsley is indeed in place and does mobilize the prostate, the handle of the Lowsley is kept vertical and handed to the first assistant.

The incision

An inverted-U-shaped incision is made from one ischial tuberosity to the other, the horizon-tal part of the incision being 1.5 cm above the anal margin (Figure 11.2.2).

Dividing the anobulbar raphe

Once the skin has been incised, the anobulbar raphe appears as a vertical muscular structure

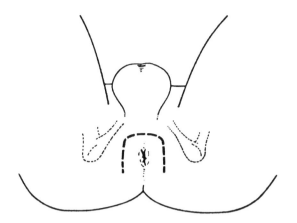

Figure 11.2.2 The incision. (Modified from reference 4, with permission from *Contemporary Urology*, Medical Economics Company.)

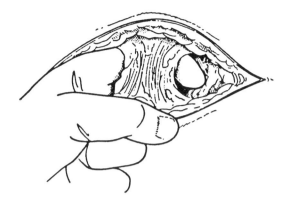

Figure 11.2.4 Controlling the anobulbar raphe. (Modified from reference 4, with permission from *Contemporary Urology*, Medical Economics Company.)

with the tissue surrounding the anal margin on both sides. After incision of this fatty tissue on both sides, the fascia superficialis is easily entered, and by dissecting with the Metzenbaum scissors on both sides the plane on each side of the anobulbar raphe is developed (Figure 11.2.3). Introduce a forefinger into

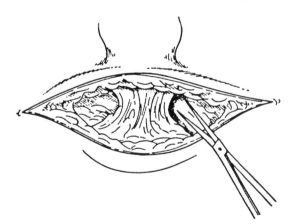

Figure 11.2.3 Developing the ischiorectal fossa. (Modified from reference 4, with permission from *Contemporary Urology*, Medical Economics Company.)

each ischiorectal fossa and, by blunt dissection, introduce the left forefinger behind the anobulbar raphe from one side to the other (Figure 11.2.4). The raphe can be divided using the scissors or a Bowie knife (Figure 11.2.5). Once the

raphe has been incised, the inferior aspect of the incision is sewn to a surgical towel in order to protect the anus.

Exposing the anterior rectal wall
Once the raphe has been divided, the anal sphincter appears as a transverse red muscle under which appears the white glistening anterior rectal wall. By lifting the anal sphincter upwards with two retractors (Figure 11.2.6) the anterior rectal wall can be brought progressively down on each side of the median line by using a Kittner or the knife handle. Small vessels interposing between the levators and the anterior rectal wall can be coagulated and divided.

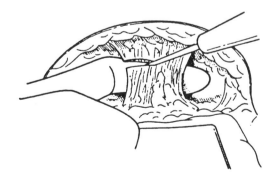

Figure 11.2.5 Dividing the raphe. (Modified from reference 4, with permission from *Contemporary Urology*, Medical Economics Company.)

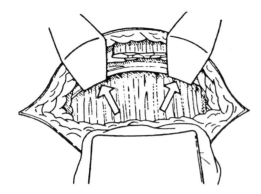

Figure 11.2.6 Exposing the anterior aspect of the rectal wall. (Modified from reference 4, with permission from *Contemporary Urology*, Medical Economics Company.)

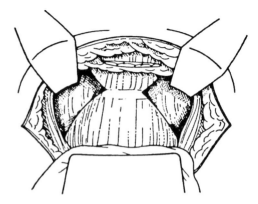

Figure 11.2.7 Freeing the rectum and dividing the rectourethralis muscle. (Modified from reference 4, with permission from *Contemporary Urology*, Medical Economics Company.)

Exposing and dividing the rectourethral muscle

In pursuing the dissection of the two anterolateral aspects of the rectal wall on each side of the median line with the Kittner and the knife handle, deep in the incision the surgeon can feel the posterior aspect of the prostate, which can be easily identified by means of the movements transmitted by the Lowsley tractor manipulated by the first assistant. With the Lowsley tractor kept vertical, the prostatic apex is hidden behind the rectourethralis muscle, a muscular structure that binds the anterior aspect of the rectum to the apex of the prostate. At this stage, it is useful to introduce the left forefinger into the rectum so that the right forefinger can easily identify the anterior rectal wall and the rectourethral muscle. The development of the interprostatorectal space on each side of the median line can usually be achieved without major difficulty and, having totally separated the rectourethral muscle, this structure can be divided at the prostate apex, using either the knife or the Metzenbaum scissors (Figure 11.2.7). Once the rectourethralis muscle has been divided, the posterior aspect of the prostate apex is easily identified by the appearance of the glistening, white Denonvilliers' fascia.

Incising Denonvilliers' fascia

The incision of Denonvilliers' fascia can be done in one of two ways:

- vertically, which theoretically preserves the neurovascular bundles[6]; or
- horizontally (Figure 11.2.8), which is usu-

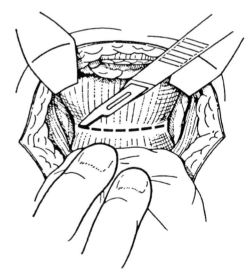

Figure 11.2.8 Incising Denonvilliers' fascia. (Modified from reference 4, with permission from *Contemporary Urology*, Medical Economics Company.)

ally associated with trauma to the neurovascular bundles, but usually gives better exposure for the rest of the surgery.

Once the posterior aspect of Denonvilliers' fascia has been incised, it is possible to develop, using the handle of the knife, the space between the two layers of Denonvilliers' fascia. At this point, the anterior rectal wall literally drops into the interior part of the incision, where it can be safely retracted by interposing a surgical towel between the blade of a retractor and the anterior rectal wall.

Dissecting the urethra at the prostate apex

Once the posterior aspect of the prostate and the base of the seminal vesicles have been identified, the apex itself is easily dissected using the curved cisors (Figure 11.2.9). A right-angle

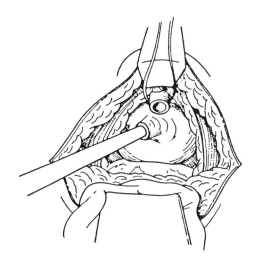

Figure 11.2.10 Incising the posterior aspect of the urethra. (Modified from reference 4, with permission from *Contemporary Urology*, Medical Economics Company.)

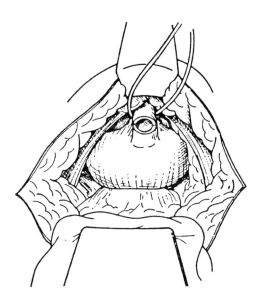

Figure 11.2.9 Dissecting the apex of the prostate and the urethra. (Modified from reference 4, with permission from *Contemporary Urology*, Medical Economics Company.)

clamp can usually be passed behind the urethra, which can then be isolated using a vascular loop. The Lowsley tractor is withdrawn, the posterior aspect of the urethra is incised and, once the urethral lumen has been identified, three 2/0 PDS sutures placed in the distal pos-

terior lip of the urethra. The anterior aspect of the urethra is then divided using the knife or the scissors and three 2/0 PDS sutures are placed in the distal anterior lip of the urethra. The bladder is emptied using a Foley catheter and, when the bladder is empty, the catheter is removed and the straight prostatic tractor introduced into the bladder (Figure 11.2.10).

Dissecting the anterior aspect of the prostate

Pressing down on the Young straight prostatic tractor exposes the anterior aspect of the prostate, which can be freed from the surrounding structures by blunt dissection with the Kittner. The vessels that appear at the anterior aspect of the prostate can easily be clipped and divided using the curved clip applicators and scissors (Figures 11.2.11 and 11.2.12).

Defining the bladder neck

By turning the Young tractor from left to right and from right to left it is easy to palpate its wings in the bladder and to define the bladder neck. Considering that the dissection of the anterior aspect proceeds under the prostatic fascia, it is not surprising that dissection with the Kittner and the handle of the knife leads

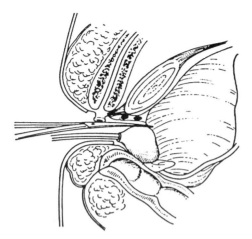

Figure 11.2.11 Dissecting the anterior aspect of the prostate. (Modified from reference 4, with permission from *Contemporary Urology*, Medical Economics Company.)

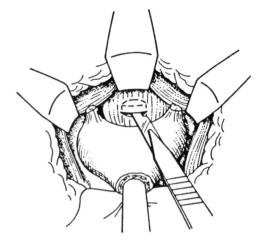

Figure 11.2.13 Incising the bladder neck. (Modified from reference 4, with permission from *Contemporary Urology*, Medical Economics Company.)

directly to the avascular plane separating the base of the prostate from the base of the bladder. At this point, it may sometimes, in extremely favourable cases, be possible to isolate the urethral mucosa at the bladder neck, and to pass behind the bladder neck a right-angle clamp and then a vessel loop. If this is not possible, which is more usually the case, it is easier to incise the bladder neck using the knife (Figure 11.2.13).

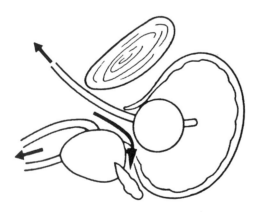

Figure 11.2.12 Dissecting the intervesicoprostatic plane. (Modified from reference 4, with permission from *Contemporary Urology*, Medical Economics Company.)

Dissecting between the prostate and the bladder base

Once the bladder neck has been incised, the straight Young tractor is removed, a Foley catheter is introduced into the bladder neck, and the balloon is inflated to 25–30 ml. A Penrose drain is introduced into the prostatic urethra, where it will be used to bring the prostate downwards (with less risk of disrupting the anterior commissure than with the Young tractor). The Foley catheter is handed to the first assistant who pulls it forwards and upwards to delimit the posterior aspect of the bladder; the surgeon pulls down on the Penrose drain (Figure 11.2.14), taking care not to break the anterior prostatic commissure by using too strong traction. The divergent traction between the Foley catheter and the Penrose drain helps the surgeon to define the plane between the prostate base and the posterior aspect of the bladder, and to pass a right-angle clamp behind the posterior aspect of the bladder neck. The plane of dissection between the bladder base and the vasa and seminal vesicles can, therefore, now be easily entered. However, the proper plane of dissection is sometimes somewhat difficult to define. The dissection should proceed layer by layer until the vasa and semi-

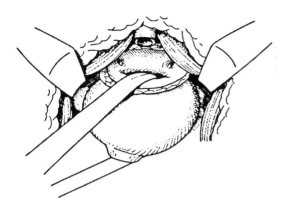

Figure 11.2.14 Using the Penrose drain to exert traction on the prostate. (Modified from reference 4, with permission from *Contemporary Urology*, Medical Economics Company.)

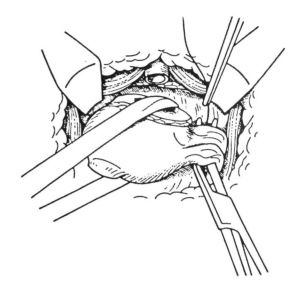

nal vesicles are exposed, remembering not to penetrate too deeply into the detrusor in order to avoid injury to the seminal ureters. It is wise to ask the anaesthesist to inject intravenously a vial of indigocarmin, which will help in identifying the ureteric orifices, if necessary.

Dividing the lateral pedicles, vasa and seminal vesicles

Once the bladder neck has been divided, and the plane between the bladder base and the vasa and seminal vesicles identified, the next step is to divide the lateral pedicles. Using the traction on the Penrose drain, it is easy to identify, on the right- and left-hand sides, the lateral pedicles which can be usually isolated on a right-angle clamp, double clipped using the right-angle clip applicators, and divided (Figure 11.2.15).

The next step is to divide the vasa, which should be dissected, clipped and divided as far away as possible in the perineal cavity in order to avoid their adherence to the medial aspect of the seminal vesicles. Once the vasa have been divided, it is easy to pass the right-angle clamp between them (in order to perforate the posterior aspect of Denonvilliers' fascia) and to introduce the Penrose drain between the vasa (in order not to break the anterior prostatic commissure). These actions will help to bring the

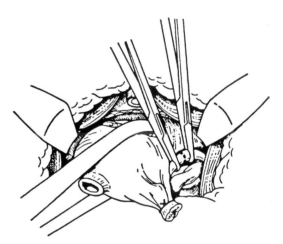

Figure 11.2.15 Controlling and dividing the lateral pedicles. (Modified from reference 4, with permission from *Contemporary Urology*, Medical Economics Company.)

specimen a little more out of the perineal cavity and thus make the following steps easier. At this time, the surgeon has an excellent handle on the specimen and the seminal vesicles. Seminal vesicles can now be dissected, taking care to clip every small vessel before dividing them. The specimen is then removed in its entirety.

It may happen that the traction on the seminal vesicles will disrupt them. This is not a problem because the vesicles can usually be removed separately; it is easy to grasp the seminal vesicles using Duval forceps, and to dissect them in the depth of the perineal cavity to their tip.

Anastomosing the bladder to the urethra

After checking the quality of haemostasis, if the bladder neck has been preserved an end-to-end vesicourethral anastomosis is performed. In the other cases it may be necessary to close the 'racquet handle' by using 2/0 absorbable synthetic sutures. The vesicourethral anastomosis itself is done using 6–8 synthetic absorbable sutures over a 20- or 22-gauge Foley catheter. The anastomosis is usually done under direct vision, and must be perfectly water and air tight (Figure 11.2.16).

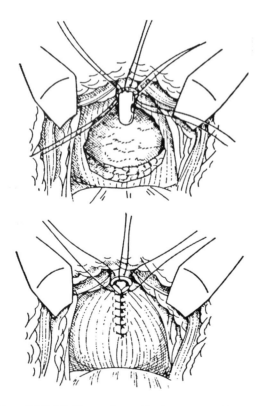

Figure 11.2.16 The vesicourethral anastomosis. (Modified from reference 4, with permission from *Contemporary Urology*, Medical Economics Company.)

Once the anastomosis has been performed, a Penrose or a suction drain is placed in the perineal cavity. The levators and then the anobulbar raphe are reapproximated using figure-of-eight synthetic absorbable 2/0 sutures. The subcutaneous tissues are sutured using a 3/0 Vicryl running suture, and the skin of the perineum is usually closed using a subcuticular 3/0 Vicryl running suture. A compressive dressing is then applied.

INTRAOPERATIVE COMPLICATIONS

There are three types of complication that may occur during radical perineal prostatectomy:

- a rectal tear,
- uncontrollable bleeding, and
- rupture of the anterior prostate commissure.

A rectal tear is most likely to occur during the division of the rectourethralis muscle or when liberating the rectum from the posterior aspect of the prostate and seminal vesicles. The rectal tear should be recognized and repaired immediately using a two-layer running absorbable suture. It is not mandatory to perform a colostomy. The patient will resume normal alimentation 1 week later.[8]

Major bleeding can occur when developing the plane at the anterior aspect of the prostate if the dissection is carried too far up and away such that it interferes with the dorsal venous complex. Haemostasis can usually be achieved by suture ligature, compression and traction on the Foley balloon. In most cases, the vesicourethral anastomosis will induce a spectacular reduction in the bleeding.

Rupture of the anterior prostate commissure may occur if the traction applied with the Penrose drain is too vigorous. In this case, further dissection may be awkward unless one manages to pass a right-angle clamp into the triangle between the vasa in order to perforate the posterior aspect of Denonvilliers' fascia, thus allowing the Penrose drain to be passed between the vasa and seminal vesicles and a good handle on the entire specimen to be obtained.

POSTOPERATIVE CARE

The patient is seated in the late afternoon on the day of surgery and will be ambulant the next day. Normal alimentation is resumed on the day following surgery. The Penrose drain is mobilized and removed at the latest on postoperative day 4. The patient can be discharged home, with his urethral catheter still in situ, on day 4 or 5.

CONCLUSION

In these times of cost containment, the radical perineal prostatectomy technique is undoubtedly making a spectacular comeback. Because the surgery itself is probably less aggressive than the retropubic approach, the patient can usually be discharged on postoperative day 2 or 3.

However, the major issue is the quality of the control of the disease: is the radicality of perineal prostatectomy equal to that of retropubic prostatectomy in terms of the margins of the resection? On this matter the jury is still out.[9,10]

REFERENCES

1. Lerner SE, Fleischmann J, Taub HC, Chamberlin JW, Kahan NZ, Melman A, Combined laporoscopic pelvic lymphnode dissection and modified belt radical perineal prostatectomy for localized prostatic adenocarcinoma. *Urology* 1994; **43**: 493–8.
2. Parra RO, Isorna S, Perez MG, Cummings JM, Boullier JA, Radical perineal prostatectomy without pelvic lymphadenectomy: selection criteria and early results. *J Urol* 1996; **155**: 612–15.
3. Thomas R, Steele R, Smoth R, Brannan W, One stage laparoscopic pelvic lymphadenectomy and radical perineal prostatectomy. *J Urol* 1994; **152**: 1174–7.
4. Resnick MI, Radical perineal prostatectomy redux. *Contemp Urol* 1991; **3**: 44–53.
5. Trasher JB, Paulson DF, Reappraisal of radical perineal prostatectomy. *Eur Urol* 1992; **22**: 1–8.
6. Weldon VE, Tavel FR, Potency-sparing radical perineal prostatectomy: anatomy, surgical technique and initial results. *J Urol* 1988; **140**: 559–62.
7. Angermeier KW, Jordan GH, Complications of the exaggerated lithotomy position: a review of 177 cases. *J Urol* 1994; **151**: 866–8.
8. Lassen PM, Kerase WS, Rectal injuries during radical perineal prostatectomy. *Urology* 1995; **45**: 266–9.
9. Weldon VE, Tavel FR, Neuwirth H, Cohen R, Patterns of positive specimen margins and detectable prostate specific antigen after radical perineal prostatectomy. *J Urol* 1995; **153**: 1565–9.
10. Walther PJ, Radical perineal vs. retropubic prostatectomy: a review of optimal application and technical considerations in the utilization of these exposures. *Eur Urol* 1993; **24**: 34–8.

11.3

Laparoscopic pelvic lymphadenectomy for prostate cancer

Malcolm J Coptcoat, Abhijit Darshane

CONTENTS • **Anatomy of the pelvic lymphatics** • **The extent of the dissection** • **Indications for pelvic lymphadenectomy** • **Endoscopic techniques** • **Complications**

A surgical procedure is only as good as the pathophysiological foundation that it rests upon. It is no coincidence that many surgical procedures introduced over the last 10 years have not been retained in routine clinical practice. This is undoubtedly due to a better understanding of the questions that a precise technique attempted to answer. It is also partly due to the attraction towards technology. There is a universal first sensation that something complex and difficult to learn must be relevant, but in the end, all great principles are distilled and simplified. This has been the story of the laparoscopic pelvic lymphadenectomy (LPL). It is not yet time to write its obituary, but its relevance as a routine procedure is waning, while its legacy will be carried forward. That legacy is a better understanding of the way to stage localized prostate cancer, the relevance of involved pelvic lymph nodes and a simplified lymphadenectomy technique.

Staging of a cancer must have a concrete purpose other than to provide prognostic insight in clinical trials. In this case the identification of involved pelvic lymph nodes is important to prevent patients undergoing unnecessary radical treatment. An investigation is only relevant when

the answer may change the management of that patient, but unfortunately the negative predictive value of a pelvic lymphadenectomy for future metastatic disease remains unnecessarily high. This is why the indications for an LPL have changed. Associated lymph node disease has historically been the most sensitive indicator of metastatic disease.[1,2] This, however, reflected a situation much later in the natural history of a patient's disease. The corollary of this dictum is not true. An absence of lymph node involvement does not exclude the possibility of metastatic disease. And so, given the weakness of a lymphadenectomy to predict the ultimate outcome for a patient when one considers the morbidity of an open lymphadenectomy, it is clear why there has been a need to find either a non-invasive or at least a minimally invasive alternative.

Magnetic resonance imaging, computer tomographic (CT) scanning and lymphangiography have been investigated, but their unacceptably low sensitivity and specificity have been major drawbacks.[3-6] Similarly, ultrasound- and CT-guided fine-needle aspiration biopsies are operator-dependent techniques that are ineffective in the absence of gross lymphadenopathy. For these reasons, the histopathological evaluation of surgically procured lymphatic tissue remained a gold standard on which appropriate therapeutic decisions were based.[6] The minimally invasive nature of an LPL has provided a very reasonable compromise since its inception some six years ago.[7,8] There is now a wide experience with this technique, but in this time two further refinements have occurred. The first of these is the surgical technique itself. Nodes can be approached endoscopically via either a transperitoneal or a retroperitoneal route. Also the rebound effect among those unfamiliar with more advanced endoscopic techniques has been the very reasonable development of a minilaparotomy for the pelvic lymphadenectomy. The second refinement, which has provided enormous insight into the development and progression of prostate cancer and our ability to monitor such events, concerns the predictive value of clinical staging as determined by transrectal ultrasound (TRUS), serum prostate-specific antigen (PSA) and biopsy material from both the prostate and the seminal vesicles. The use of these preoperative indicators has changed the application of any form of lymphadenectomy, and the number of patients now undergoing an LPL has greatly diminished.

ANATOMY OF THE PELVIC LYMPHATICS

The anatomy of the pelvic lymphatics is shown in Figure 11.3.1. The common iliac nodes are grouped around the artery inferior to the aortic bifurcation and anterior to the fifth lumbar vertebra of sacral promontory. They drain the external and internal iliac nodes and send efferents to the lateral aortic nodes. The common iliac nodes are usually in medial, lateral and intermediate (anterior) chains, the lateral being the main route.

The external iliac nodes are arranged in three subgroups: lateral, medial and anterior to the external iliac vessels; the anterior is inconstant. The medial nodes are considered the main channel of drainage, collecting from the inguinal nodes, the deeper layers of the infraumbilical abdominal wall, the adductor region of the thigh, the glans penis or clitoris, the membranous urethra, the prostate, the vesical fundus, the cervix uteri and upper vagina. Their efferents pass to

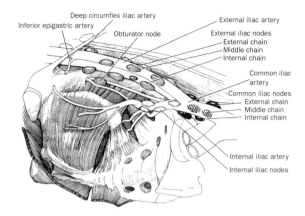

Figure 11.3.1 Diagram of the pelvic lymphatics.

the common iliac nodes.

Inferior epigastric and circumflex iliac nodes are associated with their vessels and drain the corresponding areas, being outlying members of the external iliac group and inconstant in number. The internal iliac nodes surround the vessels, receiving afferents from all the pelvic viscera, deep parts of the perineum, and gluteal and posterior femoral muscles. Efferents pass to the common iliac nodes. Sacral nodes along the median and lateral sacral vessels, and an obturator node sometimes occurring in the obturator canal, are outlying members of the internal iliac group.

There is considerable bypassing in the iliac groups of lymph nodes. Lymphangiographic studies have demonstrated the connections between the right and left groups.

Collecting vessels from the ductus deferens end in the external iliac nodes, while those from the seminal vesicle go to the internal and external iliac nodes. Prostatic vessels end mainly in internal iliac and sacral nodes; a vessel from the posterior surface accompanies the vesical vessels to the external iliac nodes, and one from the anterior surface gains the internal iliac group by joining vessels of the membranous urethra.

THE EXTENT OF THE DISSECTION

The extent of the dissection recommended in an LPL is based on the expected lymphatic drainage of the cancer. It is also influenced by the historical development of the open pelvic lymphadenectomy. The earlier approach of such an open lymphadenectomy was an extensive dissection lateral to the genitofemoral nerve, taking all fibrolymphatic tissue of the external iliac vessels, extending proximally to the common iliac vessels and medially to skeletonize the obturator vessels and nerve, as well as the internal iliac artery and branches. Finally, the dissection included the presacral and lateral sacral lymph nodes. The distal extent of the dissection included Cloquet's inguinal node and extended inferiorly to the point where the circumflex vein crosses over the external iliac artery.[9]

Over the last 10 years, many urological surgeons have become less radical and have recommended a modified open pelvic lymphadenectomy that includes primarily the nodal and fibro-fatty tissue within the obturator fossa surrounding the obturator vessels and nerve. The lateral and medial borders of this dissection include the external iliac vein and hypogastric artery, respectively. The cranial and cordial limits are the bifurcation of the iliac vessels and Cloquet's node or Cooper's ligament, respectively.

A major reason in urology for this modification was that 86–94% of the positive nodes from prostate cancer were within the region of the obturator and internal iliac artery, with no more than 6–14% of cases showing skip lesions, involving only the presacral or common iliac regions.[2] A second reason is that postoperative complications are more significant, especially when followed by radiotherapy.[10] Developments such as these in open surgery have influenced our technique for the LPL.

INDICATIONS FOR A PELVIC LYMPHADENECTOMY

The correlation between advanced clinical stage disease and an increased likelihood of lymphatic metastases was well documented by Flocks and colleagues[2] in 1959. They specifically demonstrated that in cases where examination indicated periprostatic extension involving the seminal vesicles, lymphatic metastases were discovered in over 50% of cases. This was a retrospective study, and it is well known with our experience of understaging localized prostate cancers that a preoperative assessment of periprostatic extension and, in particular, seminal vesicle involvement is poor. The serum PSA does have some preoperative predictive power in determining the likelihood of extraprostatic disease. Lange et al[11] reviewed the PSA data from several studies. These collectively showed that lymph node involvement was present in approximately 65% of cases with a preoperative PSA value between 20 and 50 ng/ml. However, over recent years the consensus has been that such patients with a high PSA are unlikely to do well following radical surgery. At King's College Hospital, London, no patient with a serum PSA of less than 10 ng/ml demonstrated lymphatic metastases following an LPL or open lymphadenectomy and only 6% of patients demonstrated lymphatic metastases with a PSA over 10 and less than 20 ng/ml. This is becoming a more reasonable group on which to consider radical treatment, and the predictive power of the PSA in conjunction with stage and Gleason score has been further refined by Oesterling's group.[12] The objective of this study was to determine if the preoperative variables of PSA, primary Gleason grade from the biopsy specimen and a local clinical stage as determined from digital rectal examination could accurately predict the pelvic lymph node status in patients with clinically localized prostate cancer. The records of 1632 patients who underwent bilateral pelvic lymphadenectomy were reviewed. Using logistic regression analysis, serum PSA was found to be the best predictor of lymph node metastases ($p < 0.0001$). The predictive power of serum PSA could be enhanced considerably by taking into account the Gleason grade and local clinical stage. A statistical model using all three variables was developed, and this should allow an estimate on an individual basis of the probability of lymph node involvement preoperatively. Using a conservative cut-off point of less than 3% as an acceptable false-negative rate, it was seen that 61% of the patients with clinical stages T1A to T2B disease and 29% of those with clinical stage T1A to T2C could have been spared either an open or laparoscopic staging bilateral pelvic lymphadenectomy. This single paper[12] has probably had the largest impact recently in determining the indications for any form of lymphadenectomy.

We have previously known that seminal vesicle involvement is commonly associated with positive nodal disease. Stock et al[13] have very reasonably put forward the suggestion that seminal vesicle biopsies (SVBs) should always be taken preoperatively. They looked at 120 patients with clinical stage T1B to T2C prostate cancer with a negative bone scan and negative pelvic CT scans. These all underwent TRUS-guided SUBs (three from each side). Ninety-nine of these patients also underwent an LPL. A positive SVB was found in 15% of patients. Again a logistic regression analysis was performed to test the effect of grade, PSA and stage on these results. In a very similar trend that predicted nodal involvement it was also found that combined grade and PSA were significant predictors of a positive SVB. Patients with a combined Gleason grade of 7 or greater had a higher positive SVB rate of 37.5% compared with 7% of patients with a lower grade. Patients with a PSA value greater than 10 ng/ml had a positive SVB rate of 21% compared with 6% for patients with values under 10 ng/ml. LPL detected positive pelvic nodes in 10% of patients. The effect of a positive SVB, combined Gleason grade, PSA and stage on detection of positive nodes were tested using a step-wise logistic regression analysis. In this case the SVB was the most significant predictor of positive nodes ($p < 0.0001$). Positive nodes were found in 50% of patients with a positive SVB compared with 0% of patients with a negative SVB. Positive nodes were found in 35% of patients with a combined Gleason grade of 7 or greater compared with 2% of patients with a combined grade less than 7. LPL dissection revealed positive nodes in 3% of patients with PSA levels less than 20 ng/ml compared with 24% of patients with PSA levels greater than 20 ng/ml.

This certainly adds a further parameter to our staging protocol for patients considered suitable for radical treatment. It could be reasonably argued that finding a positive SVB by TRUS-guided biopsy should exclude an LPL because, even with the greater instance of positive nodes, the presence of invasion into the seminal vesicle is in itself a poor prognostic factor, and is associated with a poor outcome following either radical surgery or radical radiotherapy. However, SVB is technically demanding and often painful for the patient, and few centres at present consider it a routine part of the work-up towards radical surgery.

The specific indications for an LPL at King's College Hospital are for patients with clinically localized prostate cancer who are being considered for a radical prostatectomy. If the patient has a clinical stage T2B cancer or less, Gleason score 6 or less and a PSA less than 10 ng/ml then an LPL is not undertaken and a total perineal prostatectomy is the curative operation of choice. An LPL is indicated for patients with a T2B stage or less but with a Gleason score of 7 or greater or a PSA value over 10 ng/ml. The LPL is undertaken as a separate day-case procedure, with a total perineal prostatectomy usually chosen 1 week later if the nodes are negative on paraffin sections. It has been our policy to perform a radical retropubic prostatectomy in grade T2C patients and above, in which case an open lymphadenectomy with frozen sections will precede the definitive prostatectomy. Previous radiotherapy to the pelvis is not a contraindication to a LPL. Jarrard and Chodak[14] reported the feasibility of LPL in six patients with a previous history of external beam radiotherapy for prostate cancer who were considered possible candidates for a salvage prostatectomy following a biochemical failure. Blood loss was minimal and there were no serious perioperative problems.

ENDOSCOPIC TECHNIQUES

Although the early laparoscopic pelvic lymphadenectomy cases were all undertaken via a transperitoneal route, there is now considerable experience with extraperitoneal access. The equipment used, sites of the ports and extent of the dissection are very similar for both types of operation. They differ only in the initial route of access. This will be described below. It had been considered unnatural to use the transperitoneal route for dissection of an extraperitoneal compartment, and it was expected that unnecessary complications would arise. As will be discussed later, the incidence of postoperative bowel obstruction has been very rare, and is easily compensated for by the fact that lymphocoele formation is quickly absorbed into the peritoneum and does not form a collection, as has often been the case with an extraperitoneal route whether carried out by open surgery or endoscopically. Several authors have undertaken comparative studies of LPL with an open lymphadenectomy: in all cases approximately the same number of nodes could be removed (mean of approximately five on each side), with the additional negative characteristic that the operation itself took longer, but with the positive characteristic that the procedure could often be carried out as a day case, and, if not, needed only a one-night stay in hospital, and was always followed by a very rapid return to normal activities.[7,8,15–17]

LPL technique

The most significant change in our technique has been in the method used for entry into the peritoneum. First, Veress needle insertion has proved to be sometimes frustrating in inexperienced hands. Secondly, many patients had undergone previous abdominal surgery and possible adhesions make a blind entry difficult. Thirdly, and most importantly, a major vessel (common iliac artery and vein) laceration has occurred in one patient from the 'blind' introduction of the first port, despite having a protection shield. For these reasons it is now our practice to use the Hasson technique.[18]

A subumbilical transverse incision (2.5 cm) is made just below the umbilicus. By staying in the midline, it should be possible to make an avascular 'open' entry into the peritoneum. Long-stay vicryl sutures are placed on each end of the rectus sheath incision, which can be used to produce a snug air-tight fit around the

Hasson cannulae, and subsequently to close the sheath at the end of the procedure.

1. Under a general anaesthetic with muscle paralysis and assisted ventilation, the patient is put in a supine position with a 20–25° head-down tilt. No catheter is required if the patient's bladder has recently emptied and the length of the procedure is expected to be less than 90 min. Hip flexion is not required. Heparinization is not recommended, but thromboembolic deterrent stockings should be worn for deep venous thrombosis (DVT) prophylaxis.
2. Formation of the pneumoperitoneum: a Hasson cut-down technique should be used for the first port. This should be inserted well away from a scar so that adhesions can be seen and taken down.
3. Three 10-mm ports and one 5-mm port are placed as shown in Figure 11.3.2. The

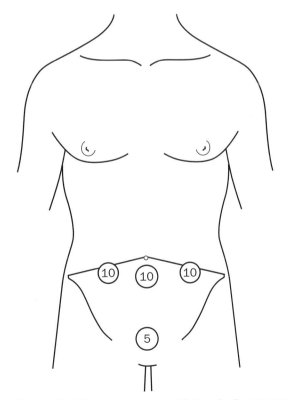

Figure 11.3.2 Laparoscopic pelvic lymphedenectomy: port sites (3 × 10 mm + 1 × 5 mm). The telescope or stapler can be interchanged between the 10-mm ports.

subumbilical port is used for the telescope. The two lateral ports along the edge of the rectus sheath are for manipulative and dissecting instruments. The central port 3–4 cm above the symphysis pubis is for the Endoclip Applier. The ports should be fixed using either grips or purse-string sutures. The use of 10-mm ports for the subumbilical and lateral ports allows greater options for introducing the telescope, Endoclip Applier and 10-mm instruments.

4. The operator stands on the contralateral side of the patient, while the camera-holder is on the ipsilateral side.

5. Monitors should be at the bottom corners of the operating table.

6. The landmarks of dissection are the umbilical ligament medially, the pubic bone anteriorly and the external iliac vessels laterally (Figure 11.3.3). The vas or round ligament courses across this triangle and sometimes requires division for easier access to the obturator fossa.

7. The dissection is begun by incising the peritoneum along the medial border of the external iliac vein, and fibro-fatty tissue is removed from around the vessel until it can be clearly exposed between the inguinal ligament and a region 2–3 cm proximal to its bifurcation. The dissection then begins in the obturator fossa, and all fibro-fatty tissue is removed until the obturator nerve is exposed. The obturator artery and vein can usually be left intact (Figure 11.3.4).

The circumflex vein and an aberrant obturator artery (10%) sometimes run across this space, and these usually have to be clipped and cut. The use of diathermy in the obturator fossa should be minimized in order to prevent obturator nerve injury.

The dissection always stays lateral to the medial umbilical ligament, and care must be taken closer to the iliac bifurcation, where the ureter is crossed by the ligament. Many of the lymphatics are small and can be sealed with diathermy, but larger vessels require clips. Ideally, the fibro-fatty tissue will have been removed in discrete blocks, but sometimes this comes away in several pieces. The number of pieces should be noted by a nurse, and these can be left to one side in the paracolic gutter until they are all placed in a retrieval bag.

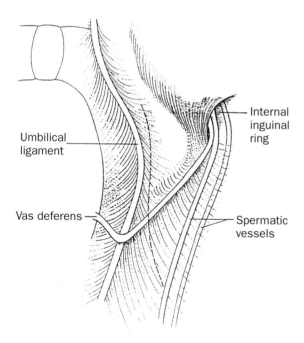

Figure 11.3.3 Peritoneal incision (dotted lines) between the umbilical ligament (medially) and the external iliac vein (laterally) that will lead to the obturator fossa. The vas must usually be divided.

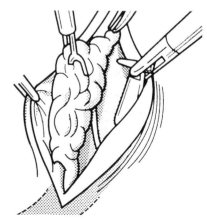

Figure 11.3.4 Laparoscopic photograph of the dissected obturator fossa.

8. The fibro-fatty tissue dissected should be placed in a retrieval bag inserted through a post from the opposite iliac fossa. The neck can be held open with two sets of forceps while a third places the tissue inside the bag. Specialized bags are available, but the finger of a surgeon's glove suffices. It is advisable to mark the retrieval bags as left and right for future audit of the dissection.

9. Both sites should be irrigated and aspirated. If there is any oozing, a swab can be pressed over the area. Usually no drain is required.

10. After completing the dissection on the opposite side, by the same method, the instruments can be removed and the ports taken out under direct vision. All carbon dioxide is evacuated.

11. To prevent wound herniation, all wounds require a deep fascial suture. The skin can be sutured with a subcuticular absorbable suture or steristripped. The patients require two to three hours to recover, and can usually then be discharged if they can demonstrate effective micturition and do not feel discomfort or nausea.

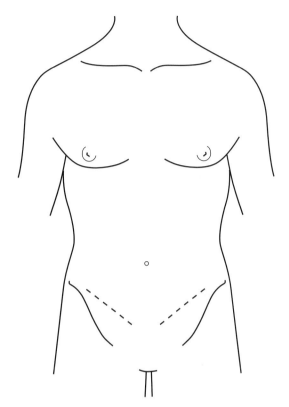

Figure 11.3.5 Extraperitoneal minilaparotomy: incisions.

The minilaparatomy alternative

The LPL must now be compared with the cheaper and more easily learnt minilaparotomy (Figure 11.3.5) approach.[19] Brant et al[20] have compared the results of 51 patients who had undergone a minilaparotomy pelvic lymphadenectomy (MPL) with 60 LPL patients. Of the MPL patients, only one had to stay overnight in hospital, and all left within 24 hours. The cost of the MPL was 50% of the cost of an LPL, with no interoperative or postoperative morbidity. The MPL took, on average, only 35 minutes. The MPL is more easily undertaken through two separate 'inguinal' incisions. This is only relevant to those surgeons who carry out a lymphadenectomy in association with a total perineal prostatectomy or radiotherapy. It makes sense to use a midline incision if a retropubic prostatectomy is to be the next step.

The MPL involves an extraperitoneal access, which alone carries a certain intuitive surgical correctness. The endoscopic lymphadenectomy can be carried out both transperitoneally or extraperitoneally, and several reports suggest that both rates are equally successful, but with fewer complications associated with the extraperitoneal route.[21] Perhaps surprisingly, the incidence of postoperation small bowel adhesions to the pelvic floor, presenting as subacute obstruction, is unusual and similar for both routes of access.[22] This is almost certainly related to the initial access and, as is described above in the authors' technique for LPL, can be circumvented by using a Hasson 'open' access technique.

COMPLICATIONS

The laparoscopic pelvic lymphadenectomy can usually be carried out as a day-case procedure.

Only 6% of the patients in King's College Hospital have required overnight stay; the reason for this was persistent nausea. Some of our elderly patients receive peroperative opiate analgesia, and this was identified as a cause of their nausea. Further eradication of this problem has come with the introduction of ondansetron. This is not given routinely, but only to those patients who still feel nauseous two to three hours after the procedure. Complications can otherwise be those general to laparoscopy and those specific to this procedure.

Recent reports of the complications of an LPL have confirmed our early optimism.[23,24]. An interesting observation by Chow[25] demonstrated that the diagnosis of small bowel obstruction or hernia into trocar sites, urinoma, lymphocoele or haematuria could be made using CT scanning.

Ruckle et al[26] reported a 14% specific complication rate, which included two patients with a DVT, an obturator nerve palsy, a retroperitoneal abscess and an accidental cystotomy. The King's College Hospital experience of this procedure has an 8% complication rate. DVTs have not been experienced in our series, possibly due to the universal use of thromboembolic-deterrent stockings. One patient required immediate open exploration because of arterial bleeding during dissection. This was identified at the junction between the supposedly obliterated umbilical artery and the internal iliac artery. It was a reminder not to take the dissection so proximally in the future, since this is also the point at which the ureter may be cut accidentally, where it crosses beneath the obliterated umbilical artery. Winfield et al[27] reported a 6% incidence of peroperative haemorrhage. Two of these four cases required urgent exploration. This slightly high incidence probably reflects the variety in radicalism of the lymphadenectomy. The morbidity of a laparoscopic pelvic lymphadenectomy is, however, much less than that of an open procedure.[28]

One King's College Hospital patient went into urinary retention, and this will always be a possibility if routine catheterization is used in elderly men. One would have imagined that carbon dioxide absorption through the dissection sites would be high, but the continual measurement of end-tidal carbon dioxide levels and correction with assisted ventilation has not led to any such complications. Minor complications such as the formation of a pneumoscrotum do occur occasionally, but these all settle within a few hours of the procedure and do not seem to cause the patient any discomfort.

SUMMARY

Our refined indications for radical surgery and radiotherapy have, to a large extent, made the prognostic significance of lymphatic spread much less. As a surgical technique, the LPL can be viewed as a very reasonable alternative to an open lymphadenectomy. It can become part of a urologist's repertoire without the need for great expertise. However, many urologists will probably choose a modified minilaparotomy (extraperitoneal) because it does not require the technology of laparoscopy.

The reduced role of any form of a lymphadenectomy, given our better understanding of PSA, Gleason score, clinical stage, seminal vesicle biopsy and perhaps also reverse-transcriptase polymerase chain reaction (RT-PCR) for mRNA, as described by Olssen's group,[29] does suggest that the retropubic approach for radical surgery is now rarely necessary. It is not a coincidence that there is now a renewed interest in the total perineal prostatectomy for localized prostate cancer.

REFERENCES

1. Cline WA Jr, Kramer SA, Farnam R et al, Impact of pelvic lymphadenectomy in patients with prostatic adenocarcinoma. *Urology* 1981; **27**: 129.
2. Flocks RH, Culp D, Porto R, Lymphatic spread from prostatic cancer. *J Urol* 1959; **81**: 194.
3. Mukamel E, Hannah J, Barbaric Z et al, The value of computerized tomography scan and magnetic resonance imaging in staging prostatic carcinoma: comparison with the clinical and histologic staging. *J Urol* 1986; **136**: 1231.
4. Benson KH, Watson RA, Spring DB et al, The value of computerized tomography in evaluation of pelvic lymph nodes. *J Urol* 1981; **126:** 63.
5. Leoning SA, Schmidt JD, Brown RC et al, A comparison between lymphangiography and pelvic node dissection in the staging of prostate cancer. *J Urol* 1977; **117:** 752.
6. Paulson DF, Piserchia PV, Gardner W, Predictors of lymphatic spread in prostatic adenocarcinoma: Uro-oncology Research Group study. *J Urol* 1980; **123:** 697.
7. Schuessler WW, Vancaillie TG, Reich H et al, Trans-peritoneal endosurgical lymphadenectomy in patients with localised prostate cancer. *J Urol* 1991; **145:** 988.
8. Schuessler WW, Pharand D, Vancaillie TG, Laparoscopic standard pelvic node dissection for carcinoma of the prostate: Is it accurate? *J Urol* 1993; **150:** 898–901.
9. Golimber M, Morales P, Al-Askari D et al, Entendedpelvic lymphadenectomy for prostate cancer. *J Urol* 1979; **121:** 617.
10. Paulson DF, The prognostic role of lymphadenectomy in adenocarcinoma of the prostate. *Urol Clin North Am* 1980; **7:** 615.
11. Lange PH, Ercole CJ, Lightner DJ et al, The value of serum prostate-specific antigen determinations before and after radical prostatectomy. *J Urol* 1989; **141:** 873.
12. Bluestein DL, Bostwick DG, Bergstralh EJ, Oesterling JE, Eliminating the need for bilateral pelvic lymphadenectomy in select patients with prostate cancer. *J Urol* 1994; **151:** 1315–20.
13. Stock RG, Stone NN, Ianuzzi C, Unger P, Seminal vesicle biopsy and laparoscopic pelvic lymph node dissection: implications for patient selection in the radiotherapeutic management of prostate cancer. *Int J Radiat Oncol Biol Phys* 1995; **33:** 815–21.
14. Jarrard DF, Chodak GW, Prostate cancer staging after radiation utilising laparoscopic pelvic lymphadenectomy. *Urology* 1995; **46:** 538–41.
15. Rukstalis DB, Gerber GS, Vogelzang NJ et al, Laparoscopic pelvic lymph node dissection: a review of 103 consecutive cases. *J Urol* 1994; **151:** 670–4.
16. Guazzoni G, Montorsi F, Bergamaschi F et al, Open surgical revision of laparoscopic pelvic lymphadenectomy for staging of prostate cancer: the impact of laparoscopic learning curve. *J Urol* 1994; **151:** 930–3.
17. Kerbl K, Clayman RV, Petros JA et al, Staging pelvic lymphadenectomy for prostate cancer: a comparison of laparoscopic and open techniques. *J Urol* 1993; **150:** 396–8 [discussion: 399].
18. Hasson HM, A modified instrument and method for laparoscopy. *Am J Obstet Gynecol* 1971; **110:** 886–7.
19. Perrotti M, Gentle DL, Barada JH et al, Minilaparotomy pelvic lymphnode dissection minimizes morbidity, hospitalisation and cost of pelvic lymph node dissection. *J Urol* 1996; **155:** 986–8.
20. Brant LA, Brant WO, Brown MH et al, A new minimally invasive open pelvic lymphadenectomy surgical technique for the staging of prostate cancer. *Urology* 1996; **47:** 416–21.
21. Das SL, Laparoscopic staging pelvic lymphadenectomy: extraperitoneal approach. *Semin Surg Oncol* 1996; **12:** 134–8.
22. Fowler JM, Hartenbach EM, Reynolds HT et al, Pelvic adhesion formation after pelvic lymphadenectomy: comparison between transperitoneal laparoscopy and extraperitoneal laparotomy in a porcine model. *Gynecol Oncol* 1994; **55:** 25–8.
23. Kavoussi LR, Sosa E, Chandhoke P et al, Complications of laparoscopic pelvic lymph node dissection. *J Urol* 1993; **149:** 322.
24. Burney TL, Campbell EC Jr, Naslund MJ, Jacobs SC, Complications of staging laparoscopic pelvic lymphadenectomy. *Surg Laparosc Endosc* 1993; **3:** 184–90.
25. Chow CC, Daly BD, Burney TL et al, Complications after laparoscopic pelvic lymphadenectomy: CT diagnosis. *Am J Roentgenol* 1994; **163:** 353–6.
26. Ruckle H, Hadley R, Lui P, Stewart S, Laparoscopic pelvic lymph node dissection: assessment of intraoperative and early postoperative complications. *J Endourol* 1992; **6:** 117–19.

27. Winfield HN, Donovan JF, See WA et al, Laparoscopic pelvic lymph node dissection for genitourinary malignancies: indications, techniques and results. *J Endourol* 1992; **6:** 103–12.

28. McLaughlin AP, Saltzstein SL, McCollough DL et al, Prostatic carcinoma: incidence and location of unsuspected lymphatic metastases. *J Urol* 1976; **115:** 89.

29. Katz AE, de Vries EM, Begg MD et al, Enhanced reverse transcriptase–polymerase chain reaction for prostate specific antigen as an indicator of true pathological stage in patients with prostate cancer. *Cancer* 1995; **75:** 1642.

12

Radiation therapy in the treatment of localized/organ-confined prostate cancer

Arthur T Porter, Kimberly B Hart

CONTENTS • **Technical background** • **Historical background** • **Treatment of cancer in the PSA era**
• **Improving the outcome of radiation therapy** • **Dose escalation** • **High linear energy transfer radiation**
• **Brachytherapy** • **Hormone therapy**

The treatment of early stage prostate cancer is a controversial issue for several reasons. Localized prostate cancer is a heterogeneous disease. Substantial differences in disease evolution and progression are seen among patients with similar disease stages. The comorbidities in this population are considerable because of advanced age. Patients are also faced with multiple treatment options, including radical prostatectomy, radiation therapy, and watchful waiting.

Radiation therapy, the use of ionizing radiation to destroy malignant tissue, has been used in the treatment of prostate cancer since the 1960s. Radiation acts at the cellular level to cause breakage of DNA within a cell, leading to a loss of reproductive integrity and cell death. The goal of radiation therapy in early stage prostate cancer is to sterilize tumor cells effectively while causing minimal damage to normal tissues. Technical advances in the last three decades have led to great strides in this regard. This chapter describes the evolution of radiation therapy in the treatment of early stage prostate cancer, and explores its role in the treatment of this disease.

TECHNICAL BACKGROUND

Radiation can be produced by naturally occurring isotopes such as cobalt-60 or artificially created isotopes. In a linear accelerator, high-frequency electromagnetic waves accelerate charged particles through a linear tube. The high-energy electron beam can then be made to strike a target to produce high-energy X-rays for treating deep tumors. The energy is important in radiation therapy for prostate cancer because high-energy beams penetrate further into tissue and give better beam characteristics for treating these deep-seated tumors. Radiation can also be introduced into the prostate directly using interstitial implantation of radioactive isotopes into the prostate itself, a technique referred to as brachytherapy.

The goal of radiation therapy is to deliver the highest possible radiation dose to the tumor volume while minimizing the dose received by the surrounding normal tissues. Therefore, the delivery of radiation requires meticulous treatment planning. Treatment-planning techniques have evolved from the relatively primitive use of bony landmarks on plain X-ray films to three-dimensional treatment planning using computed tomography (CT)-based systems, which allow accurate identification of the tumor volume and the surrounding normal tissues. External beam irradiation is generally delivered via multiple ports to achieve a homogeneous distribution to the tumor volume. Lead or lead substitute materials can be created to allow the treatment volume to conform to the volume of the tumor. Brachytherapy techniques have also changed considerably in the last decade. Retropubic surgical implantation of the prostate has been replaced by transperineal implantation using ultrasound guidance.

HISTORICAL BACKGROUND

Patients treated for early stage prostate cancer have several treatment choices, including surgery and radiation therapy. Historical comparisons have been made in an attempt to prove the superiority of surgery over radiation therapy. However, radiotherapy and surgical series cannot generally be matched in terms of patient populations and prognostic indicators. The original criteria for prostatectomy required that patients be less than 70 years old, be in good health, have a discrete nodule which was not high grade, and be free of metastatic disease.[1,2] The rationale was that only tumors confined to the prostate were candidates for cure.[3] Patients selected for radiation therapy were usually significantly older, had more coexisting illnesses and had an unknown extent of extracapsular disease and pelvic nodal metastasis. In the Massachusetts General Hospital Series, 54% of patients treated with radiation therapy had T2b/T2c disease and 33% had prostate-specific antigen (PSA) values above 15 ng/ml compared with 41% and 11% of surgical patients.[4] Therefore, it is problematic to compare clinically staged radiation patients with pathologically staged surgical patients.

The only randomized study to compare radiation therapy and surgery was the Veterans Administration (VA) Uro-oncologic group study.[5] In this study, patients with disease confined to the prostate by rectal examination (T1–T2) and with no evidence of metastatic disease were randomized to radical prostatectomy or megavoltage radiation therapy. The study concluded that, at 5 years, radical surgery led to a distinct disease-free survival advantage over radiation therapy. However, this study had significant flaws. Time to first recurrence was used as the endpoint of the study rather than disease-free survival. Two prostatectomy patients with pathological T3 disease were dropped from the analysis. The early presence of hepatic and pulmonary metastasis in the radiation therapy group likely indicates improper staging. The radiation therapy survival quoted was significantly lower than that seen in comparable historically relevant radiation therapy groups. For example, the results of radiation therapy delivered at Stanford University during the same period are superimposable on the surgical results in the VA study with an actuarial survival of 60% at 14 years.[6]

The 1988 National Cancer Institute consensus conference concluded that 'sufficient long term follow-up does not exist to demonstrate the ability of radiation therapy to provide 15-year survival free of cancer'.[7] However, the long-term results of radiation therapy for early stage prostate cancer are comparable to surgery in the pre-PSA era. The Stanford University experience involved 25 years of follow-up. Sufficient time has elapsed to identify clinical failures, without the benefit of PSA. The overall survival data for prostate cancer treated with radiation therapy in the pre-PSA era are presented in Tables 12.1 and 12.2.

TREATMENT OF PROSTATE CANCER IN THE PSA ERA

The widespread use of PSA measurement radically changed the concept of 'cure' in patients treated for prostate cancer. Disease-free survival has come to be defined as biochemical freedom from disease and the achievement of a low PSA, rather than being defined in terms of palpable clinical recurrence, regardless of the method of treatment. The prognostic significance of PSA is evident for local recurrence,

Table 12.1 Overall survival after radiation therapy (pre-PSA era): single institutions

Study	Clinical stage	No. of patients	10-year overall survival (%)	10-year FFR (%)	15-year overall survival (%)	15-year FFR (%)
Mallinkrodt	T1A (A2)	41	66	68	–	–
	T2 (B)	185	55	50	–	–
Stanford	T1	282	60	63	35	50
	T2	183	55	45	33	37

FFR, freedom from relapse.

Table 12.2 Overall survival after radiation therapy (pre-PSA era): patterns of care study

Cohort survival	Clinical stage	No. of patients	Freedom from (%)		Survival (%)
			Any failure	Local recurrence	
1973					
5 year	T1	60	84	97	57
10 year		–	81	97	40
15 year		–	64	83	–
5 year	T2	306	66	94	45
10 year		–	71	65	–
15 year		–	35	25	–
1978					
5 year	T1	116	82	92	63
10 year		–	72	85	–
5 year	T2	415	63	87	47
10 year		–	52	71	–
1983					
5 year	T1	116	92	100	–
	T2	96	71	88	–

metastatic relapse or any relapse. The post-treatment PSA level is useful for monitoring the presence of recurrent disease, and has led to detection of residual disease at an average of 5 years sooner than clinical methods.[8–10] PSA has taught that the cure of clinically localized prostate cancer is seen less frequently than previously believed, and that total eradication of pelvic disease is less likely to be achieved.[11–13]

The kinetics of PSA decline differ between radiation and surgical series. After surgery, decline in PSA occurs with a half-life of 3 days.[14] With radiation, serum PSA values decline after treatment, but the extent and kinetics have not been described. Radiation neither immediately eradicates the tumor nor eliminates the prostate. Postradiation clearance of PSA occurs as the radiation lethality incurred during treatment is slowly expressed during an extended period of time as tumor cells divide.[15] Therefore, slow decline of PSA does not preclude future recurrence; the initial half-life with which serum PSA declines after radiation has no role as a prognostic indicator. In Ritter's series,[15] 50% of patients had PSA values in the normal range within 1.5 months of treatment, whereas 90% had PSA values in the normal range at 18 months of follow-up.

Because the PSA baseline level represents the contribution of irradiated normal epithelium after treatment, the definition of biochemical failure after radiation differs between radiation and surgical series. High-dose radiation decreases the protein synthesis within any tissue. Thus, the normal range of PSA values is judged to be too liberal for determining biochemical failure. Conversely, to hold to the prostatectomy criterion on a PSA level of 0–0.5 ng/ml is also too strict.[16] Biochemical freedom from disease after the treatment of prostate cancer with radiation has been defined at nadir values of PSA well below the normal range. Kavadi's group[16] reported that the actuarial incidence of relapse or rising PSA was 17%, 70%, 70% and 71% for PSA nadir values of <1, 1–2, 2–4 and >4 ng/ml, respectively.[14] Mean PSA nadir was also correlated with the pretreatment PSA level. For initial PSA values of <4, 5–10, >10, 11–30 and >30 ng/ml, the corre-

sponding mean PSA nadirs were 0.8, 1.3, 2.4 and 5.4 ng/ml. Kavadi stated that the 3-year recurrence rates associated with PSA nadir values of <1, 1–2, 3–4 and >4 ng/ml were 10–15%, 30%, 55% and 60%, respectively.[16] Zietman concluded that cure is unlikely unless the serum PSA falls to a level of <1 ng/ml.[17] In the Wayne State University experience, the incidence of rising PSA was 10% for those patients with a PSA nadir of <1.0 ng/ml and 100% for a PSA nadir of >2.0 ng/ml.[18]

Pretreatment PSA has been found to be a predictor of clinical outcome in both radiation series (see Table 12.2). Zagars[19] reported that the higher the PSA value above 20 ng/ml, the greater the likelihood of disease relapse. An initial PSA value of <4 ng/ml was associated with a 8% risk of relapse in contrast to a 54% risk of relapse for patients with an initial PSA of >20 ng/ml. Kuban et al,[20] in examining the predictive value of pretreatment PSA, found an initial PSA of 0–4 ng/ml to be associated with 70% freedom from biochemical relapse versus a 0% incidence of freedom from relapse in those patients with an initial PSA of >20 ng/ml. Hart et al[18] reported the biochemical disease-free rates to be 100%, 50% and 17% for patients with pretreatment PSA values of <15, 16–20 and >20 ng/ml, respectively. Zietman et al[17] concluded that men with early stage disease and a pretreatment PSA of <15 ng/ml had a 65% freedom from biochemical failure.

Surgical series demonstrate a similar correlation between pretreatment PSA and freedom from biochemical relapse (Table 12.3). A series from Stanford University relating initial PSA to findings at radical prostatectomy found a 35% rate of seminal vesicle invasion and a 22% rate of nodal spread among patients with an initial PSA of >16 ng/ml.[21] With an initial PSA of >80 ng/ml, 50% of patients had seminal vesicle involvement and 90% had positive nodes. In the Johns Hopkins series, only 25% of men with PSA values of >15 ng/ml had organ-confined disease; 22% had seminal vesicle involvement and 36% had positive pelvic nodes. The 5-year freedom from biochemical progression was 92% for those patients with pretreatment PSA values of <4 ng/ml, in contrast to only 45% in

Table 12.3 Correlation between pretreatment PSA and disease-free survival in radiation therapy patients

Study	Pretreatment PSA (ng/ml)	5-year disease-free survival (%)
Zagars et al[16]	4.0	90
	4.0–20	60
	>20	45
Kuban et al[20]	0–4	80
	4–10	74
	10–20	70
	>20	45
Kabalin et al[34]	10–20	72
	20–50	25
	>50	16

those patients with initial PSA values of >20 ng/ml.[22]

Several researchers have created mathematical models to predict the incidence of extracapsular disease and nodal metastasis in patients with prostate cancer by incorporating PSA, clinical stage and Gleason score. Forty percent of patients predicted to have organ-confined disease by digital rectal examination, PSA and Gleason score will have disease outside the prostate.[23] The preoperative Gleason score is useful in predicting the pathologic stage in those with scores of 2–4 and 8–10. However, for the 75% of men with a Gleason score of 5–7, pathologic stage is difficult to predict from this score. Partin et al[24] created a nomogram based on PSA, Gleason score and clinical stage to identify those patients with advanced disease. Capsular penetration, seminal vesicle involvement and lymph node involvement were best predicted by a combination of these variables.[25] Roach et al[26] have expanded upon this nomo-

gram to create a mathematical formula for predicting the incidence of lymph node metastasis:

$$\text{Node positivity} = \tfrac{2}{3}\,\text{PSA} + (\text{Gleason score} - 6) \times 10.$$

Using this formula, the lowest calculated risk of positive nodes is 0% and the highest is 65%. Bluestein et al[27] have also developed a chart using the PSA values, Gleason scores and stages of 1632 patients who underwent lymph node dissection.

Spevach et al[28] tested the above mathematical models by comparing the calculated incidence of lymph-node positivity with the actual incidence of positive lymph nodes in patients undergoing lymphadenectomy. He found the Bluestein model to have the best sensitivity and the lowest false-negative rate (96% and 1.1%, respectively). There was reported to be some selection bias in the Roach model due to the high percentage of low-stage tumors (61% were less than T2A) involved in creating the formula.

Mathematical models can be useful in predicting the incidence of lymph-node metastasis and extracapsular disease, but have not yet been tested in clinical settings.

IMPROVING THE OUTCOME OF RADIATION THERAPY

Radiation therapy techniques have been refined over the past three decades in an attempt to improve the cure rates for localized prostate cancer with respect to field size and treatment planning methods. The original approach of Bagshaw et al[29] and del Regato[30] was to treat a small volume of the prostate and periprostatic tissues using megavoltage irradiation. In an attempt to increase the cure rate, Bagshaw[31] then suggested the addition of radiation therapy to pelvic nodes. The prostate, seminal vesicles and pelvic lymph nodes were treated to a dose of 4500 cGy followed by a boost dose to the prostate to give a total dose of 6000–6500 cGy. Perez et al[32] reported a 85–90% control rate for patients with stage A2 or stage B prostate cancer using this technique.

In 1977, the Radiation Therapy Oncology Group[33] instituted a trial (RTOG 77-06) to determine the value of elective pelvic node irradiation in the management of tumor limited to the prostate without evidence of nodal involvement. Patients were randomized to localized prostate irradiation alone versus elective pelvic irradiation in addition to localized irradiation. There was no difference in survival or local control with the addition of pelvic radiation. However, only 4% of patients could actually have been expected to harbor microscopic disease without distant metastasis and, therefore, to benefit from nodal treatment. Nevertheless, this study led to a greater acceptance of localized treatment fields in patients treated with radiation therapy.

The advent of PSA level monitoring, and the realization that radiation therapy was not curing as many patients as believed by clinical criteria of failure, led to radical changes in the way radiation therapy was used. Recent studies have focused on the high incidence of local relapse in localized prostate cancer treated with radiation therapy.[34,35] Standard treatment approaches have been insufficiently accurate to include the total prostate volume.[36] Plain film images were used to define the prostate, its location and the field size and shape. Simulation images were created using bony landmarks and intravesicle contrast. Therefore, the entire prostate volume may not have been encompassed and the tumor may have been underdosed.[37] The treatment volume may have been inaccurately defined, leading to an inability to calculate sufficiently accurately the dose to the prostate required. However, the proximity of the prostate to critical normal structures, such as the bladder and rectum, has limited the ability to deliver effective dose levels in excess of 70 Gy by means of conventional radiotherapy techniques.[38,39]

Three-dimensional CT-guided treatment planning

Three-dimensional conformal radiation therapy (3D-CRT) was developed to correct some of the shortcomings of conventionally planned radiation therapy. 3D-CRT challenges the standard four-field box technique for superiority of tumor coverage and critical structure sparing. Although some authors maintain that a truly conformal beam arrangement must contain non-coplanar beams, at the Karmanos Cancer Institute/Wayne State University, this technique describes any multiple-beam arrangement that uses sophisticated computer-aided devices to plan and deliver prescribed radiation doses conforming to the three-dimensional configuration of the tumor while minimizing the dose to normal tissues. The rapid decrease in dose to the surrounding normal tissues as a function of distance from the target allows the exclusion of surrounding normal tissue from the volume carried to high doses. Therefore, the dose to the tumor can be escalated beyond that possible with conventional two-dimensional systems, with a reasonable rate of normal tissue complications.[40,41]

At the Karmanos Cancer Institute/Wayne

State University, 95% of early stage prostate patients are treated with 3D-CRT. Patients are immobilized in custom cradles and are given contrast medium orally. A retrograde uretero-gram is performed to identify the lower margin of the prostate. This is an integral component of the conformal approach. Roach et al[42] have reported that the inferior margin of the prostate was inaccurately defined in 25% of patients if the ischial tuberosities were used to delineate the prostate apex. Initial volumes include the prostate and seminal vesicles with a 1.5-cm margin to allow for treatment set-up variation and prostate motion. A boost is delivered to the prostate using either axial or non-axial fields.[43] Adequacy of the target and doses to the sur-rounding normal tissues are evaluated by examining the isodose distributions on mid-plane axial, sagittal and coronal CT images and dose–volume histograms (DVHs). The DVH presents the percentage of the total organ vol-ume receiving a given percentage of the total dose. DVH projections are done for the tumor, bladder, rectum and any other site for which the dose is to be estimated.

Conformal treatment has resulted in a favor-able biochemical outcome for a large percent-age of patients with early stage prostate cancer. Corn et al[44] noted that PSA normalization was observed in 96% of patients treated confor-mally, versus only 85% of conventionally treated patients with a normal PSA considered as <4 ng/ml. The PSA normalization rate to <1.5 ng/ml was 75% versus 55%. Leibel et al[40] reported that 97% of patients with T1c and T2a disease and 86% with T2b disease had normal-ization of PSA values at 3 years after conformal treatment. The superior PSA response in con-formal treatment has been attributed to more accurate targeting of the entire prostate volume, particularly the inferior portion of the gland.[14–16] In an evaluation of prostate specimens, Stamey et al[21] found the most common site of positive margins to be at the apex.

Treatment-related toxicity has also been reduced using conformal techniques. Acute tox-icities commonly reported include fatigue, uri-nary frequency or dysuria, diarrhea, proctalgia, and occasionally rectal bleeding. These symp-toms are commonly reported in one-third to one-half of patients.[45,46] The pathogenesis of acute effects is related to rapidly dividing epithelium and correlates with treatment time and fraction size. Acute gastrointestinal and genitourinary side effects appear to be decreased in patients receiving conformal radi-ation therapy, particularly with regard to the duration of symptoms (Table 12.5). The RTOG trials reported grade 1 and grade 2 gastroin-testinal and genitourinary side effects of 10–12%.[47] In contrast, conformal techniques have led to a decrease of 30% in acute bladder and rectum symptoms.[48] The dose to bladder and rectum was reduced by 14% using confor-mal techniques in the Fox Chase and Mallickrodt experience, resulting in a 35% decrease in the presence of acute symptoms compared to conventional radiation.[49,50]

Persistent or late effects affect structures the radiation sensitivity of which may be exceeded, including the rectum, anus, rectosigmoid, small intestine, bladder, and prostatic urethra, and potency. Late side effects are ascribed to vascu-lar damage, which may be secondary to the turnover kinetics of affected tissues. This may be a result of damage or depletion of the stro-mal population. Late effects depend on fraction size and total dose, as well as on the volume of the affected organ treated. The RTOG reported a 7.7% rate of grade 3 or 4 urinary toxicity and a 3.3% rate of grade 3 and 4 gastrointestinal toxi-city.[51] 3D-CRT fields decrease the volume of rectal tissues receiving a high radiation dose by 50%. Sandler et al[52] have reported a 3% rate of grade 3 or 4 gastrointestinal or genitourinary toxicity in patients treated conformally.

Potency preservation, related to the effect of radiation-induced end-arteritis of internal pudendal and penile arteries, has not been impacted by conformal radiation therapy. The potency rates quoted in the literature range from 33% to 60%, regardless of the method of treatment.[53–55] The truly potent patient has a greater change of maintaining potency than does the borderline patient.

Table 12.4 Correlation between pretreatment PSA and freedom from progression: surgical patients

Study	Preoperative PSA (ng/ml)	5-year disease-free survival (%)
Partin et al[22]	<4.0	92
	4.0–10	83
	10–20	56
	>20	45
Catalona[21]	<4.0	95
	4.1–9.9	93
	>10	71

Table 12.5 Acute radiation therapy toxicity

Study	Treatment modality	Toxicity (%)	Comments
Genitourinary toxicity			
Bagshaw et al[46]	Conventional	24	
RTOG[47]	Conventional	13 (grade 1 or 2)	60% had no symptoms after 6 months
Viyakumar et al[48]	Conformal	10	
Soffen et al[49]	Conventional	80 (grade 1 or 2)	Fewer treatment interruptions and shorter duration of symptoms in conformal group
	Conformal	65 (grade 1 or 2)	
Gastrointestinal toxicity			
Bagshaw et al[46]	Conventional	43	
RTOG[47]	Conventional	10 (grade 1 or 2 proctitis and diarrhea)	60% persisted at 1 year
Viyakumar et al[48]	Conformal	8	
Soffen et al[49]	Conventional	55	Fewer treatment interruptions and shorter duration of symptoms in conformal group
	Conformal	42	

DOSE ESCALATION

A significant proportion of patients with localized prostate cancers have biopsy-proven local recurrences. Freiha and Bagshaw[56] reported that 61% of patients have positive biopsies at 18 months after radiation, with a higher positive biopsy rate among those with high stage and grade disease. There was a strong correlation between positive biopsy and subsequent disease progression in the 72% of patients with positive biopsies. However, disease also progressed in 24% of patients with negative biopsies, demonstrating that a negative biopsy does not guarantee the absence of disease. Kuban et al[57] stated that the local failure rates at 5 and 10 years were 8% and 24% in patients with negative postradiation biopsies in contrast to 44% and 75% for patients with positive biopsies. Crook et al[58] correlated the results of routine transrectal ultrasound biopsies with digital rectal examinations, PSA and ultrasound in men treated with radiation for carcinoma of the prostate. Over 50% of the biopsies showing residual tumor at 1 year following radiation eventually converted to negative. PSA was found to be a more accurate measure of failure in this series.

Several retrospective studies have suggested a relationship between local control and dose. Hanks et al,[59] in their patterns of care studies, noted an actuarial 7-year local recurrence rate of 36% for doses of 60–64.9 Gy, 32% for 65–69 Gy, and 24% for 70 Gy or greater. Local relapse correlates with an increased risk of metastatic dissemination.[60–62] The temporal relationship of local recurrence with distant metastasis correlates with the hypothesis that distant metastases may be derived from persistent clonogens that acquire metastatic potential after failure to eradicate the primary tumor.[63] Therefore, a cause–effect relationship may exist between local control and metastatic disease. In the Memorial Sloan–Kettering I study of 125 patients, the 20-year, distant-metastasis-free survival rate was 70% for those patients with locally controlled disease versus 13% for those patients who relapsed locally.[64]

In view of the high percentage of local recurrence, interest has developed in dose escalation. There appears to be a volume-dependent dose–response curve for prostate cancer above a dose of 70 Gy.[65] Doses up to 80–81 Gy using 3D-CRT have been delivered using photon irradiation at the Memorial Sloan–Kettering Cancer Center and the Karmanos Cancer Institute/Wayne State University.[66] In the Karmanos experience, patients with stage T3 or T4, or Gleason's grade 8 or higher tumors were treated with doses of 78 and 82.8 Gy in phase I/II dose-escalation trials.[67] Sixty percent of patients were free of clinical and biochemical recurrence at a median of 20 months of follow-up. All reported acute gastrointestinal and genitourinary toxicity was grade 2 or less. No grade 3 or 4 complications have been reported. The next step will be to apply the techniques of dose escalation to patients with localized prostate cancer, in order to improve treatment outcome.

HIGH LINEAR ENERGY TRANSFER

The rate at which charged particles deposit energy per unit distance is known as linear energy transfer (LET). Fast neutrons and protons are densely ionizing particles characterized by a high LET. These particles may offer a biologic advantage in the treatment of prostate cancer by providing a way to increase the dose delivered to the tumor. The relative biologic effectiveness (RBE) of an ionizing radiation is the ratio of the dose of that irradiation to the dose of a reference radiation required to produce a specific endpoint in a specific tissue. Therefore, if the RBE of the tumor is equal to that of the normal tissues, the therapeutic gain of neutrons compared to photons is 1.0. If the tumor RBE is greater than that of normal tissue, a therapeutic gain would result in an advantage for the patient.[68] The published RBE for prostate cancer is 3.5.[69] High LET particles are more effective than standard radiation under hypoxic conditions and are less cell-cycle dependent. These particles produce tissue injury that is less repairable.

Neutrons were initially investigated by the

RTOG. The first neutron study compared mixed neutron and photon irradiation to photons alone.[69] The prostate and regional lymph nodes received 5000 cGy with an additional boost of 2000 cGy to the prostate and periprostatic tissues. Patients treated with mixed beam received 5000 cGy 'photon equivalent' followed by a 2000-cGy 'photon equivalent' boost. At 60 months, the local/regional actuarial failure rate was 7% in the mixed group versus 38% in the photon-alone group. The disease-specific survival rate for the neutron-treated patients was 82% compared with 54% in the photon group.

The second RTOG study (No. 85-23) randomized patients to 7020 cGy of photons versus 2040 NcGy.[70] The 5-year local regional failure rate was 11% for the neutron group compared with 32% in the photon group. The PSA relapse rate was 17% versus 45%, respectively. However, the rate of late complications was significant. There were 24% grade 3 and 4 rectal toxicities in the neutron group, many requiring surgical intervention, compared with 8% in the photon group. On this basis, the RBE for bladder and rectum was calculated to be 3.5, the same as that for the cancer.[69] Differences in beam collimation capabilities contributed to the high neutron toxicity rate. No grade 3 or 4 complications were seen when the facilities included a fully rotational gantry and shaped fields.[71]

Currently, neutron irradiation is being used for prostate cancer at the University of Washington and at the Karmanos Cancer Institute. The Karmanos facility uses an isocentric treatment unit capable of 360° rotation and 12 000 independently moving tungsten rods to shape the fields. By decreasing the volume irradiated with neutrons, the rate of severe complications has been decreased, resulting in a therapeutic gain with conformal neutrons of 30%.[72,73] The rates of grade 2 chronic gastrointestinal and genitourinary toxicity are 6% and 4%, respectively.[74] No grade 3–5 toxicities were reported. At 18 months, 81% of patients with localized prostate cancer had a PSA level below 1.0 ng/ml.

BRACHYTHERAPY

Brachytherapy is a form of radiation therapy that involves the implantation of radioactive sources into the prostate. This method of treatment can deliver more radiation to the prostate and a lower dose to surrounding normal organs than can conventional radiation therapy. The higher intraprostatic dose achieved by this method could theoretically lead to more effective tumor control. The use of brachytherapy in prostate cancer has been controversial, in that the early brachytherapy experience in the 1970s appeared promising at first, but late failures turned much of the radiation oncology community away from this treatment modality. Prostate brachytherapy is presently undergoing a resurgence with the advent of transrectal ultrasound transperineal implantation in the late 1980s and early 1990s. The initial implants were performed via the retropubic approach developed by Whitmore et al in 1972.[75] A formal laparotomy was performed, with a pelvic lymph-node dissection for staging purposes. The prostate was then immobilized. Large-bore trochars were introduced via a free-hand approach for the deposition of seeds. The desired target dose was achieved by measuring the prostate intraoperatively and determining the spacing of sources and trocars using nomograms.[76] This calculation yielded the matched peripheral dose, defined as the dose of a computed contour volume that matches a mathematical ellipsoidal volume. The retropubic approach led to a very low rate of impotence and incontinence compared with the standard external beam method.[77,78] The initial reports of local control and survival were very favorable. Grossman et al[78] reported a 5-year NED (no evidence of disease) survival of 72% for patients with grade B1 and 62% for patients with grade B2 disease in the first 100 patients implanted at the Memorial Sloan–Kettering.

However, the initial appeal of retropubic implantation was soon replaced by skepticism due to the high number of late local failures. A 51% local failure rate was reported at 12 years.[78] Fuks et al[60] noted the annual hazard of local relapse to be 11.2% per year. Kuban et al[79] also reported a 29% rate of local recurrence in implanted patients, with those patients with increased stage and grade having the highest risk for relapse. The high rate of local recurrence was attributed to the inhomogeneous seed and dose distribution with a semi-blind technique of implantation. There was often an accumulation of seeds in the center of the gland with a paucity of seeds in the periphery. The degree of inhomogeneity was probably not recognized by the limited imaging technologies of the period. Patient selection criteria also contributed to the poor results. Patients with high-grade malignancy and extraprostatic extension were found to have a high rate of failure.[80–82] It has been postulated that the low dose of iodine-125 at the periphery (8 Gy/h) is insufficient to eradicate the rapidly proliferating cell lines seen in poorly differentiated tumors.[83,84] Alternatively, large tumor volumes may have led to areas of underdosage. The problems seen with retropubic implantation can therefore be attributed to multiple factors: radiobiology, inappropriate patient selection, poor dose distribution, and poor treatment planning. In 1983, Holm et al[85] revolutionized prostate implantation with their report of the use of transrectal ultrasound to verify the needle position in transperineal implantation of the prostate. This method incorporates transrectal ultrasound and computer-guided treatment planning programs to customize the dose distribution based on measurements of the target that are used to plan the placement activity and number of sources. Three-dimensional dose distributions are calculated for the prostate, rectum, and bladder in order to optimize the dose to the prostate while minimizing the dose to normal tissues. During the implantation procedure, 17- or 18-gauge needles are introduced into the perineum through parallel holes in a rigid perineal template. The dose prescribed is the minimum peripheral dose that will encompass the target on transrectal ultrasound.[86] The choice of isotope is based on the grade of the tumor. Iodine-125 is used for tumors with a Gleason score of 2–6, while palladium-103 is prescribed for tumors with a Gleason score of 7–10. It is postulated that the higher initial dose of palladium-103 will be advantageous for poorly differentiated tumors with shorter cell-cycle times.[87] Postimplant CT scans are performed to verify the accuracy of the implant. Thus far, there has been 90% success in achieving the planned target dose.[88,89]

Blasko et al[86] have described rigid guidelines for patient selection. The prostate volume must be less than 60 cm^3 and no severe pubic arch interference should be present. Patients with severe obstructive symptoms are not implanted. The cancer must be confined to the prostate. T1 and early T2 tumors are treated with implant alone, while the majority of T2b–c tumors are treated with radiation and an implant boost, unless the tumor is well differentiated and clearly confined to one lobe of the prostate.

The toxicity rates for transperineal implantation have also been reported. The maximum period of treatment-related toxicity appears within 2 months of implantation, as the initial dose rate of 8 Gy/h decreases by 50% every 60 days. Urinary symptoms consist of nocturia and dysuria. Eighty percent of patients reported grade 1–2 nocturia at 2 months after implantation.[90] This decreased to 40% by 12 months. The rates of dysuria were 48% at 2 months, decreasing to 20% by 12 months. Implantation has an increased number of urinary complications related to the prostatitis and urethritis associated with the high dose of irradiation to the prostate. The urethral dose at the center of the gland may be substantially greater than the minimum peripheral dose of 160 Gy.[91] There was also an association between transurethral resection (TUR) and serious urinary complications.[86] Suburethral necrosis, characterized by necrotic debris in the urethra with exposure to urine, was seen in 12% of patients having a TUR prior to implantation, compared with 0.4% of patients without a TUR. Total incontinence was 16% in patients with prior TUR, versus 0% in those patients who did not have a preimplantation TUR.

Twenty-five percent of patients reported a change in bowel habits within 2 months of implantation. However, by 12 months, all grade 2 bowel symptoms resolved, while 12% of patients reported grade 1 bowel toxicity.[86]

Maintenance of potency was age dependent. Eighty-five percent of those less than 70 years old remained potent after implantation. However, only 50% of patients older than 70 years remained potent.[92]

The results of transperineal implantation are preliminary in that prostate cancer has a long natural history requiring 10–15 years of follow-up to assess progression.[90] In the Memorial Sloan–Kettering experience, the rate of normalization of PSA 24 months after implantation was 94%.[92] Eighty-five percent of patients had a PSA level below 2.0 ng/ml and 74% had a PSA level below 1.0 ng/ml. Priestley and Beyer[92] reported an 80% normalization rate of PSA at 18 months. At a median follow-up of 37 months, Blasko et al[86] noted a 93% rate of PSA normalization.

The current techniques of prostate implantation produce an implant that is more homogeneous, reproducible and of larger volume than is achieved with the retropubic approach. With careful selection criteria, the local control should be improved over that previously reported. Implant alone is suitable for early confined lesions in patients with an intact prostate.

HORMONE THERAPY

Hormone therapy is increasingly being used to improve the therapeutic outcome in the treatment of prostate cancer. The most commonly used agents are the luteinizing hormone-releasing hormone (LHRH) agonist decapeptides (leuprolide (Lupron), goserelin acetate (Zoladex) and the non-steroidal antiandrogens (flutamide, Nilutamide, bicalutamide (Casodex)). The LHRH agonists cause the anterior pituitary to release LH and follicle-stimulating hormone (FSH), with subsequent downregulation of testosterone release.[93] The non-steroidal antiandrogens act at the androgen receptor, competitively inhibiting the binding of dihydrotestosterone.[93] Endocrine therapy results in a decrease in PSA and cytoreduction of the tumor volume, which should theoretically improve the effectiveness of radiation therapy.

Both direct and indirect interactions occur with radiation therapy and androgen blockade. The potential direct interactions include a slowing of the cell cycle by androgen effect, which leads to a decrease in repopulation during radiation therapy. In addition, there may be a synergistic enhancement of cell death by apoptosis that is induced by both modalities.[94] An indirect interaction is the reduction in tumor size resulting from androgen blockade, which may result in an improvement in local control. Early androgen blockade may provide less of an opportunity for tumor progression after radiation therapy.[94]

Several randomized trials have been performed to assess the effect of androgen blockade in conjunction with radiation therapy. The RTOG 94-08 study randomized patients with localized prostate cancer (T1–T2b) to radiation therapy with or without 4 months of leuprolide and flutamide. The impetus for this study can be found in the RTOG protocols 85-19[95] and 86-10.[94] RTOG 85-19 was a phase II study evaluating the efficacy of goserelin and flutamide as cytoreductive agents in patients with locally advanced carcinoma of the prostate (T2b–T3).[95] Hormone treatment was administered for 2 months prior to radiation and continued throughout radiation therapy. Clearance of primary tumor was documented in 28 of 30 patients (minimum 2-year follow-up).

This preliminary study led to RTOG 86-10, a phase III study in which patients with locally advanced prostate cancer were randomized to neoadjuvant hormone therapy with goserelin acetate and flutamide versus radiation therapy alone.[96] A significant decrease in local progression was noted in the group receiving hormone therapy. The 5-year incidence of local progression was 46% in the hormone group versus 71% in the radiation-only group. The incidence of distant metastasis in the hormone group was 34% compared with 41% in the radiation-only group. The 5-year progression-free survival rate was 36% versus 15%, respectively. This study suggested a benefit to neoadjuvant hormone therapy in patients with locally advanced prostate cancer. The Androcur study also evaluated the effectiveness of neoadjuvant hormone therapy in men with locally advanced prostate cancer.[97] Patients were randomized between radiation alone versus cyproterone acetate for 12 weeks prior to radiation therapy. The neoadjuvant treatment was effective in clinically downstaging prostate cancer, as assessed by digital rectal examination and PSA level. The biochemical disease-free rate was 47.4% in the hormone group and 21% in the radiation-alone group.

The EORTC phase III trial evaluated the long-term role of hormone therapy in patients with locally advanced prostate cancer. Patients were randomized to radiation therapy alone versus radiation in conjunction with hormone therapy (goserelin and cyproterone acetate) with continued hormone therapy for 3 years.[98] The local control rate was 95% in the hormone-treated group versus 75% in the radiation-only group. The clinical disease-free survival rates were 85% and 44%, respectively. RTOG 92-02 is also exploring the role of maintenance hormone therapy, comparing neoadjuvant hormone therapy with maintenance hormone therapy given for 2 years after radiation therapy. The study has recently closed and preliminary results should soon be available.

Hormone therapy, by reducing the tumor volume, may result in a reduction in normal tissue complications. The decrease in target volume size and improved geometric configuration reduces the amount of normal tissue exposed to high doses of radiation. Increased doses can be delivered to the prostate and seminal vesicles, while respecting normal tissue tolerance. This has important implications in dose escalation with conformal radiation therapy. Zelefsky et al[99] noted a 25% decrease in the size of the prostate volume after 3 months of neoadjuvant hormone therapy. The volume of rectum receiving 95% of the prescribed dose was decreased from 36% to 30%. Similarly, the volume of bladder receiving 95% of the prescribed dose decreased from 53% to 35%. Forman et al[100] reported an average decrease in the prostate volume of 37% after 3 months of neoadjuvant hormone therapy. The average bladder and rectal volume receiving high-dose irradiation was also decreased.[100]

CONCLUSIONS

The treatment of localized prostate cancer is a complex issue in that patients are faced with numerous options. In addition, substantial differences are seen in the natural history of this disease in patients with similar disease stages. The PSA era has demonstrated the inability of all current treatments to cure a large number of patients. Future directions for treatment will require the identification of patients at high risk of treatment failure and the development of improved methods of eradication of disease.

REFERENCES

1. Jewett HJ, Eggleston JC, Yawn DH, Radical prostatectomy in the management of carcinoma of the prostate: probable causes of some therapeutic failures. *J Urol* 1972; **107:** 1034–40.
2. Culp OS, Meyer JJ, Radical prostatectomy in the treatment of cancer of the prostate. *Cancer* 1973; **21:** 1113–18.
3. Walsh PC, Jewett HJ, Radical surgery for prostatic cancer. *Cancer* 1980; **45:** 1906–11.
4. Zietman AL, Coen JJ, Shipley WV, Eferd J, Radical radiation therapy in the management of prostatic adenocarcinoma: the initial PSA value as a predictor of treatment outcome. *J Urol* 1994; **151:** 640.
5. Paulson DF, Lin GH, Hinshaw W, Stephani S, Radical surgery versus radiotherapy for adenocarcinoma of the prostate. *J Urol* 1982; **128:** 502–3.
6. Bagshaw MA, Current conflicts in the management of prostate cancer. *Int J Radiat Oncol Biol Phys* 1985; **12:** 1721–7.

7. The Management of Clinically Localized Prostate Cancer, National Institute of Health Consensus Development Conference. *J Urol* 1987; **13:** 1369–73.

8. Parten AW, Carter HB, Chan DW et al, Prostate specific antigen in the staging of localized prostate cancer: influence of tumor differentiation, tumor volume and benign hyperplasia. *J Urol* 1990; **143:** 747–52.

9. Zagars GK, Prostate specific antigen as an outcome variable for T_1 and T_2 prostate cancer treated by radiation therapy. *J Urol* 1994; **152:** 1786–91.

10. Pisansky TM, Cha SS, Earle JD, Prostate specific antigen as a pretherapy prognostic factor in patients treated with radiation therapy for clinically localized prostate cancer. *J Clin Oncol* 1993; **11:** 2158–66.

11. Paulson DF, Impact of radical prostatectomy in the management of clinically localized disease. *J Urol* 1994; **152:** 1826–30.

12. Trapasso JF, de Kernion JN, Smith RB, Dorey H, The incidence and significance of detectable levels of serum PSA after radical prostatectomy. *J Urol* 1994; **152:** 1821–5.

13. Zagars GK, von Eschenbach AC, Ayala AG, Prostate specific antigen: an important marker for prostate cancer treated by external beam radiotherapy. *Cancer* 1993; **72:** 538–48.

14. Kavadi VS, Zagars GK, Pollack A, Serum prostate specific antigen after radiation therapy for clinically localized prostate cancer: prognostic implications. *Int J Radiat Oncol Biol Phys* 1994; **30:** 279–87.

15. Ritter MA, Messing EM, Shanahan TG et al, Prostate specific antigen as a predictor of radiotherapy response and patterns of failure in localized prostate cancer. *J Clin Oncol* 1992; **10:** 1208–17.

16. Zagars GK, Pollack A, Kavadi VS, von Eschenbach AC, Prostate specific antigen and RT for clinically localized prostate cancer. *Int J Radiat Oncol Biol Phys* 1995; **32:** 293–306.

17. Zietman AL, Coen JJ, Shipley WV, Willett CG, Eferd JT, Radical radiation therapy in the management of prostate adenocarcinoma: the initial prostate specific antigen value a predictor of treatment outcome. *J Urol* 1994; **151:** 640–5.

18. Hart KB, Shamsa F, McLaughlin W, Forman JD, Jeffrey D, Forman MD, Correlation of post-treatment histologic and biochemical results with long-term outcome in prostate cancer patients following radiation therapy. Submitted.

19. Zagars GK, Prostate specific antigen as a prognostic factor for prostate cancer treatment by external beam radiotherapy. *Int J Radiat Oncol Biol Phys* 1992; **23:** 47–53.

20. Kuban DA, El-Mahdi AM, Schellhammer PF, Prostate specific antigen for pretreatment prediction and post-treatment evaluation of outcome after definitive irradiation for prostate cancer. *Int J Radiat Oncol Biol Phys* 1995; **32:** 307–16.

21. Stamey TA, Kabalin JN, McNeal JE et al, Prostate specific antigen in the diagnosis and treatment of adenocarcinoma of the prostate. *J Urol* 1989; **141:** 1076–80.

22. Partin AW, Pound CR, Clement JQ, Epstein J, Walsh PC, Serum PSA after radical prostatectomy – the Johns Hopkins experience. *Urol Clin North Am* 1993; **20:** 713–25.

23. Carter HB, Coffey DS, Prostate cancer: the magnitude of the problem in the United States. In: *A Multidisciplinary Analysis of Controversies in the Management of Prostate Cancer* (Coffey DS, Resnick MI, Dorr FA, Carr JP, eds). Plenum Press: New York, 1988: 1–7.

24. Partin AW, Carter HB, Chan DW et al, Prostate specific antigen in the staging of localized prostate cancer: influence of tumor differentiation, tumor volume and benign hyperplasia. *J Urol* 1990; **143:** 747–50.

25. Partin AW, Yoo J, Carter HB et al, The use of prostate specific antigen, clinical stage and Gleason score to predict pathologic stage in men with localized prostate cancer. *J Urol* 1993; **150:** 110–14.

26. Roach M, Marquez C, Yuo H-S et al, Predicting the risk of lymph node involvement using the pre-treatment prostate specific antigen and Gleason score in men with clinically localized prostate cancer. *Int J Radiat Oncol Biol Phys* 1993; **28:** 33–7.

27. Bluestein DL, Bostwick DG, Bergstralh EJ, Osterling JE, Eliminating the need for bilateral pelvic lymph adenectomy in selected cases of prostate cancer. *J Urol* 1994; **151:** 1315–20.

28. Spevach L, Killon LT, West JC, Rooker GM, Brewer EA, Cuddy PG, Predicting the patient at low risk for lymph node metastasis with localized prostate cancer: an analysis of four statistical models. *Int J Radiat Oncol Biol Phys* 1996; **34:** 543–5.

29. Bagshaw MA, Ray GR, Pistemma DA, Casletling RA, Meares EM, Ext beam radiation therapy of $1°$ carcinoma of the prostate. *Cancer* 1975; **36:** 723–8.

30. del Regato JA, Radiotherapy is the conservative treatment of operable and locally inoperable carcinoma of the prostate. *Radiology* 1967; **88**: 761–6.
31. Bagshaw MA, Patential for radiotherapy alone in prostate cancer. *Cancer* 1985; **55**: 2079–85.
32. Perez CA, Pilepich MV, Garcia D, Simpson JR, Zwnuska F, Hederman MA, Definitive radiation therapy in carcinoma of the prostate localized to the pelvis: experience at the Mallinkrodt Institute of Radiology. *NCI Monographs* 1988; **7**: 85–95.
33. Asbell SO, Krall JM, Pilepich MV, Elective pelvic irradiation in stage A_2, B carcinoma of the prostate: analysis of RTOG 77-06. *Int J Radiat Oncol Biol Phys* 1988; **15**: 1307–16.
34. Kabalin JN, Hodge KR, McNeal JE, Freiha FS, Stamey TA, Identification of residual cancer in the prostate following radiation therapy: the role of transurethral ultrasound guided biopsy and prostate specific antigen. *J Urol* 1989; **142**: 326.
35. Perez CA, Hanks GE, Leibel SA, Zietman AL, Fuks Z, Lee WR, Localized carcinoma of the prostate. Review of management with external beam radiation therapy. *Cancer* 1993; **72**: 3156–60.
36. Leibel SA, Zelefsky MJ, Kutcher GJ et al, Three-dimensional conformal radiation therapy in localized carcinoma of the prostate: interim report of a phase I dose escalation study. *J Urol* 1994; **152**: 1792–8.
37. Ten Haken RK, Perez-Tamayo C, Tesser RT et al, Boost treatment of the prostate using shaped fields. *Int J Radiat Oncol Biol Phys* 1989; **16**: 193–7.
38. Smit WGJM, Helle PA, Van Putte WLJ et al, Late radiation damage in prostate cancer patients treated by high dose external beam radiation therapy in relation to rectal dose. *Int J Radiat Oncol Biol Phys* 1996; **18**: 23–9.
39. Greskovich FJ, Zagars GK, Sheramn NE, Johnson DE, Complications following external beam radiation therapy for prostate cancer: an analysis of patients treated with and without staging laparatomy. *J Urol* 1991; **146**: 798–802.
40. Leibel SA, Kutcher GJ, Mohan R et al, Three-dimensional conformal radiation therapy at Memorial Sloan Kettering Cancer Center. *Semin Radiat Oncol* 1992; **2**: 274–89.
41. Leibel SA, Ling CC, Kutcher GJ et al, The biologic basic of conformal 3-D radiation therapy. *Int J Radiat Oncol Biol Phys* 1991; **21**: 534–47.
42. Roach M, Pickett B, Holland J et al, The role of the uretrogram during simulation for localized carcinoma of the prostate. *Int J Radiat Oncol Biol Phys* 1993; **25**: 299–307.
43. Mesina CF, Sharma R, Rissman LS et al, Comparison of a conformal non-axial boost with a 4 field boost technique in the treatment of adenocarcinoma of the prostate. *Int J Radiat Oncol Biol Phys* 1994; **30**: 427–30.
44. Corn BW, Hanks GE, Schultheiss TE, Conformal treatment of prostate cancer with improved targeting: superior prostate specific antigen. *Int J Radiat Oncol Biol Phys* 1995; **32**: 325–30.
45. Shipley WV, Zietman AL, Hanks GE et al, Treatment related sequelae following external beam radiation for prostate cancer: a review with an update in patients with T1 and T2 tumors. *J Urol* 1994; **152**: 1799–805.
46. Bagshaw MA, Ray GR, Cox RS, Complications associated with radiation therapy in prostate cancer. In: *Complications of Urologic Surgery* (Smith R, Erlick R, eds). WB Saunders: Philadelphia, 1991: 88–9.
47. Pilepich MV, Krall J, George FW, Asbell SO et al, Treatment related morbidity in Phase III RTOG studies of extended field irradiation for carcinoma of the prostate. *Int J Radiat Oncol Biol Phys* 1984; **10**: 1861–7.
48. Vijaykumar S, Awan A, Kavuson T et al, Acute toxicity during external beam radiotherapy for localized prostate cancer: comparison of different treatment techniques. *Int J Radiat Oncol Biol Phys* 1993; **25**: 359–64.
49. Soffen EM, Hanks GE, Hunt MA, Epstein BE, Conformal static field radiation therapy treatment of early prostate cancer VS. non-conformal techniques: a reduction in acute morbidity. *Int J Radiat Oncol Biol Phys* 1992; **24**: 485–8.
50. Emami B, Purdy JA, Manolis JM et al, 3-D static conformal radiotherapy: preliminary results of a prospective clinical trial. *Int J Radiat Oncol Biol Phys* 1991; **21**: 197.
51. Lawton CA, Won Minhee, Pilepich MV et al, Long term treatment sequelae following external beam irradiation for adenocarcinoma of the prostate: analysis of RTOG 7506, 7706. *Int J Radiat Oncol Biol Phys* 1991; **21**: 935–9.
52. Sandler H, McLaughlin PW, Ten Haken R et al, 3-D conformal radiotherapy for the treatment of prostate cancer: low risk of chronic rectal morbidity observed in a large series of patients. *Int J Radiat Oncol Biol Phys* 1993; **27**(suppl 1): abstr 14.
53. Banker FL, The preservation of potency after treatment of prostate cancer with external beam

irradiation. *Int J Radiat Oncol Biol Phys* 1988; **15:** 219–21.

54. Hanks GE, Asbell S, Krall JM et al, Outcome for lymph node dissection negative T16, T2 prostate cancer treated with external beam radiotherapy in RTOG 77-06. *Int J Radiat Oncol Biol Phys* 1993; **27**(suppl 1): 106.

55. Bagshaw MA, External radiation therapy of carcinoma of the prostate. *Cancer* 1980; **45:** 1912–21.

56. Freha FS, Bagshaw M, Carcinoma of the prostate, results of post-radiation biopsy. *Prostate* 1984; **5:** 19–25.

57. Kuban DA, El Mahdi AM, Schellhamer P, The significance of post-irradiation prostate biopsy with long term follow-up. *Int J Radiat Oncol Biol Phys* 1992; **24:** 409–14.

58. Crook J, Robertson S, Collin R, Gerard M, Zeleski V, Esche B, Clinical relevance of transrectal ultrasound biopsy and PSA after radiation therapy for carcinoma of the prostate. *Int J Radiat Oncol Biol Phys* 1993; **27:** 31–7.

59. Hanks GE, Martz RL, Diamond JJ, The effect of dose on local control of prostate cancer. *Int J Radiat Oncol Biol Phys* 1988; **15:** 1299–305.

60. Fuks Z, Leibel SA, Wallner KE et al, The effect of local control on metastatic dissemination in carcinoma of the prostate: long term results in patients treated with ^{125}I implants. *Int J Radiat Oncol Biol Phys* 1991; **21:** 534–47.

61. Kuban DA, El-Mahdi AM, Schellhamer PF, Sites of failure in patient with local recurrence after definitive RT for prostate cancer. *Cancer* 1989; **63:** 2421–5.

62. Zagars GK, von Eschenbach AC, Ayala AG et al, The influence of local control on metastatic dissemination of prostate cancer treated by external beam megavoltage. *Radiat Ther Cancer* 1991; **68:** 2370–7.

63. Leibel SA, Fuks Z, The impact of local tumor control on the outcome in human cancer. In: *Current Topics in Clinical Radiobiology of Tumors* (Beck-Bornholdt H-P, ed). Springer-Verlag: Berlin, 1993: 113–23.

64. Leibel SA, Fuks Z, Zelefsky MJ et al, The effects of local and regional treatment on metastatic outcome in prostate cancer with lymph node involvement. *Int J Radiat Oncol Biol Phys* 1994; **28:** 7–16.

65. Perez CA, Pilepich MV, Zwnuska F, Tumor control in definitive irradiation of localized carcinoma of the prostate. *Int J Radiat Oncol Biol Phys* 1986; **12:** 523–31.

66. Forman JD, Orton CG, Warmelink C, Preliminary results of a hyperfractionated dose escalation trial. *Radiother Oncol* 1993; **27:** 203–8.

67. Forman JD, Duclos M, Porter AT, Orton CG, Hyperfractionated conformal RT in locally advanced prostate cancer: results of a dose escalation study. *Int J Radiat Oncol Biol Phys* 1996; **34:** 655–62.

68. Forman JD, Kocheril PK, Hart K et al, Estimate of the relative biologic effectiveness for pelvic neutron irradiation in patients treated for carcinoma of the prostate. Submitted.

69. Laramore GE, Krall JM, Thomas FJ, Griffin TW, Maor MH, Henrickson FT, Fast neutron radiotherapy for locally advanced prostate cancer. *Int J Radiat Oncol Biol Phys* 1985; **11:** 1621–7.

70. Russell RJ, Caplan RJ, Laramore GE et al, Photon versus fast neutron external beam radiotherapy in the treatment of locally advanced prostate cancer. *Int J Radiat Oncol Biol Phys* 1993; **28:** 47–54.

71. Austin-Seymour M, Caplan R, Russell K et al, Impact of multi leaf collimator on treatment morbidity in localized carcinoma of the prostate. *Int J Radiat Oncol Biol Phys* 1994; **30:** 1065–71.

72. Forman JD, Warmelink C, Devi S et al, Alternating conformal neutron and proton radiation therapy for locally advanced carcinoma of the prostate. *Am J Clin Oncol* 1995; **18:** 231–8.

73. Sharma R, Warmelink C, Yudelev M, Mesina CF, Maughan RL, Forman JD, Description of a 3-D conformal neutron and photon radiation therapy techniques for prostate carcinoma. *Med Dosim* 1995; **20:** 45–51.

74. Forman JD, Duclos M, Sharma R et al, Conformal mixed neutron and photon irradiation in localized and locally advanced prostate cancer: Preliminary estimates of the therapeutic ratio. *Int J Radiat Oncol Biol Phys* 1996; **35:** 259–66.

75. Whitmore WF Jr, Hilaris B, Grabstaid H, Retropubic implantation of ^{125}I in the treatment of carcinoma of the prostate. *J Urol* 1972; **108:** 1918–20.

76. Anderson LL, Spacing nomograph for interstitial placement of ^{125}I seeds. *Med Phys* 1976; **3:** 48–51.

77. Gottesman JE, Failure of open radioactive ^{125}I implantation to control localized prostate cancer. *J Urol* 1991; **146:** 1317–20.

78. Grossman HB, Batala M, Hilaris B et al, ^{125}I implantation for carcinoma of the prostate. *Urology* 1982; **11:** 591–8.

79. Kuban DH, el-Mahdi AM, Schellhammer PF, ^{125}I interstitial implantation for prostate cancer. What have we learned 10 years later? *Cancer* 1989; **63:** 2415–20.

80. Deblasco DS, Hilaris BS, Nori D et al, Permanent interstitial implantation of prostate cancer in the 1980s. *Endocuriether/Hyperthermia Oncol* 1988; **4**: 193–201.

81. Delaney TF, Shipley WV, O'Leary MP et al, Pre-op radiation therapy, lymphadenectomy and ^{125}I implantation for patients with localized carcinoma of the prostate. *Int J Radiat Oncol Biol Phys* 1986; **12**: 1779–85.

82. Giles GM, Brady LW, ^{125}I implantation after lymphadenectomy in early cancer of the prostate. *Int J Radiat Oncol Biol Phys* 1987; **12**: 2117–25.

83. Mitchell JB, Beford JS, Dose rate effects in synchronosis mammalian cells in culture. *Radiat Res* 1977; **71**: 547–60.

84. Marchise MJ, Hall EJ, Encapsulated ^{125}I in radiation oncology: II-PLDR and plateau phase cell cultures. *Am J Clin Oncol* 1984; **7**: 613–16.

85. Holm JJ, Juul N, Pedersen JF et al, TP ^{125}I seed implantation in prostate cancer guided by trans rectal sound. *J Urol* 1983; **130**: 283–6.

86. Blasko JC, Gumm PD, Ragde J, Brachytherapy and organ preservation in the management of cancer of the prostate. *Semin Radiat Oncol* 1993; **3**: 240–9.

87. Ling CC, Permanent implants using Au-198, Pd-103 and I-125. Radiobiologic considerations based on L–Q model. *Int J Radiat Oncol Biol Phys* 1992; **23**: 81–7.

88. Kaye RW, Olson DJ, Lightner DJ, Payne JT, Improved technique for prostate seed implantation: combined ultrasound and fluroscopic guidance. *J Endocrinol* 1992; **6**: 61–6.

89. Blasko JC, Ragde H, Schumacher D, Transperineal percutaneous transrectal versus template guidance. *Endocuriether/Hyperthermia Oncol* 1987; **3**: 131–9.

90. Johansson J, Adami H, Anderson S, Bergstrom R, Holmberg L, Krusemo VB, High 10 year survival rate in patients with untreated prostate cancer. *J Am Med Assoc* 1992; **267**: 2191–6.

91. Wallner K, Roy J, Zelefsky M, Fuks Z, Harrison L, Short term freedom from disease progression after ^{125}I prostate implantation. *Int J Radiat Oncol Biol Phys* 1994; **30**: 405–9.

92. Priestley JB, Beyer DC, Guided brachytherapy for treatment of confined prostate cancer. *Urology* 1992; **40**: 27–32.

93. Crawford DE, Nabort W, Hormone therapy of advanced prostate cancer. Where we stand today. *Oncology* 1991; **5**: 21–7.

94. Pollack A, Zagars GK, Kopplin S, Radiation therapy and androgen ablation for clinically localized high risk prostate cancer. *Int J Radiat Oncol Biol Phys* 1995; **32**: 13–20.

95. Pilepich MV, Al-Sarraf M, John MJ, McGowan DG, Krall JM, Phase II RTOG study of hormonal cytoreduction with flutamide and goserelin in locally advanced carcinoma of the prostate treated with definitive radiation therapy. *Am J Clin Oncol* 1990; **13**; 461–4.

96. Pilepich MV, Sause WT, Shipley WV et al, Androgen deprivation with radiation therapy compared to radiation alone for locally advanced prostatic carcinoma: a randomized comparative trial of the Radiation Therapy Oncology Group. *Urology* 1995; **45**: 616–22.

97. Porter AT, Elhilali M, Manyi M et al, Neoadjuvant therapy prior to curative radiotherapy in locally advanced prostate cancer patients. Canadian Urologic Oncology Group: Unpublished.

98. Bolla M, Gonzales D, Warde P et al, Immediate hormonal therapy improves locoregional control in patients with locally advanced prostate cancer: results of a randomized Phase III trial of the EORTC Radiotherapy and Genitourinary Cooperative Groups. *J Clin Oncol* 1996; **15**: 238 (abstr).

99. Zelefsky MJ, Leibel SA, Kutcher GJ, Harrison J, Happersett L, Fuks Z, Neoadjuvant hormones improve therapeutic ratio in patients with bulky carcinoma of the prostate treated with conformal radiation therapy. *Int J Radiat Oncol Biol Phys* 1994; **29**: 755–61.

100. Forman JD, Kumar R, Haas G, Montie J, Porter AT, Mesina CF, Effect of neoadjuvant hormonal therapy on prostate size. *Cancer Invest* 1995; **13**: 8–15.

13

Neoadjuvant hormone treatment in localized prostate cancer: a critical appraisal

Frans MJ Debruyne, Wim PJ Witjes

CONTENTS • **Historical background** • **Phase II studies** • **Randomized phase III trials**
• **Neoadjuvant hormone treatment in perspective** • **Conclusion**

The concept of neoadjuvant treatment of local-ized prostate cancer is well known among uro-logists and radiotherapists. Indeed, if one were to ask urologists today if they have ever used this form of treatment prior to radical prostatec-tomy or radiotherapy, the vast majority would admit that they have. However, if one were subsequently to ask urologists about the scien-tific clinical evidence for the efficacy of this approach, a more hesitant answer would prob-ably be given, because no such evidence is yet available, certainly for the use of hormone treat-ment before radical prostatectomy. But still urologists all over the world use hormone ther-apy and will continue to do so in the near future. One can argue for or against this form of treatment on the basis of assumptions, hypothe-ses, theoretical arguments and/or clinical ex-perience. What counts, however, is clinical evidence. In this chapter we aim to give a crit-ical review of the currently available inform-ation on the use of neoadjuvant hormone treatment prior to surgery for localized prostate cancer, with the goal of giving, as far as is pos-sible, clear guidelines for practising urologists of when and when not to use this treatment approach.

HISTORICAL BACKGROUND

The idea of applying hormone therapy before definitive treatment of localized prostate cancer is not new. Even though in the 1970s and 1980s urologists were not interested in discussing and evaluating the concept, hormone therapy has been used and applied since the scientific basis for hormone treatment of prostate cancer was established by the pioneering research of Huggins et al in 1941.[1] In 1944, Vallett[2] pub-lished the first paper on a series of patients who had undergone radical perineal prostatectomy subsequent to bilateral orchiectomy, and shortly after (1947) Colston and Brendler[3] reported on patients who were given oestro-gens prior to radical perineal prostatectomy. However, these publications concerned only small numbers of patients and a short follow-up period. Moreover, these analyses were retro-spective and did not give real and substantial arguments for the long-lasting efficacy of hor-mone therapy.

In 1949, Guttierez[4] and Parlow and Scott[5] reported on the first large series of patients treated prospectively, but again did not provide conclusive evidence for an improved outcome of surgery following hormone treatment. The last important publication before 20 years of silence about neoadjuvant hormone treatment appeared in 1969 when Scott and Boyd[6] reviewed 25 years of experience with this form of treatment, demonstrating 10- and 15-year survivals of 52% and 19%, respectively, in patients with stage C (T3) prostate cancer. However, their results were confounded, as most patients continued to receive hormone treatment after radical prostatectomy.

In the subsequent 20 years neoadjuvant hormone treatment did not maintain its place in the management of localized prostate cancer. Radical prostatectomy was not (yet) generally accepted as an effective treatment option for localized disease because of the high morbidity and even mortality associated with it. Moreover, many patients subjected to radical prostatectomy proved to have tumours that were at stages beyond curability. The irreversibility of orchiectomy and the occasionally serious toxicity and mortality of oestrogen therapy further decreased the role of hormone treatment in localized disease. During these years the majority of prostate cancer patients were still diagnosed when the disease was at a locally advanced or metastatic stage, and even when the tumour was considered localized urologists tended to advocate radiotherapy rather than radical surgery.

In the early 1980s, thanks to the innovative anatomical and surgical work by Walsh et al,[7] interest in radical retropubic prostatectomy was revived. At the same time it became increasingly evident that radiotherapy gave rather disappointing results, and this also resulted in renewed enthusiasm among urologists for surgery as the method of first choice for the curative treatment of localized disease.

In the mid-1980s reversible and less toxic hormone therapy became available with the development of luteinizing-hormone-releasing hormone (LHRH) analogues and antiandrogens. This combined form of androgen deprivation, called combined androgen blockade (CAB), was widely employed for metastatic prostate cancer and became almost standard therapy. This led, almost spontaneously, again

to the idea of pretreating patients with hormones before surgery or radiotherapy. Labrie et al[8] were among the first to focus attention again on neoadjuvant treatment prior to radical prostatectomy; they even called it a 'surgical innovation', which of course it was not. What was novel was the combination of reversible CAB with a far better surgical technique for radical prostatectomy as instigated by the work of Walsh et al.

Regimens for neoadjuvant hormone treatment before radical prostatectomy

In the first years of neoadjuvant treatment, irreversible or toxic hormone manipulation was used prior to radical prostatectomy. As mentioned above, all the initial studies used either surgical castration or high doses of oestrogen. Surgical castration is irreversible and is not easily accepted by patients. By the mid-1960s the life-threatening toxicity of even low(er) doses of oestrogens, particularly during the first months of treatment, were well documented. The first new development in hormone treatment came from the development of steroidal and non-steroidal (pure) antiandrogens. Both have been used as monotherapy in a neoadjuvant setting. In the early 1990s, Tunn et al[9] and Goldenberg, Bruchovsky and co-workers[10,11] reported phase II studies of the steroidal antiandrogen cyproterone acetate (CPA), and Flamm et al[12] described a group of patients pretreated with flutamide, the first non-steroidal antiandrogen developed. It was rather surprising to note that at the same time Fair et al[13] reported the results of a phase II trial of 3 mg diethylstilbeostrol (DES), a drug that is known to be rather toxic, and hence less appropriate than CPA. In addition, LHRH analogues were used as monotherapy or in combination with steroidal or non-steroidal antiandrogens. Different authors published their phase II results, as summarized in Table 13.1. Less common regimens were also used, such as the combination of hormone therapy and cytotoxic chemotherapy used by Köllerman et al[14] and the use of Estracyt (a com-

Table 13.1 Downstaging in clinical stage T3 (C) prostatic carcinoma after neoadjuvant treatment: overview of phase II studies

Study	Clinical downstaging (No. of patients)	(%)	Pathological downstaging (No. of patients)	(%)
Flamm et al[12]	0/21	0	7/21	29
Morgan and Myers[24]	29/36	81	3/36	8
MacFarlane et al[25]	10/12	83	3/12	25
Köllerman et al[14] 1993	49/103	48	40/103	39
Schulman[17] 1994	9/15	60	4/15	27
Voges et al[26]	64/70	91	9/64	14
Narayan et al[27]	14/30	47	3/14	21

bination of oestrogens coupled to a cytotoxic substance) by Van Poppel et al.[15]

In summary, a variety of hormone approaches has been used in a neoadjuvant setting, all aimed at obtaining insight into the effects and efficacy of this treatment.

PHASE II STUDIES

The results of the various phase II studies were difficult to compare, not only because they used different forms of hormone treatment, but also because the length of preoperative treatment differed from study to study. On average, 3 months of therapy were used, but in some cases pretreatment was as short as 8 weeks[16] and in others treatment was continued for up to 12 months or more.[17] The available phase II data are summarized in Table 13.2. The studies gave more or less similar results, but some of the conclusions drawn are conflicting.

The studies showed a clear shrinkage of the prostate and its tumour. An 80% reduction in

Table 13.2 Overview of randomized phase III studies

Study	No. of patients	Positive margin (%) Neoadjuvant therapy	RP	p
Labrie et al[28]	142	13	38	<0.01
Van Poppel et al[15]	127	PSL 32	PSL 43	NG
		API 31	API 27	NG
		BAS 18	BAS 10	NG
Soloway et al[29]	282	18	48	<0.01
Goldenberg et al[10]	213	28	65	<0.01
Witjes et al[30]	354	27	46	<0.01

API, apical; BAS, basal; NG, not given; PSL, posterolateral; RP, radical prostatectomy.

the tumour was reported by Têtu et al.[18] Using ultrasound images, these authors found that the tumour was more sensitive to volume reduction than the associated normal prostate or the benign prostatic hyperplasia (BPH) component. On average, a total reduction in prostate volume of 30%, as measured by ultrasound, was noted.[19] This reduction in volume was associated with a substantial reduction in the level of prostate-specific antigen (PSA), which is a logical consequence of hormone treatment. On average, in 40% of patients an undetectable PSA level was observed, although it rapidly became clear that the lowest PSA nadir was not reached in all patients after 3 months of hormone therapy. This reduction in PSA elicited much discussion, with speculation that the lowering of the PSA level was only artificial and could not be translated into a better treatment outcome.[20]

The data on downstaging and downgrading of tumour were even more conflicting. Clinical downstaging was evident in about 30% of patients, which is understandable as a consequence of the clinical interpretation of tumour and volume reduction. More difficult to understand was why pathological downstaging should occur, as was indeed described in some of the phase II studies. This aspect has been discussed extensively, as it is difficult to understand how neoadjuvant treatment could change a pT3 stage tumour to one of stage pT2 or less. It was difficult to believe that neoadjuvant hormone treatment can 'suck' cancer cells located outside the prostate (pT3) into the prostate (pT2 or lower). It became apparent that this downstaging phenomenon could be a consequence of the difficult pathological interpretation of the phenotypical changes that occur in the prostate and prostate cancer cells under hormone treatment.[21] The phenotype changes are well known but, for the pathologist unaware of this, sometimes difficult to recognize. Pycnosis, cell atrophy, vacuolization of cancer cells and an increase in the stromal components in the prostate may obscure persisting cancer cells outside the prostate, thus giving a false impression of tumour downstaging. When using special stains for PSA and/or cytokeratins this pathological misinterpretation can be reduced

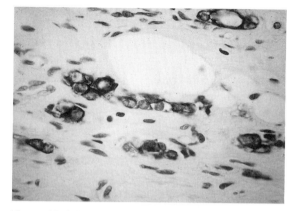

Figure 13.1 Use of cytokeratin staining in the interpretation of prostatic carcinoma tissue.

(Figure 13.1), but this detailed specific pathological evaluation was not used systematically in any of the initial phase II trails.

The same error of interpretation could have played a role in pathological grading where a pretreatment biopsy was compared with a radical prostatectomy specimen after hormone treatment. Grading, particularly that using the Gleason classification and score, is very difficult after hormone treatment, and this explains the discrepancy in the 'downgrading' results described. Some authors described downgrading, while others failed to demonstrate it or even described a higher grade after hormone treatment.[22,23]

The issue of the use of an improved surgical technique was also addressed in many of the phase II studies. It was emphasized that neoadjuvant treatment could facilitate surgery and enhance the radicality of prostatectomy. Indeed, this is necessary, as at least 40% of tumours considered at preoperative staging to be organ confined proved to have associated extracapsular disease on pathological evaluation of the operative specimen. Understaging is a well-known, but very embarrassing, phenomenon in the preoperative evaluation of the patient and (local) tumour. By downsizing the prostate tumour, by reducing the stage of the tumour and by enhancing the radicality of surgery it was anticipated that neoadjuvant hormone treatment could increase the percentage of patients with organ- and specimen-confined tumours. The effects described in the different phase II studies are, however, ambiguous. A few studies showed a better and more radical operability, but others did not, and in the majority no difference was noted.[19] Moreover, there is doubt about the consequences of local surgery on neoadjuvant hormone treatment. Indeed this treatment may induce a substantial preoperative fibrosis, making surgery even more difficult. Furthermore, it may induce a greater fragility of the blood vessels surrounding the prostate, particularly the preprostatic venous plexus, causing troublesome bleeding during surgery.

No valid and unequivocal answers to the many questions surrounding neoadjuvant treatment can be obtained from the many phase II trials (see Table 13.1). On the contrary, more questions remain and more clear answers are needed, especially regarding the most important issue, namely whether neoadjuvant treatment can improve cancer-specific survival after radical prostatectomy. The debate on these issues has continued over the last 5 years. The current situation is best summarized by a quotation from Fair et al,[13] who in 1993 stated:

> Although it is not possible to state currently that any patient has received benefit from neoadjuvant hormonal therapy it is likewise not possible to be dogmatic in the assertion that neoadjuvant therapy is not beneficial.

The answers to the many questions can only be obtained by studying the outcome of prospective randomized trials. Fortunately these trials have now been conducted and the first (preliminary) results have recently become available.

RANDOMIZED PHASE III TRIALS

After several years of more or less anecdotal and not (completely) comparable phase II studies, it became evident that there was an urgent need for prospective phase III trials if an answer were ever to be obtained to the crucial question of whether neoadjuvant hormone therapy given before radical prostatectomy can improve survival.

The first randomized studies were conceived and initiated at the beginning of the 1990s in different countries and continents. From the very beginning it was clear that an average follow-up of at least 8–10 years would be necessary before any final answers would be available, meaning that any evaluation of survival data before such a period had elapsed would have to be considered as preliminary and inconclusive. For this reason many studies used so-called 'surrogate end-points', such as a rising PSA level, positive margins, local recurrence and/or distant progression of disease.

So far preliminary evaluations of five randomized trials have been presented (see Table 13.2). Unfortunately, the results from the different trials are not completely comparable because different patient inclusion criteria, forms of neoadjuvant treatment and study end-points were used, although all the trials were ultimately aimed at evaluating improvement in overall and cancer-specific survival. One of the largest trials is the one undertaken by the European Neoadjuvant Study Group, in which we participated. On the basis of the preliminary results of this trial important issues can be presented and discussed, and the results can be compared with the findings from the other phase III studies.

The European trial started in September 1991 and patient entry was stopped in December 1995. Patients with localized prostate cancer (T2–T3, N0, M0) were randomized to receive either 3 months of neoadjuvant combined androgen blockade (CAB) treatment with an LHRH analogue (Zoladex monthly depot) and a pure antiandrogen (flutamide) followed by radical prostatectomy (NEO group), or direct radical prostatectomy (DIR group). At present 354 patients have been evaluated and the findings of this analysis are used here. The patients were recruited by urologists working in leading European urological institutions (see the Appendix at the end of this chapter) all with a

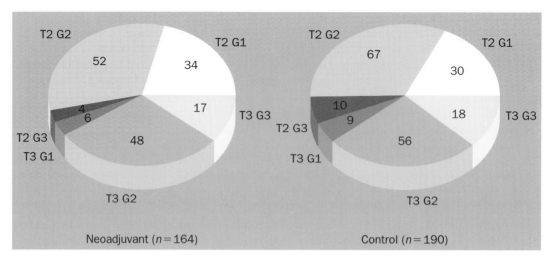

Figure 13.2 Stratification of the initial tumour stages and grades for the patients included in the European Neoadjuvant Study.[30]

large experience in radical retropubic prostatectomy. The stratification of initial tumour stages and grades was comparable in the two treatment groups (Figure 13.2).

In the NEO group, serum PSA levels decreased from a mean (±SD) of 19.9 ± 17.5 ng/ml to a mean of 0.8 ± 2.1 ng/ml after 3 months of neoadjuvant therapy. However, 40% of patients had undetectable PSA levels after 3 months of treatment. This was also the case in all other phase III studies and is in line with what was already known from phase II studies. The prostate volume decreased from a mean (±SD) of 38 ± 19 cm³ to a mean of 26 ± 15 cm³, which amounts to a 30% decrease in volume. Again, similar observations were described in the other phase III studies and the results are in concordance with most of the phase II investigations. The volume reduction and associated phenomena did not have any influence on the surgical procedure. The time required for surgery, the total blood loss and the percentage of nerve-sparing procedures were not influenced by neoadjuvant treatment (Table 13.3). Similar findings have been described by Soloway et al.[29]

The reduction in the clinical stage of tumour in the NEO group was substantial, as might be expected, and this also translated into a significant difference in pathological stage between the NEO and DIR groups. The pathological evaluation was based on the local pathologist's report. In the DIR group the pathological understaging was 54% (including positive lymph nodes). This percentage was 31% in the NEO group, which was significantly statistically different (p < 0.01). This difference in understaging between the two groups can be explained by the arguments given above, but another significant difference was found when 'pathological downstaging' was evaluated. In the NEO group 16% of patients had a pathological stage lower than the clinical stage at baseline, in contrast to only 6% in the DIR group. The meaning of this finding is only significant when it also translates into better local control and survival (see later). Pathological downstaging has also been mentioned in other randomized trials. Of particular interest are four patients (all in the clinical T2 category) in the NEO group, in whose operative specimen no remaining tumour could be found by the

Table 13.3 Mean surgery time, blood loss and percentage of patients requiring nerve-sparing procedures*

	Surgery time (min)	Blood loss (ml)	Nerve-sparing procedure (%)
NEO T2 ($n = 92$)	166	1052	38
DIR T2 ($n = 104$†)	167	1143	40
NEO T3 ($n = 69$†)	163	1168	12
DIR T3 ($n = 80$*)	149	1174	12
Total NEO ($n = 161$)	165	1102	27
Total DIR ($n = 184$)	159	1157	28

*None of the differences between the NEO group and the DIR group were statistically significant.
†Three patients not operated on (N2 disease).

pathologists (stepwise section of the whole specimen). This could indicate a complete disappearance of all tumour after 3 months of neoadjuvant MAB. This complete apoptosis of prostate cancer has also been described in all other randomized trials and in the phase II studies.

The difference in the percentages of positive operative margins between the NEO and the DIR groups was also significant in the cT2 category of our study population ($p < 0.01$), but did not reach statistical significance in the cT3 category ($p = 0.14$). Overall (cT2 + cT3), however, significance was again reached ($p < 0.01$). This difference has also been found in all the other studies and certainly reflects the effect of neoadjuvant treatment (Table 13.2). Whether this finding will also be translated into less local recurrence, less progression and better survival remains to be seen. Of interest, however, is the finding by Schulman and Sassine[31] that the significant importance of negative margins relates well to undetectable PSA levels after neoadjuvant treatment.

In our study there was also a significant difference ($p < 0.01$) in positive lymph nodes between the two groups. This is another indica-tion of a possible completely apoptotic effect on microscopic lymph-node metastasis. Again, the same difference has been observed in other randomized studies and, if clinically significant, should be reflected in time in PSA level progression. In our study the follow-up data of the time to PSA progression were available for 320 patients. In the NEO group 30/155 (19%) and in the DIR group 38/165 (23%) patients showed a progression in PSA level. The mean time to PSA progression was 32 months in both groups. The difference was not statistically significant ($p = 0.53$). In clinical stage T2 patients, 14% of the NEO group and 18% of the DIR group showed a progression in PSA. In the clinical stage T3 group the rate of PSA progression was similar in the two treatment groups. The same results have been obtained in the other randomized trials.[29]

In summary, it can be concluded that all the randomized trials show similar preliminary findings. The practical value of these results is not yet evident. However, some of these observations have already been used to obtain a better understanding of the effect and the increased efficacy of neoadjuvant hormone treatment prior to radical prostatectomy.

NEOADJUVANT HORMONE TREATMENT IN PERSPECTIVE

Having reviewed the information currently available from phase II and phase III trials and studied the role and value of neoadjuvant hormone treatment prior to radical prostatectomy, we now try to give a clear idea of the position of this form of treatment in daily urological practice. It is clear that this treatment can be given before radical prostatectomy and will influence the volume of both the prostate and the tumour and will reduce or even normalize the PSA level. The reduction in tumour volume does not lead to better surgery. On the contrary, when a substantial reduction in prostate volume is achieved surgery can be even more difficult, due to the pronounced fibrosis surrounding the prostate that is associated with volume reduction. Urologists must take this into consideration when administering neoadjuvant hormone therapy.

Normalization of the PSA level occurred more frequently in patients with clinical stage T2 lesions. Also, it is important to note that complete apoptosis (T0) after neoadjuvant hormone therapy was only observed in patients with tumours in this category. This could indicate that patients who are likely to benefit from neoadjuvant treatment are probably patients with T2 tumours. Indeed, Schulman et al[31] indicated that normalization of the PSA level was associated with a larger percentage of negative margins and, as PSA level normalization occurs more frequently in T2 lesions, it is logical to anticipate that a larger percentage of negative margins will occur for tumours in this clinical category. Indeed, in our study the difference in the number of negative margins after neoadjuvant treatment was only significant in the T2 category, and not in the T3 category.

Partin et al[32] have demonstrated that negative surgical margins are associated with a better chance of survival. It is tempting to speculate that, if neoadjuvant hormone treatment induces a larger percentage of negative surgical margins, especially for tumours in the T2 category, then this patient group is the one most likely to benefit from this form of preoperative

treatment and to have better survival. However, this assumption is not (yet) based on clinical evidence. The same reasoning could be applied to the normalization of the PSA level. If it is anticipated that normalization of the PSA level is associated with a longer survival, then patients with tumours in clinical category T2 should gain advantage from neoadjuvant therapy. All these arguments could be used to select only patients with T2 tumours for neoadjuvant hormone treatment. Only patients with this tumour category were included in the study done by Soloway et al,[29] and it is therefore important to see whether there ultimately will be a difference in outcome between these studies and other studies, such as ours, in which patients with T3 tumours were included.

The duration of neoadjuvant hormone treatment is also a point that requires further discussion. In the context of the above-mentioned arguments it is clear that, if given, neoadjuvant treatment should be continued until the lowest, or if possible undetectable, PSA level is reached. In most patients the necessary treatment period will be 3 months, as shown by the studies on intermittent hormone treatment for metastatic prostate cancer. A more rapid and complete reduction in PSA level will again be obtained in a larger percentage of patients with clinical T2 lesions. However, it remains a matter of speculation whether the PSA level can actually be used as a valid surrogate study end-point. Moreover, none of the preliminary results published so far shows a difference in PSA level recurrence between patients undergoing direct radical prostatectomy and those treated with hormones before surgery. If PSA level is a valid surrogate study end-point, this lack of difference in PSA recurrence in the two groups could also indicate that there will be no difference in survival between the groups. This would then be an argument against the use of neoadjuvant hormone treatment before radical prostatectomy.

The influence of preoperative hormone treatment on the dissimilation of tumour cells is shown by results obtained using reverse transcriptase polymerase chain reaction (RT-PCR) techniques to detect circulating cancer cells during surgery. Eschwège et al[33] clearly demonstrated that patients who had been given neoadjuvant hormone treatment did not show circulating prostate cancer cells, while patients who were subjected to direct radical prostatectomy did. The same observation was made by Su et al.[34] These results could indicate that the risk of dissemination of vital tumour cells, and hence the possible risk of preoperative tumour metastasis, could be reduced by neoadjuvant hormone treatment.

All the above-mentioned arguments leave neoadjuvant hormone treatment in an ambiguous clinical perspective. Arguments can be derived in favour of this form of treatment and an equal number can be given for this form of treatment not to be used routinely.

CONCLUSION

In recent years neoadjuvant hormone treatment for locally confined prostate cancer has been used extensively prior to radical prostatectomy, despite the fact that there is no clear and unequivocal clinical evidence that this approach has benefits for the patient. On the other hand, however, it has not been proven that this form of treatment does not yield possible advantages for the patient. The results of properly randomized clinical trials are essential in answering the main question of whether neoadjuvant treatment will directly or individually improve survival. It is still too early to derive an answer to this question from the clinical phase III trials, which until now

have only provided preliminarily results based on surrogate end-points such as positive tumour margins and rising PSA levels. The results of these analyses are conflicting. Whereas on the one hand a positive influence of neoadjuvant therapy on positive margins, pathological tumour downstaging and microscopic lymph-node metastasis has been demonstrated, on the other hand no effect on the recurrence of PSA level (which is considered the most important marker for distal metastasis and eventually survival) has been found.

This means that at present it is impossible to state that neoadjuvant treatment given prior to radical prostatectomy can be recommended as a standard treatment. Such treatment will remain experimental and investigational until the final major questions have been answered. This contrasts with the already available evidence that this form of therapy is beneficial when given before definitive radiotherapy in patients with clinical T3 prostate cancer (see Chapter 12). Thus the individual urologist will have to decide whether they will or will not adopt this approach in a specific case. However, on the basis of the current evidence, when discussing treatment options for localized disease with an individual patient, the urologist will be able to offer the use of neoadjuvant treatment (preferably, in our opinion, with combined androgen blockade (CAB) therapy) until the lowest PSA reading is reached as an option. By discussing the various arguments, the clinician and the patient will then decide whether or not to use the therapy prior to surgery.

REFERENCES

1. Huggins C, Hodges CV, Studies on prostatic cancer: the effect of castration, of estrogen and of androgen injection on serum phosphatases in metastatic carcinoma of the prostate. *Cancer Res* 1941; **1**: 293–7.
2. Vallett BS, Radical perineal prostatectomy subsequent to bilateral orchiectomy. *Del Med J* 1944; **16**: 19–20.
3. Colston JAC, Brendler H, Endocrine therapy in carcinoma of the prostate. *J Am Med Assoc* 1947; **134**: 848–53.
4. Guttierez R, New horizons in the surgical management of carcinoma of the prostate gland. *Am J Surg* 1949; **78**: 147–52.
5. Parlow AL, Scott WW, Hormone control therapy as a preparation for radical perineal prostatec-

tomy in advanced carcinoma of the prostate. *NY J Med* 1949; **49:** 629–34.

6. Scott WW, Boyd HL, Combined hormone control therapy and radical prostatectomy in the treatment of selected cases of advanced carcinoma of the prostate: a retrospective study based upon 25 years of experience. *J Urol* 1969; **101:** 86–92.

7. Walsh PC, Lepor H, Eggleston JC, Radical prostatectomy with preservation of sexual function: anatomical and pathological considerations. *Prostate* 1983; **4:** 473–85.

8. Labrie F, Belanger A, Dupont A, Emond J, Lacoursiere Y, Monfette G, Combined treatment with LHRH agonist and pure antiandrogen in advanced carcinoma of prostate. *Lancet* 1984; **ii:** 1090.

9. Tunn UW, Goldschmidt JW, Steigerwald S, Efficacy of neoadjuvant antiandrogenic treatment prior to radical prostatectomy. *J Urol* 1992; **147:** A131.

10. Goldenberg SL, Klotz LH, Srigley J et al, Randomized, prospective, controlled study comparing radical prostatectomy alone and neoadjuvant androgen withdrawal in the treatment of localized prostate cancer. *J Urol* 1996; **165:** 873–7.

11. Goldenberg SL, Bruchovsky N, Use of cyproterone acetate in prostate cancer. *Urol Clin North Am* 1991; **18:** 111–22.

12. Flamm J, Fischer M, Höltl W, Pflüger H, Tomschi W, Complete androgen deprivation in patients with stage T3 cancer of the prostate. *Eur Urol* 1991; **19:** 192–5.

13. Fair WR, Aprikian A, Sogani P, Reuter V, Whitmore WF, The role of neoadjuvant hormonal manipulation in localized prostatic cancer. *Cancer* 1993; **71:** 1031–8.

14. Köllerman MW, Sprenk P, Mühlfait V, Kahla H, Köllerman J, Downstaging of stage C prostatic carcinoma by inductive chemo-hormonal treatment. *Eur Urol* 1993; **24:** 337–42.

15. Van Poppel H, De Ridder D, Elgamal AA et al, Neoadjuvant hormonal therapy before radical prostatectomy decreases the number of positive surgical margin in stage T2 prostate cancer: Interim results of a prospective randomized trial. The Belgian Uro-Oncological Study Group. *J Urol* 1995; **154:** 429–34.

16. Aprikian AG, Fair WR, Reuter VE et al, Experience with neo-adjuvant diethylstilbestrol and radical prostatectomy in locally advanced prostate cancer. *Br J Urol* 1994; **74:** 630–6.

17. Schulman CC, Neoadjuvant androgen blockade prior to prostatectomy: A retrospective study and critical review, *Prostate* 1994; **5**(suppl): 9–14.

18. Têtu B, Srigley J, Boivin JC et al, Effect of combination endocrine therapy (LHRH-agonist and flutamide) on normal prostate and prostatic adenocarcinoma. *Am J Surg Pathol* 1991; **15:** 111–20.

19. Witjes WPJ, Oosterhof GON, Schaafsma HE, Debruyne FMJ, Current status of neoadjuvant therapy in localized prostate cancer. *Prostate* 1995; **27:** 297–303.

20. Oesterling JE, Andrews PE, Suman VJ, Zincke H, Myers RP, Preoperative androgen deprivation therapy: artificial lowering of serum prostate specific antigen without downstaging the tumor. *J Urol* 1993; **149:** 779–82.

21. Murphy W, Soloway M, Barrows G, Pathologic changes associated with androgen deprivation therapy for prostate cancer. *Cancer* 1991; **68:** 821–8.

22. Hellström M, Häggman M, Brändstedt S et al, Histopathological changes in androgen deprived localized prostatic cancer. A study in total prostatectomy specimens. *Eur Urol* 1993; **24:** 461–5.

23. Ferguson J, Zincke H, Ellison E, Bergstrahl E, Bostwick DG, Decrease of prostatic intraepithelial neoplasia following androgen deprivation therapy in patients with stage T3 carcinoma treated by radical prostatectomy. *Urology* 1994; **44:** 91–5.

24. Morgan WR, Myers RP, Endocrine therapy prior to radical retropubic prostatectomy for clinical stage C prostate cancer. Pathologic and biochemical response. *J Urol* 1991; **145:** A414.

25. MacFarlane MT, Abi-Aad A, Stein A, Danella J, Belldegrun A, deKernion JB, Neoadjuvant hormonal deprivation in patients with locally advanced prostate cancer. *J Urol* 1993; **150:** 132–4.

26. Voges GE, Mottrie AM, Stöckle M, Müller SC, Hormone therapy prior to radical prostatectomy in patients with clinical stage C prostate cancer. *Prostate* 1994; **5**(suppl): 4–8.

27. Narayan P, Lowe BA, Carroll PR, Thompson IM, Neoadjuvant hormonal therapy and radical prostatectomy for clinical stage C carcinoma of the prostate. *Br J Urol* 1994; **73:** 544–8.

28. Labrie F, Dupont A, Cusan L, Downstaging of localized prostate cancer by neoadjuvant therapy with flutamide and lupron: the first controlled and randomized trial. *Clin Invest Med* 1994; **16:** 499–509.

29. Soloway MS, Sharifi R, Wajsman Z, McLeod D, Wood DP Jr, Puraz Baez A, Randomized

prospective study comparing radical prostatectomy alone versus radical prostatectomy preceded by androgen blockage in clinical stage B2 (T2bNxM0) prostate cancer. The Lupron Depot Neoadjuvant Prostate Cancer Study Group. *J Urol* 1995; **154:** 424–8.

30. Witjes WPJ, Schulman CC, Debruyne FMJ for the European Study Group on Neoadjuvant Treatment of Prostate Cancer, Preliminary results of a prospective randomized study comparing radical prostatectomy versus radical prostatectomy associated with neoadjuvant hormonal combination therapy in T_{2-3} N_0 M_0 prostatic carcinoma. *Urology* 1997; **49**(suppl): 65–9.

31. Schulman CC, Sassine AM, Neoadjuvant hormonal deprivation before radical prostatectomy. *Eur Urol* 1993; **24:** 450–5.

32. Partin AW, Piantadosi S, Sanda MG et al, Selection of men at high risk for disease recurrence for experimental adjuvant therapy following radical prostatectomy. *Urology* 1995; **45:** 831–8.

33. Eschwège P, Dumas F, Blanchet P et al, Haematogeneous dissemination of prostatic epithelial cells during radical prostatectomy. *Lancet* 1995; **348:** 1528–30.

34. Su SL, Hesson WD, Edwards TE et al, Preoperative neoadjuvant androgen deprivation therapy decreases the incidence of circulating prostate cells. *J Urol* 1996; **157:** 1628A.

APPENDIX

Institutions participating in the European Neoadjuvant Study:

University Hospital Nijmegen, Nijmegen, The Netherlands
Ospedale Civile di Alessandria, Alessandria, Italy
Städtische Kliniken Neuss, Neuss, Germany
Ospedale di Circolo e Fond, Macchi, Varese, Italy
Hôpital Foch, Suresnes, France
Glasgow Royal Infirmary, Glasgow, UK
Cliniques Universitaires St Luc, Brussels, Belgium
Las Norias, Madrid, Spain
Border Urology Clinic, Albury, Australia
Ospedale Molinette, Torino, Italy
Krankenhaus St Pölten, St Pölten, Austria
Ospedale San Luigi Gonzaga, Orbassono-Torino, Italy

Urologische Klinik Planegg, Planegg, Germany
Kaiser-Franz-Josef-Spital der Stadt Wien, Vienna, Austria
A van Leeuwenhoekhuis, Amsterdam, The Netherlands
Ospedale Santa Corona, Pietra Ligure (SV), Italy
Università di Firenze, Florence, Italy
Canisius-Wilhelmina Hospital, Nijmegen, The Netherlands
Erasme Hôpital, Université Libre de Bruxelles, Brussels, Belgium
Università di Bari, Bari, Italy
Ospedale San Rafaele, Rome, Italy
Ospedale SS Trinità, Cagliari, Italy
Fundacion Puigvert, Barcelona, Spain
Johannes-Gutenberg-Universität, Mainz, Germany

14

The role of cryosurgery in the treatment of prostate cancer

Ronald Benoit, Ralph Miller, Lori Merlotti, Jeffrey K Cohen

CONTENTS • **Patient selection** • **Risk of side-effects** • **Candidates for CSAP** • **Theory** • **Technique** • **Results** • **Complications** • **Conclusions**

The proper treatment of clinically localized adenocarcinoma of the prostate remains controversial. No prospective randomized study exists which demonstrates a benefit from treatment of localized prostate cancer. Patients who do choose active treatment for their disease will only realize any potential benefit many years after treatment. However, complications from such treatment will be experienced in the short term. The risk of immediate morbidity in exchange for the possibility of benefit in the long term have led many to advise against treatment for early stage prostate cancer. Thus patients are left to ponder the risk versus benefit equation for treatment of their prostate cancer without the aid of firm data favoring any particular treatment.

If patients do elect to undergo treatment for early stage disease, they need to decide between the many available treatment alternatives. Several treatment options now exist for similar stage disease (clinical T1–T2), including radical prostatectomy, external beam radiation, prostate brachytherapy, watchful waiting, and cryosurgical ablation of the prostate (CSAP). Radical prostatectomy remains the gold standard for treatment of organ-confined prostate cancer.[1] The disparity between pathologically and clinically confined disease establishes the failure of this modality in clinical practice.[2] Historically, older men, men with comorbidities that make radical surgery untenable, or men with extensive local disease have undergone external beam radiotherapy. Classically, treatment failure after external beam radiation was defined as recurrence on digital rectal examination or development of metastatic disease. Treatment failure is currently defined as a rising prostate-specific antigen (PSA) level or a positive biopsy. This changing definition of treatment failure has led to the recognition of a much lower rate of cancer control by external beam radiation than was previously accepted.[3] More recently, alternative treatments such as CSAP and prostate brachytherapy have been revisited and retooled to serve as minimally invasive treatment options for men with clinically localized prostate cancer. This chapter discusses the factors responsible for the re-emergence of CSAP in the treatment of prostate cancer, as well as our philosophy regarding ideal candidates for this procedure. The technique of CSAP and several innovations that may potentially improve outcomes are then reviewed. Finally, a summary of outcomes and complications attributable to CSAP is reviewed.

PATIENT SELECTION

Patient factors

For many years, men who desired a surgical option for treatment of their prostate cancer could choose either a retropubic or perineal prostatectomy. This procedure entails hospitalization for 3–7 days followed by a recovery period of 6–12 weeks. Historically, the risk of blood loss was significant and commonly necessitated the transfusion of several units of blood.[4] More recently, the need for transfusions has decreased markedly as surgeons have learned the anatomical approach to radical prostatectomy. Urinary incontinence, depending on how it is defined, has been reported to be as high as 40% after radical prostatectomy.[5] Despite the widespread use of the nerve-sparing approach to radical prostatectomy, impotence has been reported in up to 60% of patients who undergo radical prostatectomy.[5] The fear of major surgery, the risk of urinary incontinence and/or impotence after radical prostatectomy, combined with the uncertain benefit from treatment of localized disease, have led many patients and their physicians to seek other options for treatment.

External beam radiotherapy has long been an alternative to surgery for men with clinically localized prostate cancer. The risk of incontinence and impotence after radiation is lower than after surgery.[6] However, many studies have questioned the long-term cancer control provided by radiation therapy.[3] Additionally, external beam radiotherapy is a time-consuming treatment which requires 7–8 weeks of daily treatments. Recently, prostate brachytherapy has been the subject of considerable attention by both prostate cancer patients and their physicians.[7] Prostate brachytherapy appears to offer excellent cancer control for men with low-grade, low-volume (low-PSA) prostate cancer, and shows a very acceptable

side-effect profile.[8] However, long-term follow-up for current techniques of prostate brachytherapy is not yet available.

Cryosurgical ablation of the prostate is a minimally invasive surgical approach designed for the treatment of prostate cancer. Treatment requires only an overnight hospital stay and a recovery time to full activity of approximately 2 weeks. Incontinence risks are minimal and comparable to those of external beam radiation therapy.[9] Impotence, which in the best of circumstances is difficult to quantitate, is similar to other series involving radical prostatectomy.[9] These characteristics appeal to the patient interested in minimizing morbidity and undergoing a minimally invasive treatment option for their prostate cancer.

Selection characteristics

The optimal treatment modality for men with clinically localized prostate cancer depends on the characteristics of both the tumor (grade, stage, and volume of disease) and the patient (age and comorbidities). Given the generally slow growth of prostate cancer, equal importance should be given to each patient's concern regarding potential side-effects from treatment.[10] Some patients will accept higher risks of side-effects for the perception of improved cancer control, while others may choose a treatment with unknown long-term cancer-control rates with a more acceptable side-effect profile.

Historically, younger, healthier men with low-grade and low-volume tumors underwent surgery, while older men with larger tumors received external beam radiotherapy. As a result, comparison between surgery and radiation were contaminated by the selection bias that existed between these two modalities. PSA has allowed for a more precise stratification of patients and has allowed for accurate comparison between similar cohorts of prostate cancer patients. For patients with a PSA less than 10 ng/ml and a Gleason score of 6 or less, cancer control is similar regardless of the treatment option selected.[8,11–13] However, short-term results of cancer control in men with favorable pretreatment characteristics are misleading in that the disease spans one to three decades. It is at least 5–8 years after diagnosis that cause-specific cancer deaths begin to occur in men with these favorable preoperative characteristics.[10] Given the difficulty of providing definitive data on treatment outcomes using survival data alone in this cancer, PSA and post-treatment biopsy results have become accepted as surrogate markers for long-term treatment outcomes.

While cancer control appears to be similar for surgery, radiation (delivered via teletherapy or brachytherapy), or CSAP in patients with low-grade and low-stage tumors (low-risk prostate cancer), the optimal treatment option for high-risk prostate cancers is less clear. High-risk disease is defined by tumors that are clinically T2b or larger, a Gleason score of 7 or more, or PSA greater than 15 ng/ml. Surgery or radiation as single-agent therapy offers an unacceptably low rate of cancer control.[14,15] Many treatment combinations have been advanced for these high-risk cancers, including:

- androgen deprivation therapy (ADT) prior to surgery, external beam radiotherapy, or prostate brachytherapy;
- radical prostatectomy followed by adjuvant radiotherapy;
- prostate brachytherapy preceded or followed by external beam radiotherapy, with or without ADT;
- CSAP, with or without adjuvant radiotherapy.

All the above combination therapies are being studied at major centers around the world in the hope of improving outcomes for men with high-grade, high-volume (high-risk) prostate cancers.

RISK OF SIDE-EFFECTS

Complications after treatment of prostate cancer are well documented. The major concerns of most patients are urinary incontinence and impotence. Following radical prostatectomy, the incidence of impotence has been reported to be as high as 60%, depending on age, tumor stage, and the presence of comorbidities.[5] Approximately 50% of men will develop erectile dysfunction following external beam radiotherapy,[6] while prostate brachytherapy (30% impotency rate) carries the lowest risk for impotence after treatment of clinically localized disease.[16] Cryosurgical ablation of the prostate has a risk of impotence similar to that reported for radical prostatectomy, since the treatment will extend out past the capsule, and thus will freeze the neurovascular bundles. Recovery of erectile function is usually limited to the younger population.[9] Underlying all these data is the inability to quantify impotence and the demographics of the population. Most patients have concomitant vascular disease in some form, and have lived through a time when smoking was viewed as socially acceptable behavior. During World War II and the Korean conflict cigarettes were easily accessible and affordable, thus increasing their use. How this observation factors into the measurement of impotence is of significant concern, and undermines the reliability of published reports. Treatment options for erectile dysfunction are becoming more numerous and successful, thus decreasing the pretreatment concerns of the patient regarding potential loss of erectile ability after treatment.

Given the successful treatments available for the treatment of impotence, incontinence may be a more feared complication of treatment for localized prostate cancer. The published rate of urinary incontinence following prostatectomy varies from 5% to 30%.[5,17] Radiation therapy, delivered by external beam, or prostate brachytherapy has an incontinence risk of 2% in men who have not undergone prior transurethral resection of the prostate.[16] CSAP carries an incontinence risk of approximately 4% when an adequate urethral warmer is used.[9]

CANDIDATES FOR CSAP

Patients must decide which modality is the most reasonable approach for treatment of their disease, based on the characteristics of their tumor, their overall health (i.e. life expectancy), their desire for long-term cancer control, and their fear of complications from treatment. The patient's desire to avoid surgery and the time they can or are willing to commit to treatment and recovery must also be factored into this decision. To explain better how these considerations should affect a patient's decision-making process, we have set up the Allegheny Prostate Center (APC). The APC provides an educational resource for the patient, designed to minimize the emotional aspects of the decision process, and to provide patients and their families with the information they need to make an informed choice regarding treatment of their disease. Men who have been diagnosed with prostate cancer and those seeking salvage therapy after failure of their initial treatment make up the bulk of the patients seen.

Patients are interviewed and examined separately by a urologist and radiation oncologist. They bring with them a copy of their records and the slides containing their biopsies for review. Following confirmation of the slides and an examination, a round table discussion is held with the patients, family members, and all interested parties. The discussion is led jointly by the urologist and the radiation oncologist. During this discussion, the natural history of prostate cancer is discussed, emphasizing the favorable demographics – specifically, the prevalence of the disease in the fifth to eighth decades of life, cause-specific survival data, and the incidence of death related specifically to prostate cancer. All treatment options are reviewed, including:

- watchful waiting,
- radical prostatectomy,
- external beam radiotherapy – conformal,
- prostate brachytherapy,
- cryosurgical ablation of the prostate,
- androgen deprivation therapy.

The treatment course, recovery period, outcomes of treatment, and complication rates associated with each procedure are discussed. Since all treatment options are offered to patients at our institution, a menu of treatment options unbiased by physician preference is provided. The mission of the APC is patient education and research. The purpose is to allow patients to make their own determination of proper treatment based on a thorough understanding of all the complex issues surrounding the treatment of prostate cancer. We do, however, share our philosophy of treatment with the patients. Our *preference* for men with low-risk disease (PSA < 10 ng/ml, Gleason score ⩽ 6 or clinical grade T2a) and who are aged 65 years or less and in good health is radical prostatectomy. In our opinion, radical prostatectomy has the longest follow-up of all treatments of prostate cancer. If the disease is pathologically confined and the organ is removed, the patient should be cured of their disease.[11] If the disease is specimen confined with a Gleason score of 6 or less, the chance for cancer control by surgery alone is also high.[18] Men over the age of 65 years are informed of the higher complication rates associated with surgery and the decreased need for long-term control of their cancer. This is based on the fact that the median survival of men in the USA is 75 years, and the cause-specific survival for men with low-risk disease at 5 years is also very high. The argument that men who reach the age of 70 years are likely to reach the age of 80 years is misleading in as much as the majority of those men already have prostate cancer and seem to be surviving quite nicely with it. In our opinion, men over the age of 65 years with low-risk prostate cancer can undergo radiation therapy (via brachytherapy or teletherapy) and can expect excellent cancer control.

The role of CSAP is principally in the treatment of high-risk, clinically localized prostate cancer (PSA ⩾ 10 ng/ml, Gleason score ⩾ 7, clinical grade T2b or higher). Cryosurgical ablation of the prostate appears to offer the best cancer control for these tumors when compared with other treatment options, including the various combination therapies discussed previously.[19] Cryosurgery also should be the treatment of choice for men who have local failure as diagnosed by a positive biopsy 2 years after completing external beam radiation therapy.[20] Although radiation offers very acceptable cancer control for low-risk prostate cancer, many patients with high-risk prostate cancer who underwent radiation therapy have failed to achieve local control. Radical prostatectomy after external beam radiotherapy has failed to achieve cure rates greater than approximately 30% and is associated with an unacceptably high risk of morbidity.[21,22] Cryosurgical ablation of the prostate is also a viable treatment option for men under the age of 65 years who may desire a minimally invasive treatment option, fear the risk of incontinence, or who are not appropriate candidates for surgery.

THEORY

It is accepted that cell death and necrosis will be induced by rapidly bringing tissues to subzero temperatures. Cell death is an effect of ice formation and a spectrum of events secondary to hypothermia.[23] Hypothermia begins the cascade of injury marked by decreased intracellular energy stores and a breakdown in the physical and physiologic functions of the cellular membrane. Rapid hypothermia leads to intracellular dehydration and cell shrinkage. When the temperature drops below $-4°C$, ice crystals form in the extracellular space and eventually cross the cell membrane gap junctions, leading to intracellular ice, membrane rupture, and cell death. On completion of the freezing process, microscopic ice crystals coalesce into sheets of ice, creating shearing forces that account for additional destruction. Any viable cells remaining are suddenly faced with a markedly extracellular hypotonic environment (from the thawing of pure water), resulting in a sudden influx of free water by osmotic forces (membrane function remains inactivated). This causes cell swelling, rupture, and death. Finally, the freezing process causes obstruction of the vasculature, which leads to anoxia and thrombosis. This final injury completes the cytotoxic cascade of events. Tissue absorption following cryotherapy can take up to 3 months, and is marked initially by inflammation and removal of cellular debris and later by deposition of collagen and the creation of organized scar tissue. Histologically aberrant glands can be seen fol-

lowing CSAP, including basal cell hyperplasia, squamous cell metaplasia, and transitional cell metaplasia.[24] Recovery of neural function depends on the integrity of the neural sheath and may take 6–12 months.[25]

TECHNIQUE

Preoperative preparation

Patients must be free of active lower urinary tract infection prior to treatment. Prostate volume should be less than 65 g, since glands larger than this may be difficult to treat completely in a single procedure. Alternatives include preoperative ADT to reduce the size of the gland, or treating the prostate in stages. Evaluation of nodal status is done through a 'mini-lap' pelvic lymph node dissection. At our institution, nodal evaluation is excluded for men with a PSA level below 10, men over the age of 70 years, or men who have had prior ADT.

Patients are instructed to administer a Fleets (phosphate soda) enema on the night prior to surgery and at 06.00 h on the morning of surgery. Ofloxacin (300 mg) is given orally on the night prior to surgery and on arrival at the hospital on the morning of surgery. Metronidazole (Flagyl) (750 mg) is also given orally on arrival at the hospital. Patients are admitted to the same-day-surgery unit on the morning of surgery. Spinal or general anesthetic is chosen, depending on the preference of the patient and the anesthesiologist.

Technique of cryoablation

Once anesthetized, the patient is placed in the dorsal lithotomy position. Flexible cystoscopy is performed, and a suprapubic tube is placed in the dome of the bladder. On cystoscopic examination any bladder lesions, urethral obstructive lesions, or median lobe prostate tissue is noted, since these may require further treatment postoperatively. The cystoscope is removed and a urethral warming catheter is inserted. The catheter is perfused with saline solution at 40°C to maintain the viability of the urethra.

The transrectal ultrasound probe is then placed into the rectum. A biplanar piezoelectric transducer should be used for CSAP. This allows crucial three-dimensional surveillance of the freezing process. The sagittal or longitudinal scanner must utilize a linear piezoelectric (7 MHz) crystal. The linear sagittal transducer provides better definition of the structures posterior to the prostate, without the volume averaging and refractory artifacts commonly seen with mechanical sector scanning transducers. Routine volumetric analysis is performed using the formula

Volume = (Length × Weight × Height) × 0.52.

All hypoechoic areas are noted, and any areas of suspected capsular penetration are carefully documented.

We began using color flow Doppler ultrasound to monitor CSAP in March 1994. Graphic analysis of the vessels can distinguish arterial and venous waveforms. This information is used to detect areas of increased vascularity (Figure 14.1), which can act as heat sinks to prevent adequate freezing. We can then modify the cryoprobe placement such that these vessels are encompassed and ablated in the iceball, thus enhancing the cytotoxic effects of the cryotherapy. We have also recently begun injecting the areas of increased arterial blood flow with a vasoconstrictor (epinephrine), in order to decrease blood flow in these vessels and hence decrease the heat sink effect. The blood flow to the rectum can also be assessed with color flow Doppler during freezing to prevent fistula formation.

The probe access ports are placed. Each port is placed similarly and begins with a percutaneous puncture of the perineum. With a diamond-tipped needle placed in a needle guide, transrectal ultrsound (transverse transducer) is used to guide the needle into the appropriate position in the prostate. It is then advanced under visualization by the sagittal transducer to the cephalad capsule of the prostate. A stiff 0.038-inch, J-tipped guidewire is placed and the needle is removed. A modified Amplatz dilator (Cook Urological, Spencer, IN) and Teflon introducer sheath are then advanced over the wire, again using ultrasound visualization. Once in position, the dilator and wire are removed. The sheath is irrigated with saline solution to remove air and debris (which would interfere with freezing) and improve visualization. All probe sites are subsequently placed.

Integral to the selection of probe sites is the normal geometry of the iceball that forms at the probe tip. The iceballs generated by the Accuprobe system are symmetric and reproducible. The ice begins at the probe tip (≤5 mm growth past the tip in the completed iceball) and extends up the shaft for a total length of 5 cm. The maximum radius of the iceball is 2 cm, and the final iceball is egg-shaped. In a multiple probe arrangement iceballs augment the performance of any adjacent probes. Any recesses between adjacent iceballs (probes) will be filled in as a result of this augmentation, so that the final contour is smooth (this is referred to as 'ice sculpting').

The typical template involves five individually controlled probes. Two probes are placed anteriorly and three posteriorly. The two anterior probes are placed 5–8 mm from the anterior capsule at the midpoint between the urethra and the lateral capsule. The two posterolateral probes are placed such that the iceball growth will extend past the lateral capsule before reaching the rectum (the endpoint of the procedure). The posterolateral probes should also be placed as anteriorly as possible (not beyond the 2-cm radius of the iceball) in order to let the iceball grow out laterally, to encompass the neuro-vascular bundles as seen by color flow Doppler ultrasound, and, medially, to augment the performance of the other probes. A fifth probe is placed in the midline posterior to the urethra (Figure 14.2). Additional access ports can be placed outside the prostate, parallel to the neurovascular bundles, in order to triangulate areas of extracapsular extension or seminal vesicle involvement. Advancement of the posterolateral probes into the seminal vesicles can eliminate direct spread in cases of clinical stage T3c disease.

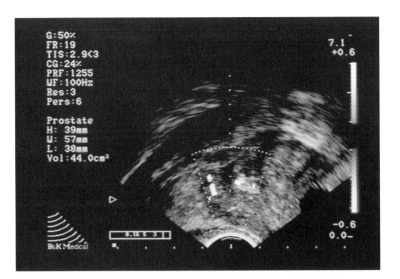

Figure 14.1 Transverse image utilizing Doppler to identify the neurovascular bundles.

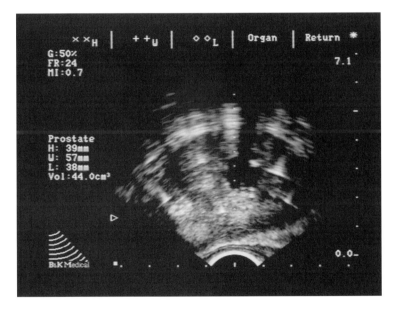

Figure 14.2 Transverse image showing probes (white dots) in the prostate gland.

Once all access ports have been established, the cryoprobes are placed in the sheaths. The pre-slit Teflon sheaths are withdrawn, and the Accuprobe circulates liquid nitrogen through the probes. This will create a small iceball at the tip of the probe, 'sticking' the probe in place and negating the chance of dislodgment. We generally stick the probes at −70°C to −100°C. The probes are suspended with rubber straps from a Bookwalter retractor ring, which is suspended above the perineum.

Objects close to the transducer cause acoustic interference, and therefore all manipulation, probe placement, and freezing are performed in an anterior-to-posterior sequence. Once all probes have been 'stuck' in place, the system is activated to circulate pressurized, supercooled liquid nitrogen at full flow through the probes

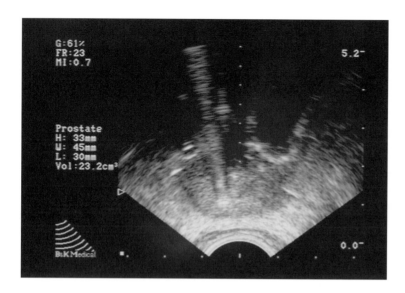

Figure 14.3 Transverse image showing anterior iceball formation and probes posterior to the iceball.

($-180°C$ to $-200°C$). As the tissue temperature drops below $-4°C$, the tissue water changes from liquid to solid. This interface reflects all sound waves, and is interpreted as a hyperechoic line. The lack of sound wave transmission beyond this interface is referred to as 'acoustic shadowing'; the iceball itself is anechoic. The early freezing process is monitored in both the sagittal and the transverse plane in order to provide a three-dimensional image (Figure 14.3).

Once the advancing edge of the iceballs from the anterior probes has reached the posterior row of probes, the posterior probes are activated. The anterior probes continue to freeze until the iceballs reach the posterior prostatic capsule. This augments the performance of the posterior probes and ensures adequate margins anteriorly. Surveillance at this point is done with the sagittal transducer because this provides better delineation of the structures posterior to the prostate. A 6-cm linear array sagittal transducer allows simultaneous visualization of the entire prostate (the ice is widest at the probe tip). The contour of the rectum does not follow a straight line; it is situated anteriorly at the apex and urogenital diaphragm, compared with a more posterior location at the base. A sagittal transducer will accurately show the relationship of the iceball to the entire rectal wall. As the treatment continues, there is an increase in blood flow around the prostate. The signals from the neurovascular bundles increase as the iceball approaches the rectum, and portosystemic shunts through the rectum can be visualized. These vascular changes are believed to be caused, in part, by microvascular obstruction in the prostate. Whether there are local factors liberated during this process is speculative, but possible. The increased peripheral flow has the potential to heat and preserve surrounding tissue. Because of this finding, we began double freezing the prostate in order to extinguish these signals by an encompassing iceball. The probes remain activated until the advancing edge of the iceball abuts the anterior rectal wall. Although the temperature of the probes is $-195°C$, the temperature at the edge of the iceball is approximately $0°C$. Extracellular ice is seen at $-15°C$ and intracellular necrosis begins at $-20°C$. However, complete freezing of the entire intracellular content is believed to occur at $-40°C$. This temperature is achieved within 2 mm of the edge of the iceball. Therefore, the iceball must extend several millimeters beyond the posterior capsule to ensure complete destruction of the prostate.

Typically, this margin is easily achieved due to the size of Denonvillier's space and the increased vascularity through the rectal wall. To ensure that adequate freezing is achieved, some centers have utilized thermocouples to monitor the temperature in and around the prostate.

After the first freeze cycle, the prostate is allowed to thaw (passively), after which the prostate is refrozen (double freeze). After the first freeze and subsequent thawing, any surviving cells are sensitized and much more susceptible to a repeat freezing process. Most prostates are longer than 4 cm, which requires pulling back the probes to treat the apical prostate and trapezoidal area. The second freezing encompasses the apical prostate and the trapezoidal area, and generally extends through the urogenital diaphragm. With prostates shorter than 4 cm, the procedure is complete after the double freeze in the initial position. The second freeze is started after the prostate has thawed passively to a sufficient degree that it is again completely visible on ultrasound (disappearance of the iceball).

Once the freezing process has been completed, the probes are thawed and then removed. Manual pressure is applied to the perineum for hemostasis, and the probe insertion sites are closed with simple 3:0 chromic sutures. The urethral warming catheter is left activated until the entire prostate has thawed (generally 20 min). The catheter is removed, the suprapubic tube placed to closed drainage, and the patient taken to the recovery room.

Postoperative care

The usual hospital stay is 1 day. On the morning of the first postoperative day the suprapubic tube is capped. The tube is removed when postvoid residuals are consistently less than $100 \, cm^3$; this is typically at about 2 weeks. Postoperative discomfort is minimal. Scrotal edema occurs in about a third of patients and can be dramatic, but will gradually resolve within 3 weeks. Normal activity can be resumed in 1–2 weeks. Occasionally, gross hematuria will be troublesome postoperatively. In these cases a urethral catheter is placed in order to institute continuous irrigation through the suprapubic catheter.

RESULTS

The largest published series of patients receiving cryosurgery for prostate cancer is from Allegheny General Hospital.[9,13] Two-year PSA and biopsy results have been reported. A total of 448 procedures were performed on 383 patients. Negative biopsy rates were 89.5% for previously untreated patients ($n = 83$), 87.1% for patients who had undergone previous androgen deprivation therapy ($n = 31$, and 100% for patients who had received previous radiotherapy ($n = 5$). Of patients with at least 21 months of follow-up, 75.8% had a PSA less than 1.0 ng/ml and 54.6% had a PSA less than 0.4 ng/ml.

Impressive results were also achieved for patients with clinical stage C lesions. The median PSA in this group of 96 patients was 13.4 ng/ml. The postprocedure PSA at 3 months was 0.98 ng/ml. Seventy-five patients (78%) had a negative biopsy 3 months after the procedure. Fourteen patients underwent repeat therapy, and nine of these patients converted to a negative biopsy, bringing the overall negative biopsy rate to 94.4%. Of the eight patients who had 2-year biopsies, seven (86%) remained negative. Equally impressive were the results for patients with high-risk prostate cancer, regardless of clinical stage, defined as those patients with a PSA greater than 10 ng/ml and a Gleason score of 7 ($n = 46$) or higher, or a PSA greater than 20 ng/ml and a Gleason score of 2–6 ($n = 24$). No patients underwent preoperative ADT. Nine patients underwent a second procedure. The negative biopsy rate in these patients was 65.1%. The mean preprocedure PSA was 22.9 ng/ml in the patients with a subsequent negative biopsy, and 33.4 ng/ml in patients with a subsequent positive biopsy. The mean postprocedure PSA was 0.66 ng/ml in the negative-biopsy cohort (at 24 months) and 12.7 ng/ml in the positive-biopsy cohort (at 3 months).

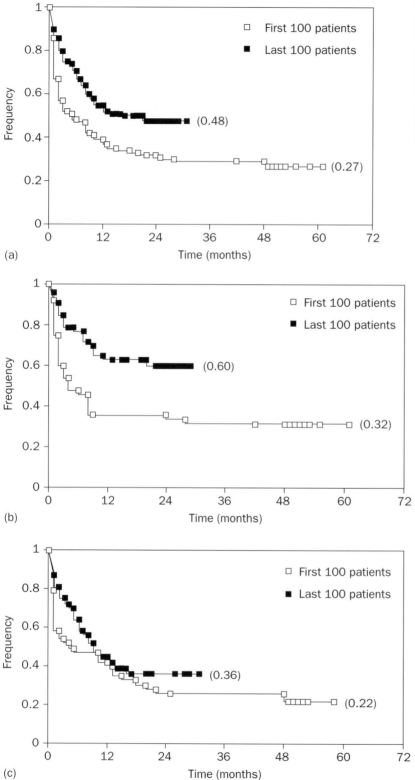

Figure 14.4 The proportion of patients showing a PSA level of ⩽0.4 ng/ml versus time after cryosurgery. Data are for the first 100 and last 100 patients treated at Allegheny General Hospital in a series of 383 patients. (a) Low- and high-risk groups combined; (b) low-risk group; (c) high-risk group.

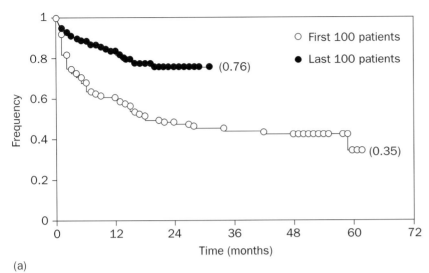

(a)

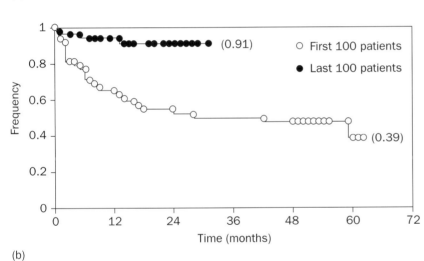

(b)

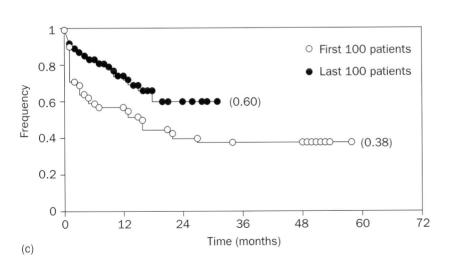

(c)

Figure 14.5 The proportion of patients showing a PSA level of ≤1.0 ng/ml versus time after cryosurgery. Data are for the first 100 and last 100 patients treated at Allegheny General Hospital in a series of 383 patients. (a) Low- and high-risk groups combined; (b) low-risk group; (c) high-risk group.

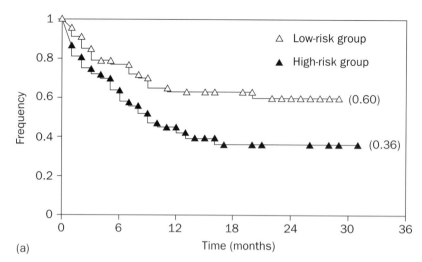

(a)

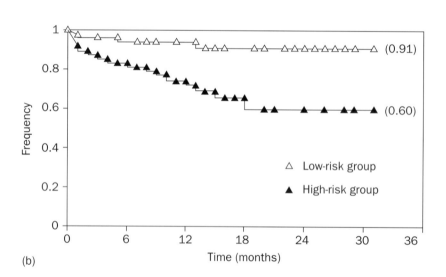

(b)

Figure 14.6 The proportions of low- and high-risk patients showing PSA levels of (a) ≤0.4 and (b) ≤1.0 ng/ml versus time after cryosurgery. Data are for the last 100 patients treated at Allegheny General Hospital in a series of 383 patients.

The wide variation in the mean PSA of the negative- and positive-biopsy cohorts suggests the presence of metastatic disease in the patients with positive biopsies. Cryosurgery followed by external beam radiotherapy also appears to be effective in the treatment of high-risk prostate cancer. At Allegheny General Hospital, 26 patients have undergone this combination therapy. The mean time from cryosurgery to radiation therapy was 14.5 months. The mean preprocedure PSA was 17.4 ng/ml in these men, while the postproce-

dure PSA was 0.49 ng/ml. Negative biopsies were achieved in 81% of patients treated.

In order to understand better the effects of cryosurgery, two factors need to be understood: the learning curve and the selection bias. The learning curve can best be demonstrated by comparing the PSA levels after cryosurgery in the first 100 and last 100 patients (clinical stage T1–T3) treated in our series of 383 patients. Figure 14.3 shows the proportion of patients with a PSA level of 0.4 ng/ml or less versus the time after treatment. For low- and high-risk groups combined (Figure 14.3a), there is a 21% improvement in results in the last versus the first 100 patients treated. For low-risk patients only (Figure 14.3b), this improvement is even higher (28%), although the improvement is small (<10%) for the high-risk group (Figure 14.3a). The latter result suggests a higher incidence of extraprostatic disease in the high-risk patients. Corresponding graphs for patients showing a PSA level of 1.0 ng/ml or less are given in Figure 14.4. This PSA level was chosen in order to be able to compare the results obtained using external radiotherapy. At 3 years after surgery, the last 100 patients treated showed an approximately 22% improvement in outcome compared with the first 100 patients treated (low- and high-risk groups combined) (Figure 14.4a). The improvement in the results for the low-risk patients was only 40% (Figure 14.4b), and that for the high-risk group was approximately 20% (Figure 14.4c). These differences in results are even more pronounced than those found using a PSA level of 0.4 ng/ml or less. Thus it can be concluded that the results of treatment have improved over time.

In order to assess the effects of selection bias, we examined the results obtained from Kaplan–Meir plots in the low- and high-risk groups of the last 100 patients treated (Figure 14.5). The proportion of patients showing the required PSA level (<0.4 ng/ml or <1.0 ng/ml) at 30 months was greater (24% and 29% respectively) in the low-risk group than in the high-risk group. The means of performing the cryosurgical procedure was similar in the last 100 patients, and thus the difference in the outcomes suggests a difference between the two groups. We conclude that the high-risk group has a higher incidence of extraprostatic disease.

Of the patients in the low-risk group, 60% achieved and maintained undetectable levels of PSA after 30 months' treatment. While this result is not as good as that obtained with prostatectomy, it is better than the outcomes obtained with external beam radiotherapy (91% and 60% of patients achieved a PSA level of 1.0 ng/ml or less at 30 months after radical prostatectomy, and external beam radiother-

apy, respectively). This comparison is flawed in that, as it is a relatively new technique, the results of cryotherapy have been collected over a shorter period of time than have the comparable results for prostatectomy and radiation therapy. However, our experience has been that, at 24 months after treatment, the PSA curves level off and remain constant. The vast majority of the failures (>90%) occur soon after treatment. The fact gives support to the comparison made here, although a prospective randomized trial is needed to validate it.

COMPLICATIONS

Complications after cryosurgery are relatively minimal. The most prevalent was urethral sloughing, which occurred in approximately 10% of patients. If an adequate urethral warmer is not used, urethral sloughing will occur in 19–51% of patients. Urethral sloughing appears to be more common in patients who have not undergone previous treatment for prostate cancer than in those who have been treated with androgen deprivation therapy or radiation therapy prior to cryosurgery. Urinary incontinence occurs at a rate of approximately 3% in patients who have not undergone a previous transurethral resection of the prostate and in whom an adequate urethral warmer was used.

Impotence is difficult to quantify after any treatment for localized prostate cancer. Published rates of impotency after cryosurgery range from 41% to 86%. The theoretical advantage of cryosurgery is the ability of the iceball to extend outside the prostate. The neurovascular bundles of the prostate should be frozen if the prostate is adequately treated. Younger men may have the ability to recover from this nerve injury, while older men may not. This is consistent with reports that younger men (<65 years old) will maintain their erections 33% of the time, while men older than 65 years will maintain their erections in only 15% of cases. Urethrorectal fistula has occurred in 0.4% of cases. There has only been one death in the published reports of cryosurgery. This death was the result of emphysematous cystitis and necrotizing fasciitis in a diabetic patient.

Patients who undergo cryosurgery as salvage therapy after failure of radiation therapy to control local disease appear to be at highest risk for complications after cryosurgery. Incontinence has been reported to be as high as 44% in this group, although this was at only 3 months after treatment. Urinary retention at 3 months in this cohort was 17%.

CONCLUSIONS

Cryosurgical ablation of the prostate is an efficacious treatment for men with clinically localized disease. It is best reserved for men with high-risk, clinically localized prostate cancer (defined as PSA >10, Gleason score ≥7, or clinical stage ≥T2b). Cryosurgery appears to offer improved rates of cancer control over other types of single or combination therapies for this high-risk prostate cancer, and is associated with

a very acceptable side-effect profile. Men with low-risk prostate cancer who choose to avoid radical surgery or radiation, desire a minimally invasive treatment option, or are not candidates for radical surgery due to other medical problems are also candidates for CSAP. The technique is effective as measured by biopsy and PSA. Ultimately, survival data will determine the effectiveness of this modality. Cryosurgery is the only reasonable option for men with clinically localized residual carcinoma in whom radiation therapy has failed. It should be reserved for men who will benefit from the effects of local control of their residual cancer.

This technique remains in its infancy and awaits further technological developments to improve outcomes. At present, CSAP is a reasonable, safe, and effective treatment for men with prostate cancer. The attraction of a minimally invasive, controllable, and reproducible treatment insures a place for this modality in the treatment of prostate cancer.

REFERENCES

1. Gibbons RP, Correa RJ, Brannen GE, Weissman RM, Total prostatectomy for clinically localized prostate cancer: long-term results. *J Urol* 1989; **141:** 564–6.
2. Partin AW, Yoo J, Carter HB et al, The use of prostate specific antigen, clinical stage and Gleason score to predict pathological stage in men with clinically localized prostate cancer. *J Urol* 1993; **150:** 110–14.
3. Stamey TA, Ferrari MK, Schmid HP, The value of serial prostate specific antigen determinations 5 years after radiotherapy: steeply increasing value characterize 80% of patients. *J Urol* 1993; **150:** 1856–9.
4. Haab F, Boccon-Gibod L, Demass V, Kemmis Toublan M, Perineal versus retropubic radical prostatectomy for T1, T2 prostate cancer. *Br J Urol* 1994; **74:** 626–9.
5. Fowler FJ, Barry JJ, Lu-Yao G, Ramon A, Wasson J, Wennberg JE, Patient-reported complications and follow-up treatment after radical prostatectomy. *Urology* 1993; **42:** 622–9.
6. Shipley WU, Zietman AL, Hanks GE et al,

Treatment related sequelae following external beam radiation for prostate cancer: a review with an update in patients with stages T1 and T2 tumor. *J Urol* 1994; **152:** 1799–805.
7. D'Amico AV, Coleman CN, Role of interstitial radiotherapy in the management of clinically organ-confined prostate cancer: the jury is still out. *J Clin Oncol* 1996; **14:** 304–15.
8. Blasko JC, Wallner K, Grimm PD, Ragde H, Prostate specific antigen based disease control following ultrasound guided 125-iodine implantation for stage T1/T2 prostatic carcinoma. *J Urol* 1995; **154:** 1096–9.
9. Cohen JK, Rooker GM, Shuman BA, Miller RJ Jr, Merlotti L, Cryosurgical ablation management alternative for localized prostate cancer. In: *Textbook of Endourology* (Smith AD, ed). Quality Medical Publishing: St Louis, 1996: 1217–33.
10. Chodak G, The role of watchful waiting in the management of localized prostate cancer. *J Urol* 1994; **152:** 1766–8.
11. Walsh PC, Partin AW, Epstein JI, Cancer control and quality of life following anatomical radical

retropubic prostatectomy: results at 10 years. *J Urol* 1994; **152:** 1831–6.

12. Leibel SA, Zelefsky MJ, Kutcher GJ, Burman CM, Kelson S, Fuks Z, Three-dimensional conformal radiation therapy in localized carcinoma of the prostate: interim report of a phase I dose-escalation study. *J Urol* 1994; **152:** 1792–7.

13. Cohen JK, Miller RJ Jr, Rooker GM, Benoit RM, Merlotti L, Four year PSA and biopsy results after cryosurgical ablation of the prostate (CSAP) for localized adenocarcinoma of the prostate. *J Urol* 1997; **157:** 419A.

14. Benson MC, Kaplan SA, Olsson CA, Prostate cancer in men less than 45 years old: influence of stage, grade and therapy. *J Urol* 1987; **137:** 888.

15. Bagshaw MA, Cox RS, Hancock SL, Control of prostate cancer with radiotherapy: long-term results. *J Urol* 1994; **152:** 1781–5.

16. Stock RG, Stone NN, Iannuzzi BA, Sexual potency following interactive ultrasound-guided brachytherapy for prostate cancer. *Int J Radiat Oncol Biol Phys* 1996; **35:** 267–72.

17. Milam DF, Franke JT, Prevention and treatment of incontinence after radical prostatectomy. *Semin Urol Oncol* 1995: **23:** 224–7.

18. Epstein JI, Incidence and significance of positive margins in radical prostatectomy margins. *Urol Clin N Am* 1996; **23:** 651–63.

19. Miller RJ Jr, Cohen JK, Merlotti LA, Percutaneous transperineal cryosurgical ablation of the prostate for the primary treatment of stage C adenocarcinoma of the prostate. *Urology* 1994; **44:** 170–4.

20. Pisters LL, von Eschenbach AC, Technique, results, and complications of 'modern' prostate cryotherapy. *AUA Update Ser* 1996; **15:** 297–304.

21. Rogers E, Ohori M, Kassabian VS, Wheeler TM, Scardino PT, Salvage radical prostatectomy: outcome measured by serum prostate specific antigen levels. *J Urol* 1995; **153:** 104–10.

22. Pontes JE, Montie J, Klein E, Huben R, Salvage surgery for radiation failure in prostate cancer. *Cancer* 1993; **71:** 976–80.

23. Baust JG, Chang AH, Cryosurgery: underlying mechanisms of damage and new concepts in cryosurgical instrumentation. In: *Proceedings from the Ninth World Congress of Cryosurgery*, June 1995.

24. Masson D, Bidair M, Shabaik A, Wilson S, Schmidt JD, Pathologic changes in prostate biopsies following cryoablation therapy. *J Urol* 1995; **153:** 484A

25. Trumble TE, Whalen JT, The effects of cryosurgery and cryoprotectants on peripheral nerve function. *J Reconstruct Microsurg* 1992: **8:** 53–8.

15 Treatment: Hormonal manipulation

15.1 ANTIANDROGENS • 15.2 TESTICULAR ANDROGEN ABLATION •
15.3 COMBINED ANDROGEN BLOCKADE

15.1

Antiandrogens

Barry JA Furr, Amir V Kaisary

CONTENTS • **Steroidal antiandrogens** • **Non-steroidal antiandrogens** • **Discussion** • **Conclusions**

Over the last few years, prostate cancer has been acknowledged as the most common cancer in men apart from skin malignancies. It is also the second leading cause of cancer-related death in men. Since the place of androgen deprivation in the management of advanced prostate cancer was demonstrated by Huggins and Hodges in 1941,[1,2] orchidectomy has been the gold standard that has been utilized. Medical castration achieved with maintenance luteinizing hormone releasing hormone (LHRH) analogue therapy is equivalent to surgical orchidectomy.[3] In recent years, many drugs that interfere with the production and/or the function of androgens have been introduced. Androgen blockade in prostatic cells aims at intracellular inhibition of nucleic acid or protein synthesis. This is accomplished by inhibiting the binding of dihydrotestosterone (DHT) to its receptor. Two types of antiandrogens are known: steroidal and non-steroidal.

The clinically available steroidal antiandrogens have progestational properties, and also act by suppressing gonadotrophins, thus lowering plasma testosterone. They lead to a decrease in libido and potency. These drugs include

cyproterone acetate, chlormadinone acetate and megestrol acetate.

Clinically available non-steroidal compounds are pure antiandrogens, and have no antigonadotrophic effects. They interfere with androgen action by binding competitively to the prostatic intracellular androgen receptors. They also block androgen receptors in the brain, which leads to an increase successively in LHRH, luteinizing hormone (LH) and testosterone secretion. The rise in plasma testosterone is self-limiting for reasons that are not fully understood.

Six antiandrogens have now been used clinically (Figure 15.1.1), and another steroidal compound, WIN 49,596, has been evaluated in extensive preclinical studies.[4-6]

STEROIDAL ANTIANDROGENS

Cyproterone acetate

Cyproterone acetate is a tribute to the pioneering work of Neumann and colleagues at Schering AG, and was the first antiandrogen to be used clinically. It is effective in a majority of

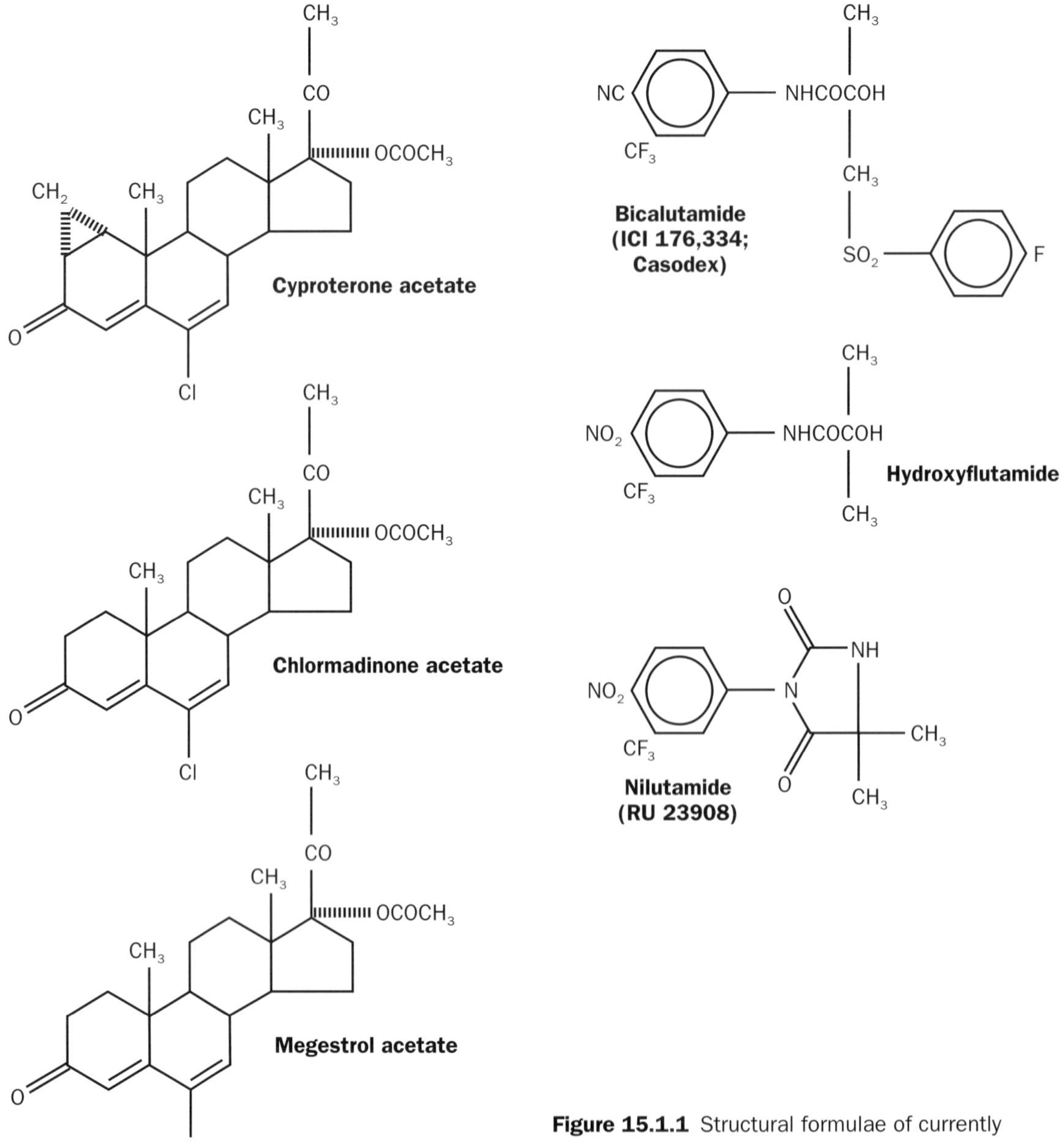

Figure 15.1.1 Structural formulae of currently available antiandrogens.

patients, and its side-effects are generally less severe than those seen with oestrogens.[7] However, thrombosis is seen in 5% of patients, fluid retention in 4%, gynaecomastia in 13% and loss of libido in the majority. The steroidal nature of the drug is probably responsible for its cardiovascular side-effects and its adverse effects on serum lipoproteins.[8] Because of its steroidal properties, there can also be effects on carbohydrate metabolism, so care is advised when prescribing the drug for diabetic patients.[9,10] Variable degrees of migraine and gastrointestinal upset have also been reported,[7] as has serious hepatic toxicity.[11–14]

Cyproterone acetate is also a potent progestin. Its progestational properties provide an advantage over surgical and medical castration and some pure antiandrogens, because it does not produce hot flushes. However, it does severely suppress libido, and causes gynaecomastia and loss of erectile potency.[15] Indeed, it has been used to treat sexual deviation. Loss of libido may not be a severe disadvantage in many very old patients, but in younger men with prostate cancer who are sexually active, it would be an unfavourable consequence of therapy. However, when used in combination with medical or surgical castration, loss of libido is inevitable, so in this situation the progestational and gonadotrophin-inhibitory properties of cyproterone acetate have less clinical relevance.

Chlormadinone acetate

Chlormadinone acetate is closely related structurally to cyproterone acetate, and is also a progestationally active antiandrogen, with properties and deficiencies essentially similar to those of cyproterone acetate. It is not used in Europe or the USA, but has a product licence in Japan, where it has been widely prescribed.[16]

Megestrol acetate

Megestrol acetate is a synthetic derivative of naturally occurring progesterone. Its exact mechanism of action has not yet been completely elucidated. It is thought to have a direct antiproliferative effect, lowering the mitotic index and inhibiting nucleic acid synthesis.[17] It blocks the pituitary secretion of gonadotrophins and suppresses adrenocorticotrophic hormone (ACTH) secretion, with a consequent suppression of adrenal function and decreases in cortisol and androgen levels.[18] In 1984, Geller and associates[19] reported a phase I–II study where megestrol acetate was applied at dosages between 40 and 160 mg/day in combination with a low dose of 0.1 mg of diethylstilboestrol (DES). This regimen was never investigated in a phase III study.

NON-STEROIDAL ANTIANDROGENS

Flutamide

Flutamide was the first available non-steroidal antiandrogen; it was discovered by Neri and colleagues at Schering–Plough. Flutamide is also effective in the treatment of prostate cancer, and appears to be better tolerated than cyproterone acetate.[7] Since it is a pure antiandrogen, it does not seem to be associated with the side-effects of thrombo-embolism and fluid retention. Moreover, since it is not a progestin, it does not suppress testes function like cyproterone acetate, and rarely causes a loss of libido.

The most frequently reported side-effect is gynaecomastia,[20,21] and gastrointestinal intolerance, particularly diarrhoea, can be a troublesome adverse event in many patients.[22,23] Reversible liver function abnormalities have been reported in some patients, and can sometimes be serious.[24] The active metabolite of flutamide, hydroxyflutamide, also has a short half-life (8–9 hours in elderly men; shorter in younger men), and so the parent drug needs to be administered three times daily.[25] This may lead to non-compliance with therapy. Since it is a pure antiandrogen, there is another perceived problem with flutamide. As well as preventing androgen from stimulating prostate growth, it antagonizes the action of androgen at the hypothalamus and pituitary gland. This leads to an increase in LH secretion. It has been suggested that the resulting increase in output of androgen by the testes requires an increased dose of antiandrogen to neutralize any stimulatory effect on the prostate gland – although this is controversial. However, when given in combination with medical or surgical castration, any rise in serum LH becomes irrelevant to clinical outcome. In addition to elevation of androgen secretion, serum oestrogen concentrations are also increased, which would tend to exacerbate any tendency to gynaecomastia.

Flutamide was investigated in several studies as a monotherapeutic agent at a dose of 250 mg three times daily. This dose seems to be purely empirical, since no phase I studies were reported. No significant differences were demonstrated in studies comparing flutamide with daily diethylstilboestrol 1 mg[26] or 3 mg.[27] However, Chang et al[28] found similar overall response rates for flutamide and DES 1 mg three times daily – but the latter had significantly longer time to treatment failure and longer survival. In 1994, Boccon-Gibod and co-workers[29] reported similar progression-free survival in 90 evaluable patients (46 of whom received flutamide and 44 orchidectomy). Most importantly, they identified a median progression-free survival rate in both groups in excess of 600 days among those patients with baseline prostate-specific antigen (PSA) 120 ng/ml. However, the numbers of patients randomized are too small to provide a high level of confidence that the treatments are truly equivalent. In 1997, Boccon-Gibod and co-workers[30] studied 104 patients who were randomized to receive flutamide or orchidectomy, and reported no significant differences in response rate. This study has been criticized by Studer.[31]

Preservation of sexual potency in patients receiving flutamide monotherapy ranged in several studies between 50%[32] and 100%.[27] Flutamide's side-effect profile was summarized in 1990 by Schroder,[33] with 10% of patients withdrawing from treatment and with diarrhoea occurring in 20%. Interestingly, loss of potency was reported in 20% of patients.

Nilutamide

Nilutamide was the second non-steroidal pure antiandrogen that became available from Roussel. It is structurally similar to flutamide, but has a longer half-life of approximately two days,[34] and so can theoretically be given once daily. Clinical trials with nilutamide have focused primarily on its combination with surgical or medical castration.[35,36] Nilutamide monotherapy has not been widely investigated. Decensi and co-workers[37] administered nilutamide at a dose of 300 mg daily (100 mg three times daily) to each of 26 previously untreated patients with metastatic prostate cancer. Partial response was demonstrated in 38.5% of patients, stable disease in 42.3% and progression in 7.7%, with 11.5% of patients being non-evaluable. Median survival was 23 months, with a progression-free survival of only 9 months. Libido and potency were maintained in 46.7%, attenuated in 20% and abolished in 33.3% of patients. A relatively high incidence of side-effects included decreased adaptation to darkness (30.8%), nausea (26.9%) and alcohol intolerance (19.2%). The visual disturbances, however, were reported by Dijkman and co-workers[38] to be mild, with a tendency to disappear after the scheduled dosage reduction from 300 mg to 150 mg or spontaneously. They only led to approximately 2% of withdrawals from therapy, and were always reversible on discontinuation of treatment. Interstitial pneumonitis is also a serious adverse event associated with nilutamide.[33] Therefore nilutamide has been cautiously proposed as a valid option in the treatment of advanced prostate cancer. After 8.5 years of follow-up of a large double-blind trial on 457 patients randomized to receive nilutamide or placebo after orchidectomy, Dijkman et al[38] reported that nilutamide was well tolerated in the long term, with no increase in the incidence of drug-specific adverse events.

Bicalutamide

Bicalutamide (Casodex) is the latest clinically available pure antiandrogen. It is well tolerated and has a half-life (nearly seven days) that is compatible with once-daily use. This certainly offers clinical advantages over existing therapies, since compliance with therapy should be less of an issue.[39] In addition, in developing bicalutamide, it was hoped that a peripherally selective antiandrogen could be identified that would prevent prostate growth but would not act at the hypothalamic–pituitary–gonadal axis to increase serum LH and thereby testosterone.

Binding affinity
Preclinical studies showed bicalutamide to bind to cytosol androgen receptors in the prostate cells of rats, dogs and men. However, it has much lower affinity than the natural androgen

and 5-α-DHT.[5,6,40–45] The majority of studies show bicalutamide to have a two- to fourfold higher affinity for the androgen receptor than hydroxyflutamide, which is the active metabolite of flutamide. However, Luo and coworkers[45] suggest that hydroxyflutamide has a higher affinity for the receptor than bicalutamide. This discrepancy could be related to methodology; this has been reviewed in reference 46. Bicalutamide was also shown to have a negligible affinity for sex hormone-binding globulin and no affinity for corticosteroid-binding globulin. This is in contrast to cyproterone acetate, which has a significant affinity for sex hormone-binding globulin and a high affinity for corticosteroid-binding globulin.[41] Bicalutamide also has no effect on steroid 5-α-reductase.[47]

Activity in tumour cell lines

An important study by Veldscholte and coworkers[48] describes the effects of bicalutamide on binding to an androgen receptor present in the human LNCaP prostate tumour cell line. In this tumour cell line, the androgen receptor has a point mutation in the steroid-binding domain. This defect does not prevent compounds such as cyproterone acetate, nilutamide and hydroxyflutamide from binding to the receptor, but the resulting receptor complex acts as if an androgen were bound and stimulates growth of the cell line: it does not prevent androgen-induced growth. Bicalutamide, however, remains a pure antiandrogen, and so inhibits growth response to the synthetic androgen R1181. Evidence that withdrawal responses to flutamide are not infrequent is now available;[49,50] there is also evidence of withdrawal responses with chlormadinone acetate, DES and megestrol acetate.[51] While such tumours might actually be stimulated by flutamide if they arise from cell clones that contain a mutated androgen receptor, they would still be responsive to bicalutamide. Tumours with this mutation have been found clinically,[52] and the presence of such mutated androgen receptors has been linked to flutamide withdrawal response.[53] However, the position may not be so simple, since some withdrawal responses

have also been observed with bicalutamide.[54,55]

The Shionogi S115 mouse mammary tumour cell line contains androgen receptors, and its growth can be stimulated by androgens.[56] Short-term androgen withdrawal results in a change from fibroblastic to epithelial morphology, a reduction in proliferation rate, an increase in density regulation, and the loss of ability to grow in suspension culture.[56] Long-term growth of these cells in the absence of androgen also results in an ordered, reproducible series of phenotypic changes, culminating in loss of both cellular and gene-sensitive markers responsive to androgen. Darbre and King[57] have described the effects of bicalutamide on this cell line. Bicalutamide (10^{-6} M) inhibited cell growth stimulation by testosterone (10^{-8} M) in monolayer cultures, and was particularly effective against testosterone (10^{-9} M). Similarly, bicalutamide at 10^{-6} M inhibited the growth of suspension culture of SC-115 cells in the presence of testosterone (10^{-9} M). Bicalutamide had no agonist activity at 10^{-6} M, since it failed to promote growth in either monolayer or suspension culture and the cells had an epithelial appearance. Moreover, bicalutamide had no stimulatory effect on mouse mammary tumour virus RNA production, whereas androgen did cause such a stimulation. Again, Luo and co-workers[45] found bicalutamide to have lower potency than reported by Darbre and King.[57]

Anti-tumour activity in animals

In immature castrated rats treated daily with testosterone propionate (0.2 mg/kg), bicalutamide produced a profound inhibition of androgen-stimulated accessory sex organ growth and was more potent than flutamide.[58] Dose–response studies show that bicalutamide produces a significant inhibition of testosterone propionate-induced accessory sex organ growth at oral doses down to 0.25 mg/kg. These findings were supported by studies in castrated immature male rats given a higher dose of testosterone propionate (0.8 or 1 mg/kg), where bicalutamide was more potent than flutamide, cyproterone acetate and WIN 49,596, a new steroidal antiandrogen.[58] However, studies by

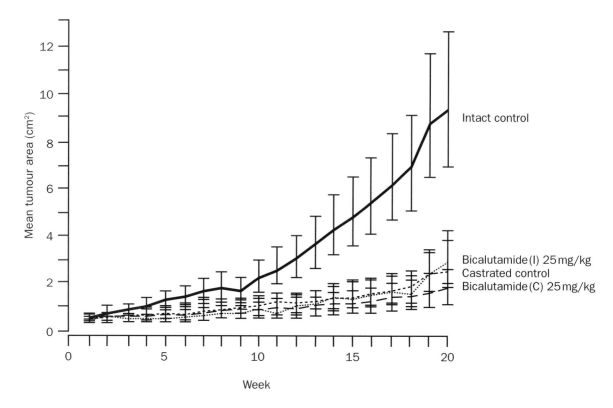

Figure 15.1.2 Effect of a daily oral dose of 25 mg bicalutamide/kg on the growth of Dunning prostate tumours: I = intact; C = castrated. (Reproduced from Furr et al,[40] with permission from the Society for Endocrinology)

Luo and co-workers[45] are again at variance, and show flutamide to be more potent than bicalutamide. A comparison of the oral activity of bicalutamide and flutamide in mature male rats dosed over 14 days showed that both drugs caused dose-related reductions in accessory sex organ weights, but that bicalutamide was around five times more potent than flutamide. Moreover, bicalutamide did not cause a significant elevation in either LH or testosterone at any dose. In contrast, flutamide caused dose-related increases in both serum LH and testosterone. These results have been confirmed and extended by a report from Snyder et al[4] and three studies by Nieschlag's group,[59–61] but yet again are at variance with the results of Luo et al.[45]

Studies in rats bearing the Dunning R3327H prostate tumour show that bicalutamide causes a significant inhibition of tumour growth, and at an oral daily dose of 25 mg/kg is as effective as surgical castration (Figure 15.1.2). There was no significant difference in tumour growth rate in castrated rats and in castrated rats given bicalutamide, indicating again that bicalutamide has no agonist properties.

It can be concluded that the majority of the independent published work confirms the view that bicalutamide is a potent antiandrogen that is peripherally selective in animals. In contrast, flutamide has lower potency and no peripheral selectivity in rats. The exceptional report[45] that shows flutamide to be more potent than bicalutamide has been comprehensively criticized.[46]

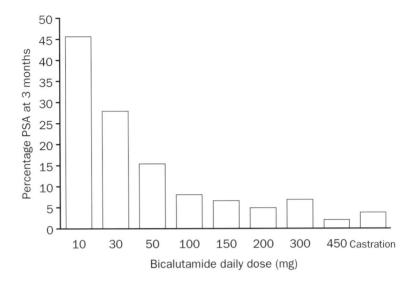

Figure 15.1.3 Effect of bicalutamide on PSA levels in prostate cancer patients in comparison with the pretreatment level. (Reproduced from Kaisary[68], with permission from Karger, Basel)

Preclinical safety, pharmacology and toxicology

In all studies, bicalutamide was well tolerated. It showed no significant effects in any safety pharmacology tests, except in dogs, where, on chronic administration, it caused a small increase in heart rate and a reduction in P–R interval at doses more than 25 times the ED50 value for prostate atrophy. Since there was neither impairment of cardiac function nor pathological findings when cardiac histology was examined in chronic toxicity studies, it is concluded that this idiosyncratic finding is of no toxicological consequence. This conclusion is supported by clinical observations, which fail to demonstrate any effect of bicalutamide on cardiac function.

In toxicity studies in rats, benign adenomas of the Leydig cells and thyroid were found, as well as some liver tumours.[62] Leydig cell hyperplasia and adenomas are common features following alteration of the endocrine milieu in rats, but are of no relevance to human exposure to the drug. This is consistent with a lack of Leydig cell hyperplasia or adenomas in testes from patients treated with bicalutamide.[63] The liver and thyroid tumours are related, and are considered to be due to the mixed-function oxidase-inducing properties of bicalutamide in the rat. It is well recognized that agents that induce mixed-function oxidases in the rat can lead to liver and thyroid tumours, but that this is of no relevance to humans.[64,65]

Clinical studies
Monotherapy
Studies in which bicalutamide was used as monotherapy at a dose of 50 mg versus castration in newly diagnosed metastatic prostate cancer showed that, although effective, it is inferior to castration in terms of time to treatment failure and time to progression.[66] Favourable results on the efficacy of bicalutamide were demonstrated at a dose of 150 mg.[67] This prompted investigation of a higher dose of bicalutamide for its potential use as monotherapy. Preliminary data demonstrate a very satisfactory response with regard to PSA levels after 12 weeks of therapy (Figure 15.1.3).

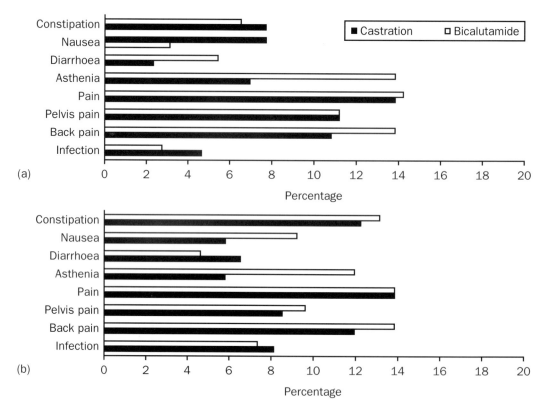

Figure 15.1.4 Adverse effects of bicalutamide 50 mg (a) and 150 mg (b) compared with castration. (Reproduced from Kaisary[68], with permission from Karger, Basel)

There is a continuing trial designed as a randomized ascending-dose study focusing primarily on tolerability, pharmacokinetics and decrease in PSA levels as a surrogate of activity. Reductions in PSA for doses of 450 mg and 600 mg are at least as great as those seen with castration.[69]

Combination therapy

The efficacy and tolerability of bicalutamide combined with an LHRH analogue (LHRH-a) have been compared with flutamide combined with an LHRH-a in a multicentre, randomized trial in 813 patients with metastatic prostate cancer.[70] The final results of this trial, at a median follow-up of 160 weeks, showed trends in both time to progression and survival that favoured the bicalutamide plus LHRH-a group, although the difference between groups for either endpoint was not statistically significant. The hazard ratio for time to progression for bicalutamide plus LHRH-a to flutamide plus LHRH-a was 0.93 (95% confidence interval (CI) = 0.79–1.10; $p = 0.41$) and that for survival was 0.87 (95% CI = 0.72–1.05; $p = 15$), thus indicating that patients in the bicalutamide group had a 13% lower risk of dying. The more favourable tolerability profile for bicalutamide was unchanged from the profile previously reported.[70]

Side-effects

Bicalutamide was well tolerated. Adverse events reported in bicalutamide clinical trials were acceptable to a majority of patients. The incidence of adverse events reported during bicalutamide monotherapy both at 50 mg and at 150 mg daily are shown in Figure 15.1.4.

DISCUSSION

Testosterone, a steroid hormone produced by Leydig cells in testicular tissue, represents the majority of circulating androgen. It passes through the prostate cell membrane, and is converted in the cytoplasm to dihydrotestosterone (DHT) through the activity of the enzyme 5-α-reductase. DHT is believed to be the primary intracellular messenger responsible for stimulating gene expression after it binds to the intracellular androgen receptor. The affinity of DHT for the androgen receptor is about seven times higher than that of testosterone. Adrenal androgens, which include androstenedione and dihydroepiandrosterone, are produced in the zona fasciculata and reticularis in the adrenal cortex. Without androgen receptor binding, androgens cannot exert their biological effects. Accordingly, androgen deprivation can be achieved in several ways, including castration (surgical or medical), androgen blockade at the target cells or 5-α-reductase inhibition. These have been applied individually or in various combinations.

Combined androgen blockade

Although castration is acknowledged as the gold standard for endocrine treatment of prostate cancer, relapse eventually occurs. It has been established that the concentration of DHT remains high within the prostate tissue after castration. Huggins and Scott[71] attempted to control this residual androgen by a combination of orchidectomy and adrenalectomy. Investigations of other means to control adrenal androgen stimulating effects were initially reported by Bracci and Di Silverio[72] and by Labrie et al.[73]

Widespread and enthusiastic evaluation of this therapeutic approach (Table 15.1.1) led to, and still causes, controversy concerning its value. In 1997, the results of a randomized multicentre open-label trial in 813 patients comparing bicalutamide with flutamide, both in combination with an LHRH agonist, showed that bicalutamide was superior to flutamide in time to progression (hazard ratio (HR) = 0.93;

Table 15.1.1 Combination therapies
Surgical castration and antiandrogens:
orchidectomy + nilutamide
orchidectomy + flutamide
orchidectomy + cyproterone acetate
orchidectomy + bicalutamide
Medical castration and antiandrogens:
leuprolide + flutamide
goserelin + flutamide
buserelin + cyproterone acetate
goserelin + bicalutamide
Oestrogens + antiandrogens

$p = 0.41$; median times 97 versus 77 weeks) and survival (HR = 0.87; $p = 0.15$; median times 180 versus 148 weeks).[70] Examination of the hazard ratio for survival, its confidence limits and p-value indicates that there is a 9.25% (non-significant) chance that bicalutamide plus an LHRH analogue confers a death risk that is lower to some extent than that for flutamide plus an LHRH analogue (Data on File, Zeneca Pharmaceuticals). Bicalutamide was also better tolerated, particularly in relation to the incidence of diarrhoea.[70] In 1998, further analysis of the trial by Sarosdy and co-workers[74] showed that, among the four combined androgen blockade (CAB) regimens, leuprolide plus flutamide appeared the least effective for overall survival (Figure 15.1.5). However, these results should be interpreted with caution, since the analyses performed were exploratory. Questions still remain with regard to possible differences between various pure antiandrogens.

A combination of a non-steroidal antiandrogen and a 5-α-reductase inhibitor could be an option in men who want their potency preserved.[75,76] Combination therapy with an antiandrogen and an LHRH analogue would be an option for men in whom potency is not a concern.

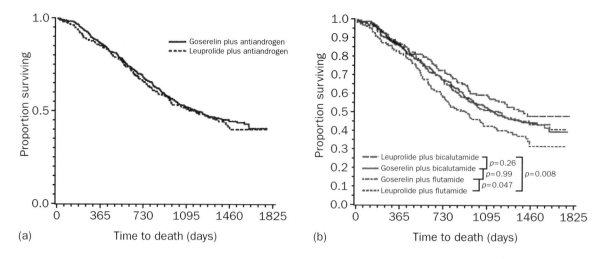

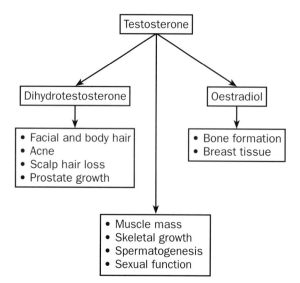

Figure 15.1.5 (a) Comparison of goserelin and leuprolide in combined androgen blockade (CAB) for advanced prostate cancer: Kaplan–Meier probability of overall survival. (b) Kaplan–Meier probability of overall survival in four CAB groups. (Reproduced from Sardosy et al[74], with permission from Elsevier Science)

Figure 15.1.6 Effects of testosterone and its metabolites in men.

Antiandrogens as monotherapy

With increasing awareness of prostate cancer and advances in its early detection, quality of life in patients treated with androgen ablation has become a prominent topic. Antiandrogens used as monotherapy would have an effect on prostate growth, since they interfere with the formation of the DHT–intracellular receptor complex. However, they could spare the effects of testosterone on sexual function and possibly skeletal mineralization and musculature (Figure 15.1.6), leading to an improved sense of well-being. Bicalutamide 150 mg monotherapy was compared by Iversen et al[77] with castration in a total of 480 patients with previously untreated non-metastatic prostate cancer. At a median follow-up of four years, there was a similar survival outcome, with significant benefits with respect to sexual interest and physical capacity. Bicalutamide 150 mg monotherapy was prospectively compared with castration in the management of 1453 patients with confirmed metastatic disease (M1) or T3/T4 non-metastatic disease with elevated PSA values. Bicalutamide 150 mg was less effective than castration with regard to survival (the difference in median time to death was 42 days). However, bicalutamide 150 mg monotherapy showed a benefit in terms of quality of life, subjective response and an acceptable tolerability

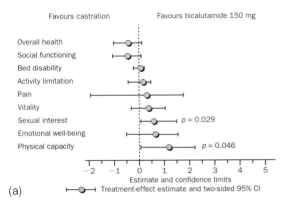

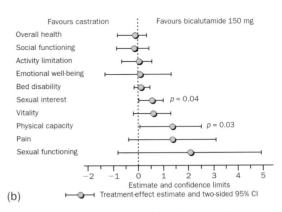

Figure 15.1.7 Analysis of quality of life at 12 months in prostate cancer patients receiving bicalutamide 150 mg: combined treatment-effect estimates and two-sided confidence intervals (CI). (a) M0 patients.[77] (b) M1 patients.[78] (Reproduced from Iversen et al[77], with permission from Elsevier Science; and Tyrrell et al,[78] with permission from Karger, Basel)

profile (Figure 15.1.7). This is an option for patients in whom castration (surgical or medical) is not acceptable or indicated.[78] The impact, particularly on sexual function, is emphasized in the report by Helgason et al,[79] who pointed out that some patients with prostate cancer are willing to abstain from treatment that may result in loss of sexual function.

CONCLUSIONS

Prostate cancer is an androgen-dependent carcinoma with a possible long latent period prior to

diagnosis and a prolonged course in those responding to androgen ablation therapy. Antiandrogens provide a therapy that has great potential in terms of patient compliance and quality of life. In addition, such therapy is an important part of the combined androgen blockade therapy approach.

The preclinical and clinical properties of bicalutamide (Casodex) give it advantages from the viewpoint of tolerability, potency and maintenance of effective antiandrogen serum concentrations. Its potential role in early prostate cancer and in long-term chemoprevention is yet to be determined.

REFERENCES

1. Huggins C, Hodges CV, Studies on prostatic cancer: (I) The effect of estrogen and of androgen injection on serum phosphates in metastatic carcinoma of the prostate. *Cancer Res* 1941; **1**: 293–7.

2. Huggins C, Stevens RE, Hodges CV, Studies on prostatic cancer: (II) The effects of castration on advanced carcinoma of the prostate gland. *Arch Surg* 1941; **43**: 209.

3. Kaisary AV, Tyrrell CJ, Peeling WB, Griffiths K. Comparison of LHRH analogue (Zoladex) with orchidectomy in patients with metastatic prostatic carcinoma. *Br J Urol* 1993; **67**: 502–8 [Erratum: 1993; **71**: 632].

4. Snyder BW, Winneker RC, Batzold FJ, Endocrine profile of WIN 49,596 in the rat: a novel androgen receptor antagonist. *J Ster Biochem* 1989; **33**: 1127–32.

5. Juniewicz RE, McCarthy M, Lemp BM et al, The effect of the steroidal androgen receptor antagonist, WIN 49,596, on the prostate and testis of Beagle dogs. *Endocrinology* 1990; **126**: 2625–34.

6. Winneker RC, Wagner MM, Batzold FH, Studies on the mechanism of action of WIN 49,596: a steroidal androgen receptor antagonist. *J Ster Biochem* 1989; **33**: 1133–8.

7. Neumann F, Jacobi GH, Androgens in tumour therapy. *Clin Oncol* 1982; **1:** 41–65.

8. Paisey RB, Kadow C, Bolton C et al, Effects of cyproterone acetate and a long acting LHRH analogue on serum lipoproteins in patients with carcinoma of the prostate. *J R Soc Med* 1986; **79:** 210–11.

9. Seed M, Godsland IF, Wynn V et al, The effects of cyproterone acetate and ethinyl estradiol on carbohydrate metabolism. *Clin Endocrinol* 1984; **21:** 689–99.

10. Harris AL, Cantwell BMJ, Side effects of endocrine therapies used to treat breast and prostate cancer. *Clin Oncol* 1985; **4:** 511–33.

11. Darkos PE, Gez E, Catane R, Hepatitis due to cyproterone acetate. *Eur J Cancer* 1992; **150:** 908–13.

12. Ohri SK, Gaer JAR, Keane PP, Hepatocellular carcinoma and treatment with cyproterone acetate. *Br J Urol* 1991; **67:** 213–21.

13. Watanabe S, Yamasaki S, Tanae A, Three cases of hepatocellular carcinoma among cyproterone users. *Lancet* 1994; **334:** 1567–8.

14. Committee on the Safety of Medicines, Hepatic reactions with cyproterone acetate ('Cyprostat' 'androcur'). Dose-related serious hepatic toxicity may occur with prolonged use. *Curr Problems Pharmacovigilance* 1995; **21:** 1.

15. Neumann F, Pharmacology and clinical uses of cyproterone acetate. In: *Pharmacology and Clinical Uses of Inhibitors of Hormone Secretion and Action* (Furr BJA, Wakeling AE, eds). Baillière Tindall: Eastbourne, 1987: 132–59.

16. Shida K, Takai S, Tsuji J et al, Clinical evaluation of chlormadinone acetate for prostatic carcinoma. *Hinyokika Kiyo* 1980; **26:** 1553–74.

17. Robustelli della Cuna G, *Comprehensive Guide to the Therapeutic use of Medroxyprogesterone Acetate in Oncology*. Farmitalia Carlo Erba Monograph: Milan, 1987.

18. Robustelli della Cuna G, et al. In: *The Role of Medroxyprogesterone Acetate in the Management of Endocrine Related Tumours* (Temongkol P, Somboonchareon S, eds). Farmitalia Carlo Erba, Thailand Branch: Bangkok, 1986.

19. Geller J, Albert JD, Nachtsehem DA, Loza D, Comparison of prostatic cancer tissue dihydrotestosterone levels at the time of relapse following orchidectomy or estrogen therapy. *J Urol* 1984; **132:** 693–700.

20. Delaere KPJ, Van Thillo EL, Flutamide monotherapy as primary treatment in advanced prostatic carcinoma. *Semin Oncol* 1991; **18**(5): 13–18.

21. Brufsky A, Fontaine-Rothe P, Berlane K et al, Finasteride and flutamide as potency-sparing androgen-ablative therapy for advanced adenocarcinoma of the prostate. *Urology* 1997; **49:** 913–20.

22. McFarlane JR, Tolly DA, Flutamide therapy for advanced prostate cancer: a phase II study. *Br J Urol* 1985; **57:** 172–4.

23. Crawford ED, Eisenberger MA, McLeod DG et al, A controlled trial of leuprolide with and without flutamide in prostatic carcinoma. *N Engl J Med* 1989; **321:** 419–24.

24. DeKernion JN, Murphy GP, Priore R, Comparison of flutamide and Emcyt in hormone-refractory metastatic prostatic cancer. *Urology* 1988; **31:** 312–17.

25. Radwanski E, Perentesis G, Symchowicz S, Zampaglione N, Single and multiple dose pharamacokinetic evaluation of flutamide in normal and geriatric volunteers. *J Clin Pharmacol* 1989; **29:** 554–8.

26. Jacobo E, Schmidt JD, Weinstein SH, Flocks RH, Comparison of flutamide and diethylstilbesterol in untreated advanced prostatic cancer. *Urology* 1976; **8:** 231–3.

27. Lund F, Rasmussen F, Flutamide versus stilbesterol in the management of advanced prostatic cancer. A controlled prospective study. *Br J Urol* 1988; **61:** 140–2.

28. Chang A, Yeap B, Davis T et al, Double-blind randomised study of primary hormonal treatment of stage D2 prostate carcinoma: flutamide versus diethylstilbesterol. *J Clin Oncol* 1996; **14:** 2250–7.

29. Boccon-Gibod L, Fournier G, Battet P et al, Flutamide versus orchidectomy in patients with metastatic prostate carcinoma. In: *Proceedings of the 11th Congress of the European Association of Urology, 1994, Berlin:* Abstract 25.

30. Boccon-Gibod L, Fournier G, Bottet P et al, Flutamide versus orchidectomy in the treatment of metastatic prostate carcinoma. *Eur Urol* 1997; **32:** 391–5.

31. Studer UE, Flutamide versus orchidectomy in the treatment of metastatic prostate carcinoma. *Eur Urol* 1997; **32:** 395–6.

32. Lundgen R, Flutamide as primary treatment for metastatic prostatic cancer. *Br J Urol* 1987; **59:** 156–8.

33. Schröder FH, Pure antiandrogens as monotherapy in prospective studies in prostatic carcinoma. In: *Treatment of Prostatic Cancer: Facts and Controversies.* EORTC, Genito-Urinary Group

Monograph 8. Wiley–Liss: New York, 1990: 93–103.

34. Tremblay D, Dupont A, Meyer BJ, Pottier J, The kinetics of antiandrogens in humans. In: *Prostate Cancer: Research into Endocrine Treatment and Histopathology* (Murphy GP, Khoury S, Kuss R et al, eds). Alan R Liss: New York, 1979: 345–50.

35. Janknegt RA, Abbou C, Bartoletti R et al, Orchidectomy and nilutamide or placebo as treatment of metastatic prostatic cancer in a multinational double-blind randomized trial. *J Urol* 1993; **149:** 77–83.

36. Ojasoo J, Nilutamide. *Drugs of the Future* 1987; **12:** 763–70.

37. Decensi AU, Boccardo F, Guarneri D et al, Monotherapy with nilutamide, a pure non-steroidal antiandrogen, in untreated patients with metastatic carcinoma of the prostate. *J Urol* 1991; **146:** 377–81.

38. Dijkman GA, Jankegt RA, De Reijki TM, Debruyne FMJ, for the International Anandron Study Group, Long term efficacy and safety of nilutamide plus castration in advanced prostate cancer and the significance of early prostate specific antigen normalisation. *J Urol* 1997; **158:** 160–3.

39. Kaisary AV, Compliance with hormonal treatment for prostate cancer. *Br J Hosp Med* 1996; **55:** 359–66.

40. Furr BJA, Valcaccia B, Curry B et al, ICI 176,334: a novel non steroidal peripherally selective antiandrogen. *J Endocrinol* 1987; **113:** R7–9.

41. Ayub M, Levell MJ, The effect of ketoconazole, related imidazole drugs and antiandrogens on (^{3}H) R1881 binding to the prostatic androgen receptor and (^{3}H) 5 alpha-dihydrotestosterone and (^{3}H) cortisol binding to plasma proteins. *J Ster Biochem* 1989; **33:** 251–5.

42. Veldscholte J, Berrevoets CA, Ris-Stalpers C et al, The androgen receptor in LNCaP cells contains a mutation in the ligand binding domain which affects steroid binding characteristics and response to antiandrogens. *J Ster Biochem* 1992; **41:** 665–9.

43. Teutsch G, Goubet F, Battmann J et al, Nonsteroidal antiandrogens: synthesis and biological profile of high affinity ligands for the androgen receptor. *J Ster Biochem* 1991; **48:** 111–19.

44. Kemppainen JA, Wilson EM, Agonist and antagonist activities of hydroxyflutamide and Casodex related to androgen receptor stabilisation. *Urology* 1996; **48:** 157–63.

45. Luo S, Martel C, Le Blanc G et al, Relative potencies of flutamide and Casodex: preclinical studies. *Endocr Rel Cancer* 1996; **3:** 229–41.

46. Furr BJA, Relative potencies of flutamide and Casodex. Preclinical studies by Luo et al. *Endocr Rel Cancer* 1997; **4:** 197–202.

47. Freeman SN, Studies on the mechanism of action of a novel, non steroidal antiandrogen, ICI 176,334. PhD Thesis, University of Leeds, 1988: 109–115.

48. Veldscholte J, Berrevoets CA, Brinkmann AO et al, Antiandrogens and the mutated androgen receptor of LNCaP cells: differential effects on binding affinity, heat-shock protein interaction and transcription activation. *Biochemistry* 1992; **31:** 2393–9.

49. Kelly WK, Scher H, Prostatic specific antigen decline after antiandrogen withdrawal: the flutamide withdrawal syndrome. *J Urol* 1993; **149:** 607–9.

50. Dupont A, Gomez JL, Cusan L et al, Response to flutamide withdrawal in advanced prostate cancer in progression under combination therapy. *J Urol* 1993; **150:** 908–13.

51. Kelly K, Endocrine withdrawal syndrome and its relevance to the management of hormone refractory prostate cancer. *Eur Urol* 1998; **34**(Suppl 3): 19–23.

52. Bentel JM, Tilley WD, Androgen receptors in prostate cancer. *J Endocrinol* 1996; **151:** 1–11.

53. Suzuki H, Akakura K, Komiya A et al, Codon 877 mutation in the androgen receptor gene in advanced prostate cancer: relation to antiandrogen withdrawal syndrome. *Prostate* 1996; **29:** 153–8.

54. Small E, Carroll PR, Prostate specific antigen decline after Casodex withdrawal: evidence for an antiandrogen withdrawal syndrome. *Urology* 1994; **43:** 408–10.

55. Nieh P, Withdrawal phenomenon with the antiandrogen Casodex. *J Urol* 1995; **153:** 1070–2.

56. Darbre PD, King JB, Steroid hormone regulation of cultured breast cancer cells. In: *Breast Cancer and Molecular Biology* (Lippman ME, Dickson R, eds). Kluwer Academic: Boston, 1988: 307–41.

57. Darbre PD, King RJB, Antiandrogen ICI 176,334 does not prevent development of androgen insensitivity in S115 mouse mammary tumour cells. *J Ster Biochem* 1990; **36:** 385–9.

58. Furr BJA, Casodex: preclinical studies. In: *Antiandrogens in Prostate Cancer* (Denis L, ed). European School of Oncology Monograph. Springer-Verlag: Berlin, 1996: 75–88.

59. Chandolia RK, Weinbauer GF, Behre HM, Neischlag EL, Evaluation of a peripherally selective antiandrogen (Casodex) as a tool for studying the relationship between testosterone and spermatogenesis in the rat. *J Ster Biochem* 1991; **38**: 367–75.

60. Chandolia RK, Weinbauer GF, Simoni M et al, Comparative effects of chronic administration of the non-steroidal antiandrogens flutamide and Casodex on the reproductive system of the adult male rat. *Acta Endocrinol* 1991; **125**: 547–55.

61. Simoni M, Weinbauer GF, Chandolia RK, Nieschlag E, Microheterogeneity of pituitary follicle-stimulating hormone in male rats: differential effects of the chronic androgen deprivation induced by castration or androgen blockade. *J Mol Endocrinol* 1992; **9**: 175–82.

62. Eri LM, Eri KJ, Tveter K, A prospective placebo controlled study of the antiandrogen Casodex as treatment for patients with benign prostatic hyperplasia. *J Urol* 1993; **150**: 90–4.

63. Jones HB, Betton GR, Bowdler AL et al, Pathological and morphometric assessment of testicular parameters in patients with metastatic prostate cancer following treatment with either the antiandrogen Casodex (ZM176,334) or bilateral orchidectomy. *Urol Res* 1994; **22**: 191–5.

64. McClain RM, The significance of hepatic microsomal enzyme induction and altered thyroid function in rats: implications for thyroid neoplasia. *Toxicol Pathol* 1989; **17**: 294–306.

65. McClain RM, Mouse liver tumours and microsomal enzyme-inducing drugs: experimental and clinical perspectives with phenobarbital. In: *Mouse Liver Carcinogenesis: Mechanisms and Species Comparisons* (Stevenson DE, McLain RM, Popp JA et al, eds). Alan R Liss: New York, 1990: 345–65.

66. Iversen P, Update of monotherapy trials with the new antiandrogen, Casodex (ICI 176,334). *Eur Urol* 1994; **26**(Suppl 1): 5–9.

67. Tyrrell CJ, Kaisary AV, Iversen P et al, A randomised comparison of Casodex (bicalutamide) 150 mg monotherapy versus castration in the treatment of metastatic and locally advanced prostate cancer. *Eur Urol* 1995; **28**: 215–22.

68. Kaisary AV, Antiandrogen monotherapy in the management of advanced prostate cancer. *Eur Urol* 1997; **31**(Suppl 2): 14–19.

69. Blackledge GRP, Monotherapy with antiandrogens. In: *New Perspectives in Prostate Cancer* (Belldegrun A, Kirby RS, Oliver T, eds). Isis Medical Media: Oxford, 1998: 245–53.

70. Schellhammer PF, Sharifi R, Block NL et al, Clinical benefits of bicalutamide compared with flutamide in combined androgen blockade for patients with advanced prostatic carcinoma: final report of a double-blind, randomised, multicenter trial. *Urology* 1997; **50**: 330–6.

71. Huggins C, Scott WW, Bilateral adrenalectomy in prostatic cancer; clinical features and urinary excretion of 17-ketosteroids and estrogen. *Ann Surg* 1945; **122**: 1031–41.

72. Di Silverio F, Role of cyproterone acetate in urology. In: *International Symposium on Androgens and Antiandrogens* (Martini L, Matta M, eds). Raven Press: New York, 1977.

73. Labrie F, Dupont A, Belanger A et al, Combination therapy with flutamide and castration (LHRH agonist or orchidectomy) in advanced prostate cancer: a marked improvement in response and survival. *J Ster Biochem* 1985; **23**: 833–42.

74. Sardosy MF, Schellhammer PF, Sharifi R et al, Comparison of goserelin and leuprolide in combined androgen blockade therapy. *Urology* 1998; **52**: 82–8.

75. Catalona WJ, Management of cancer of the prostate. *N Engl J Med* 1994; **331**: 996–1004.

76. Fleshner NE, Trachtenberg J, Combination finasteride and flutamide in advanced carcinoma of the prostate: effective therapy with minimal side effects. *J Urol* 1995; **154**: 1642–6.

77. Iversen P, Tyrrell CJ, Kaisary AV et al, Casodex (bicalutamide) 150 mg monotherapy compared with castration in patients with previously untreated non metastatic prostate cancer: results from two multicentre randomised trials at a median follow up of 4 years. *Urology* 1998; **51**: 389–96.

78. Tyrrell CJ, Kaisary AV, Iversen P et al, A randomised comparison of Casodex (bicalutamide) 150 mg monotherapy versus castration in the treatment of metastatic and locally advanced prostate cancer. *Eur Urol* 1998; **33**: 447–56.

79. Helgason AR, Adolfsson J, Dickman P et al, Waning sexual function – the most important disease specific stress for patients with prostate cancer. *Br J Cancer* 1996; **73**: 1417–21.

15.2

Testicular androgen ablation

Saad Khoury

CONTENTS • **Surgical castration** • **Oestrogen therapy** • **LHRH analogues**

The landmark observations of Huggins and Hodges in 1941 about the efficacy of androgen-ablative or -suppressive therapy in the treatment of metastatic prostate cancer established 'androgen deprivation' as the mainstay of treatment for advanced prostatic carcinoma.[1,2] Indeed, about 70% of patients so treated will show beneficial responses of an objective and subjective nature, including:

- a decrease in the size of primary and metastatic tumours;
- reduction in the levels of serum prostatic acid phosphatase (PAP) and prostate-specific antigen (PSA);
- decrease in bladder outlet and ureteric obstruction;
- a partial reversal of myeloplastic anaemia;
- relief of bone pain;
- an improvement in appetite along with a general sense of well-being.

This approach was based on the logical hypothesis that prostate cancer cells retained some of the characteristics of non-transformed prostatic epithelium and would therefore undergo atrophy after androgen deprivation.

The duration of this response ranges from a few months to several years, with most patients succumbing to the uncontrolled growth of androgen-independent disease (stage D3 – see Appendix on page 357) within 6–18 months.

Hormone treatment used in clinical practice aims either to ablate the androgens in the host or to block their action on the androgen receptors in the tumour. The current procedures of androgen withdrawal are:

- bilateral orchidectomy;
- oestrogens;
- luteinizing hormone-releasing hormone (LHRH) agonists.

These are discussed in more detail in the next chapter.

Methods of androgen withdrawal include surgical castration, oestrogen therapy and LHRH analogues.

SURGICAL CASTRATION

Hormonal consequences

Ninety per cent of circulating testosterone is derived from the testes; bilateral castration decreases the plasma testosterone level from 500 ng/100 ml to about 50 ng/100 ml in the great majority of cases (Figure 15.2.1). The fall of testosterone to castration level is very quick and ranges from 3 to 12 hours (mean: 8.6 hours). The biological half-life of testosterone is 30–60 min (mean: 45 min). This is much quicker than the time needed for oral oestrogens or the use of LHRH analogues. It should be noted that, after castration, there was

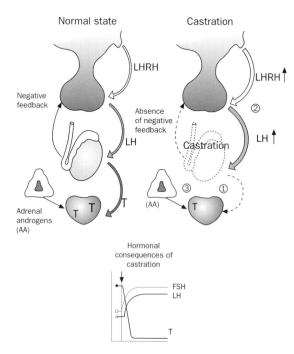

Figure 15.2.1 Castration induces suppression of testicular testosterone (95% of plasma testosterone or T). This results in a reactive rise in LHRH and LH. The 5% of circulating testosterone which persists is derived from the adrenal glands.

only a 75% reduction in the dihydrotestosterone (DHT) level present in prostate tissue, despite the finding that there was a more than 90% reduction in circulation testosterone level in the plasma after castration. This raises the key issue of whether the 25% residual DHT after castration provides a sufficient stimulus to growth of residual prostate tumour cells.

Androgen ablation by bilateral orchidectomy has long been considered the gold standard against which other forms of treatment for the management of advanced prostate cancer can be evaluated.

Orchidectomy has much to offer the patient when cost, ease of the procedure, compliance and immediate decrease of circulating testosterone are considered. Subcapsular orchidectomy is occasionally used, in which the tunica albuginea and epididymis of each testis are left intact.[3] This procedure has been criticized

because of the possibility of leaving functional testicular tissue behind. By the use of sophisticated hormone assays, it has been shown that the risk is negligible when this technique is used carefully.[4]

Castration is the procedure of choice for the uraemic patient who has ureteric obstruction secondary to prostate cancer. This procedure, if done as an emergency, could be an alternative to percutaneous nephrostomies and other procedures aiming at relief of obstruction.

Technique

Total castration

General, or preferably local, anaesthesia can be used.[4,5] Bilateral castration is generally performed via two inguinal incisions or a horizontal infrapubic incision. Testicular prostheses may be inserted at the end of the operation when desired by the patient.

Subcapsular orchidectomy

Subcapsular orchidectomy consists of removing the secretory pulp of the testis, while leaving the albuginea, which is closed.

Extra-epididymal castration

This operation achieves the same cosmetic effect as subcapsular orchidectomy and would appear to be preferable, because it avoids the risk of leaving behind a few islands of Leydig cells.

Results

Castration gives results equivalent to those of oestrogen without the disadvantages of metabolic and cardiovascular complications and feminization.

Complications

Aside from the negative psychological impact on the patient, castration has some direct side-effects.

Impotence

As with oestrogens, impotence is constant after surgical castration.

Hot flushes

Hot flushes (Figure 15.2.2) are the most frequently reported side-effects, apart from impotence. On average, more than 60% of these patients have hot flushes.[6–8] Of patients 48% still had hot flushes 5 years after treatment.

From previous studies it is known that half of these patients experience a great deal of inconvenience from the hot flushes or are greatly distressed.[9] Patients experience a sensation of warmth, spreading from the chest to the rest of the body, followed by an outbreak of sweat mostly on the forehead, chest and back.[10] Hot flushes sometimes occur several times an hour, and often at night.[11,12] Incidence, symptoms and aetiology are quite similar to the hot flushes experienced by menopausal women or women after an ovariectomy. There are numerous implications for the patient's quality of life,[13,14] for example, hot flushes and sweating during the night might cause sleep deprivation. Symptoms observed, such as nervousness, easy

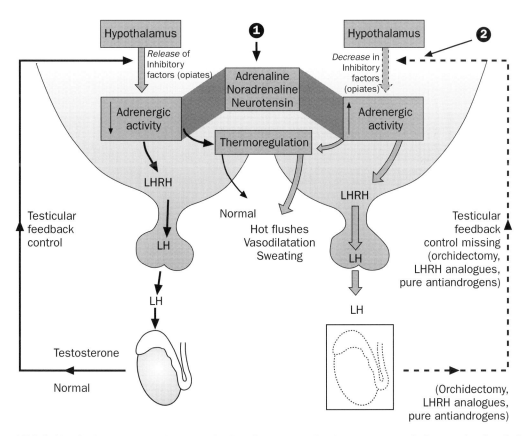

Figure 15.2.2 Hot flushes are somehow attached to the neuroendocrine counterregulation mechanism induced by low levels of the sex steroids. High hypothalamic concentrations of noradrenaline are believed to be the reason for hot flushes. Noradrenaline is the neurotransmitter for LHRH and is therefore involved in the central counterregulatory process. Thus, prevention of hot flushes is possible with substances that (1) block noradrenaline centrally (e.g. clonidine) or (2) reinstate the release of inhibitory opiates (e.g. androgens, oestrogens and progestogens).

fatiguability, depression or inability to concentrate, are considered to result from sleep deprivation after night sweats.[14] Hot flushes and outbreak of sweat could be reduced by half over a 6-month observation period using cyproterone acetate (CPA).[15]

Low-dose diethylstilboestrol 1–3 mg daily in selected patients can give the same results.

Bone mineral density
In the orchidectomized patient, bone mineral density and bone mineral content decrease significantly after treatment. This osteoporosis is of osteoplastic origin.

Prognosis

After an orchidectomy, minimum PSA values are an excellent prognostic factor with significant predictive value. In a study of 50 patients with extracapsular prostate cancer (58% stage C, 42% stage D), PSA measurement and clinical assessment were continued at 3-monthly intervals until there was evidence of clinical progression. Serum PSA level decreased in all patients to a minimum after 3–6 months. There was a statistically significant difference in the probability of disease progression for minimum PSA values at 1 ng/ml and 10 ng/ml. Of the 13 patients in group 1 (with minimum PSA values < 1 ng/ml), 11 stayed in remission during a mean follow-up duration of 45.9 months. Of 25 patients in group 2 (with minimum PSA values between 1 and 10 ng/ml), 19 developed progression after a mean remission period of 16.7 months, whereas all 12 patients in group 3 (with minimum PSA values > 10 ng/ml) progressed after a mean remission period of 12.5 months. This raises the question of whether an adjuvant treatment should be given as early as possible for group 2 and 3 patients. Group 3 patients, with their high probability of early progression, can also form a group suitable for studies of new therapeutic modalities.

The mean volume reduction of the prostate at 3 months after start of treatment was also studied. Patients in whom the volume of the prostate had regressed 50% or more at 3 months had a better prognosis compared with those who had a smaller volume reduction.

OESTROGEN THERAPY

Mechanism of action

Although the principal mechanism of action of diethylstilboestrol (DES) appears to be exercised indirectly by decreasing testicular testosterone secretion and by pituitary suppression of LH secretion, evidence also exists for a direct action of DES on both the prostate and testis. Moreover, DES increases the circulating levels of sex hormone-binding globulin (SHBG), thereby indirectly decreasing the plasma free testosterone fraction. At high doses, DES can decrease DNA synthesis (Figure 15.2.3).

Diethylstilboestrol and prostatic cancer

Clinical results
Diethylstilboestrol was the most widely used reference oestrogen for the treatment of prostatic cancer. This synthetic oestrogen is the least expensive and most effective of the oestrogens used. DES, at the dose of 3 mg/day, appears to be effective, but is less so at 1 mg/day. A dose of 5 mg, or the administration of very high doses (>100 mg), does not appear to be any more effective than 3 mg/day.

The Veterans Administration studies (VACURG) provided a most instructive contribution to our understanding of endocrine treatment in prostatic cancer.

First VACURG study[16]
The first study, which started in 1960, was directed to patients with stage A and B cancer randomized to receive either radical prostatectomy with placebo or radical prostatectomy with DES 5 mg/day.

Patients with stage C and D disease were randomized to receive placebo, DES 5 mg/day, castration with placebo or castration with DES 5 mg/day.

The results of this first study showed that the

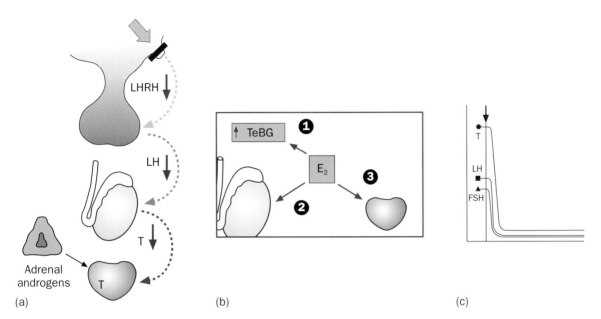

Figure 15.2.3 (a) The principal mechanism of action of oestrogens is central: they block LHRH secretion by the hypothalamus, which results in inhibition of LH secretion by the pituitary and testosterone secretion by the testis. (b) They also have a peripheral action: increase TeBG, thereby decreasing the plasma free testosterone (T), by decreasing testosterone secretion via a direct action on the testis, and antiandrogenic action on the prostate. (c) Hormonal consequences of oestrogen therapy. E_2, oestradiol; TeBG, testosterone-binding globulin.

overall survival was less favourable in stage A patients who received 5 mg DES, but no significant difference was observed in stage B patients. The survival was also less favourable in stage C patients who received castration together with 5 mg DES, in comparison with those who received placebo alone, or castration with placebo. No significant differences were observed among the various treatment schedules for stage D patients.

The study of the survival curves, taking into account cause of death, showed that stage C and D patients who received 5 mg DES, in comparison with the placebo group, had a significantly higher mortality from cardiovascular complications (most of the deaths occurred during the first year) and a lower death rate from prostatic cancer.

These results were most surprising. At the time, oestrogens were thought to have a favourable effect on cardiovascular disease, as reflected in the fact that randomized clinical studies were then being conducted to evaluate oestrogen treatment as a means of preventing the progression of cardiovascular disease.

The first VACURG study revealed another surprise: the overall survival of the patients treated with placebo was equivalent to that of the patients receiving endocrine therapy. In reality, this conclusion was biased, as most of the patients with stage C cancer (70%), and all of the patients with stage D cancer initially treated with placebo, subsequently received endocrine therapy when disease progression made this treatment necessary. The definitive results were still tabulated, however, in the form of initial randomization, i.e. placebo. For this reason, the VACURG results did not show that placebo was equivalent to endocrine therapy in terms of overall survival, but that deferred endocrine therapy was as effective as early endocrine therapy initiated at the time of diagnosis.

Second VACURG study[17]

The second VACURG study started in 1967 and was designed to demonstrate: (1) that in patients with stage A and B cancer, radical prostatectomy could offer an advantage in terms of survival over placebo alone; and (2) that low doses of DES were more effective than doses of 5 mg, in controlling progression of prostatic cancer without inducing cardiovascular complications.

Patients with stage C and D disease were randomized to receive placebo or DES 0.2 mg/day, 1 mg/day or 5 mg/day. In patients with stage C and D disease, the dose of 1 mg DES was as effective as the dose of 5 mg, and significantly more effective than the 0.2 mg dose or placebo, in the prevention of death from prostatic cancer with no concomitant association with an increased frequency of cardiovascular mortality.

Third VACURG study[18]

A third study, started by VACURG in 1969, compared the efficacy of oestrogens other than DES, or of certain progestins administered orally, with that of DES 1 mg/day. Patients were randomized to receive DES 1 mg/day, medroxyprogesterone acetate 30 mg/day, premarin 1.25 mg for one month, followed by 2.5 mg/day and medroxyprogesterone acetate 30 mg with DES 1 mg/day. The results did not reveal any significant advantage in terms of overall survival, or cancer death, for these therapeutic protocols when compared with DES 1 mg/day.

Discussion

Although the VACURG studies profoundly influenced our ideas about endocrine therapy in prostatic cancer, they nevertheless gave rise to certain invalid interpretations of the results. An erroneous conclusion was based on the concept that oestrogens were more effective than castration in the reduction of mortality from prostatic cancer – this resulted from poor interpretation of the first study in which the patients treated with oestrogens had the lowest cancer mortality rate. In fact, as the patients treated with oestrogens had an excessive cardiovascular mortality, essentially occurring during the first year of treatment, it is probable that many of these patients would have died from cancer if they had not died from cardiovascular causes during the first year of endocrine therapy. In a study by Nesbit and Baum in 1950,[19] the 5-year survival rate of patients with stage D cancer was 10% for those receiving DES 1–5 mg, 22% for those treated with castration alone and 20% for those treated by the two modalities. This suggests that castration is the most effective form and that the administration of DES 1–5 mg to castrated patients did not improve survival. Overall, adequate oestrogen therapy, or castration, appears to provide equivalent results and there is little to be gained from combining the two modalities. Castration is preferred because it is a more reliable, although more radical, method ensuring adequate suppression of plasma testosterone, avoiding the problems of patient compliance reported in several papers.

Complications of DES

Although widely used in the treatment of metastatic prostatic cancer, the clinical value of DES has been a controversial subject over recent years since the VACURG group drew attention to the cardiovascular complications, particularly thromboembolic, that can cancel out the benefit obtained by this treatment of the cancer itself. Hypertensive crises and salt and water retention were also reported.

The thromboembolic cardiovascular complications associated with oestrogen therapy for prostatic cancer are related to fluid retention, alteration of plasma antithrombin III levels, increased platelet aggregation and changes in plasma lipids. Antithrombin III is an α_2-globulin produced by the liver which seems to be the most important physiological inhibitor of coagulation. Some studies have shown that the administration of oestrogen decreases the levels of antithrombin III to zones of hypercoagulability. Patients undergoing castration have normal antithrombin III levels. DES 15 mg/day markedly decreases levels of antithrombin III in the plasma, while patients receiving DES

1 mg/day have normal antithrombin III levels. The increased platelet aggregation can be largely prevented by the use of aspirin.

Other side-effects of administration of DES, such as feminization, decreased libido, impotence, azoospermia, gastrointestinal disturbances, nausea and vomiting, have also been reported. However, these side-effects are dose dependent and are minimal with a DES dose of 1 mg/day, but this low dose does not completely suppress testicular activity and the plasma testosterone concentration may rise to above castrate levels at certain times during the day.

Oestrogens other than DES

Oestrogens other than DES have been used for the treatment of disseminated prostatic cancer but none can be considered to have achieved universal acceptance. The long-acting poly-oestradiol phosphate (Estradurin) is popular in Scandinavia. It is injected intramuscularly (80–160 mg/month), and weakly suppresses luteinizing hormone (LH) secretion. Premarin 2.5 mg three times daily, a mixture of conjugated equine oestrogens and ethinyloestradiol-17β 0.15–1.0 mg/day are generally considered to be less effective and more expensive than DES.

LHRH ANALOGUES

Structure of naturally occurring LHRH

In 1971, Schally and co-workers isolated and described the molecular structure of naturally occurring LHRH and later synthesized this

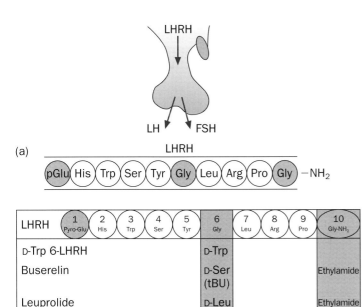

(a)

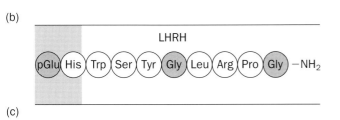

(c)

Figure 15.2.4 (a) Structure of LHRH: LHRH has an identical structure in all mammals; it is a decapeptide formed by a chain of 10 amino acids which forms a C-shaped configuration in aqueous solution. (b) LHRH analogues: LHRH agonists have a very similar structure to natural LHRH. Structural modifications are required in order to increase the lifespan of the compound and to increase its affinity for the receptor, therefore resulting in more potent peptides with a longer duration of action. (c) LHRH antagonists: modifications of the first amino acids (principally replacement of histidine in position 2) induces an antagonist activity. The molecules bind to LHRH receptors and block them without exerting any biological activity.

hormone.[20] LHRH is a linear decapeptide (Figure 15.2.4); substitutions of amino acids at different positions lead to the production of several polypeptides, some with *agonist* and some with *antagonist* abilities. Therapy at the present time is only with agonists. The synthetic analogues of this decapeptide are approximately 100 times more potent than their naturally occurring counterparts.

Mechanism of action (Figures 15.2.5 and 15.2.6)

The agonists cause an abrupt increase in LH release and subsequent testosterone release in the male after acute administration (termed the flare period); paradoxically, during chronic administration, testosterone falls to the castrate level. The exact mechanism of this action is not

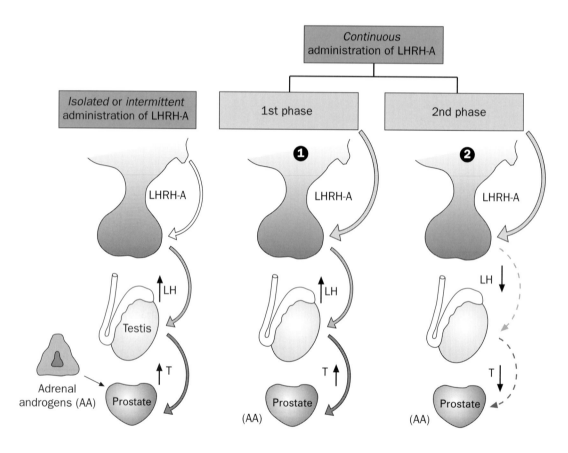

Figure 15.2.5 Isolated or intermittent administration of LHRH analogues, as under physiological conditions, induces an increased secretion of LH and testosterone. A biphasic phenomenon occurs during continuous administration: initially, there is a rise in LH and testosterone (T) (flare-up), as in (1), followed, several days later, by a fall in LH and testosterone levels which reach castration levels after 3–4 weeks (2). LHRH analogues do not affect the adrenal secretion of testosterone (T).

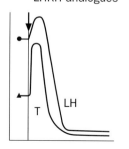

Hormonal consequences of *prolonged administration* of LHRH analogues

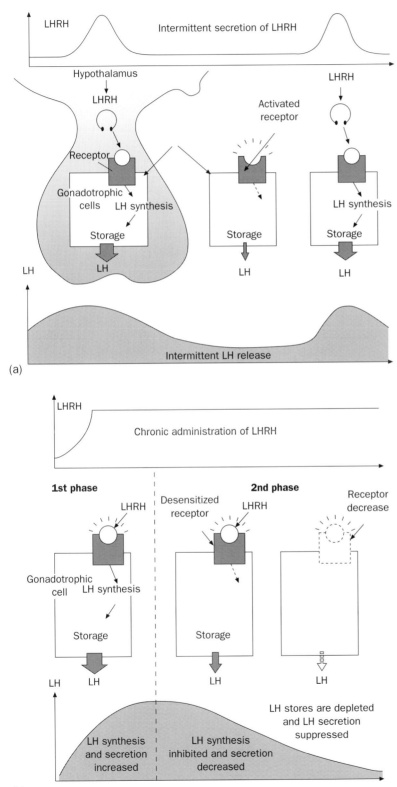

Figure 15.2.6 (a) Physiological action: LHRH is secreted by the hypothalamus and is released directly into the capillaries, reaching the anterior, pituitary via the hypothalamo-hypophyseal portal system to act directly on the gonadotrophic cells of the anterior hypophysis. LHRH binds specifically to membrane receptors situated on the surface of pituitary gonadotrophic cells. The binding of LHRH to its receptor triggers the secretion of LH and FSH. LHRH receptors only retain their activity while they are intermittently occupied, which is normally the case, because LHRH is secreted according to a pulsatile mode and has a short half-life. (b) Continuous administration: when the receptors are continuously occupied by LHRH perfusion or by an agonist, however, the hypophyseal gonadotroph receptors become desensitized resulting in inhibition of gonadotrophin secretion 10–15 days later. This results in a marked fall in LH and follicle-stimulating hormone (FSH) secretion. Furthermore, the number of LHRH receptors decreases secondarily during 'desensitization'. This phenomenon is the basis for the clinical use of LHRH agonists.

clear, and could involve alterations in the central feedback control of LH release and desensitization of the hypophysis to LHRH action.

Clinical studies

Numerous randomized comparative studies[21,22] of LHRH agonists with orchidectomy or oestrogens confirmed that there was no statistically significant difference between LHRH analogue therapy and either orchidectomy or oestrogens, with regard to objective response rate and time to first evidence of progression and actuarial survival. However, there were fewer serious cardiovascular complications and incidents of gynaecomastia with the LHRH analogue-treated group than in the oestrogen-treated group.

In the LHRH analogue groups, the reported side-effects have been mainly those expected from testosterone suppression, such as hot flushes, loss of libido and impotence. Some increase in bone pain in patients with bone metastases has been observed; this is thought to result from the initial rise in serum testosterone, although the incidence has been low (about 5%) and tended to resolve spontaneously.

As a result of the possibility of inducing spinal cord injury during the flare period in those patients with vertebral metastases, several strategies, such as initial use of antiandrogens or oestrogens, were devised to reduce the effect of this period. Despite these manoeuvres, use of LHRH analogues in patients with any form of neurological deficit suggesting tumour compression is clearly unwarranted.

Many other studies using the various agents confirmed these results and demonstrated that these agents are capable of sustaining their physiological effects on androgen production for periods longer than 2 years.[9]

The LHRH analogues goserelin, leuprolide, triptorelin and buserelin are registered in many countries for the treatment of the prostate and gastrointestinal tract; therefore other routes of administration need to be used to establish sustained plasma concentrations.

Injections, which have to be given daily, and nasal sprays, which must be taken several times a day, are less convenient and reliable than longer-acting depot preparations. Some of these analogues – goserelin, leuprolide and triptorelin – are available in such depot formulations for administration every 4 weeks. Serum testosterone concentrations are suppressed to the castrate range by 3–4 weeks after the initial administration, and remain suppressed, provided that the drugs are given on a monthly basis. Many trials have now demonstrated that this mode of administration reduces and maintains serum testosterone at the castrate level for a period of at least 7 months. Similarly several clinical trials demonstrated this agent to be as effective as either orchidectomy or DES in maintaining remission in a patient with advanced prostate cancer.[9]

All of the currently available LHRH analogues appear clinically equivalent. Efforts have now been directed at extending the duration of action of these agents: 3-month sustained-release preparations are now available.

Cost-effectiveness

Several studies have raised the issue of surgical castration in comparison to medical castration by LHRH analogues.

A recent study has compared the costs of leuprolide therapy and orchidectomy.[23] The results showed that the charges incurred by leuprolide-treated patients and by surgically-treated patients were equal by 9 months. However, by 20 months, the charges incurred by leuprolide-treated patients were twice those incurred by patients who had undergone orchidectomy. The true hospital costs of treatment followed the same trend, with leuprolide therapy being twice as expensive as surgical treatment by 15 months. For the average case with stage D2 prostate cancer, the charges for leuprolide therapy were 63% more than those for orchidectomy.

It was concluded that, although the initial high cost of orchidectomy means that leuprolide therapy is less expensive for the first 9 months, the costs of the two treatments then become equal, after which continued care becomes more expensive for leuprolide-treated patients. With an average life expectancy of 3 years for a patient with newly diagnosed stage D2 prostate cancer, the costs incurred for leuprolide therapy would be estimated at more than twice those for orchidectomy. LHRH analogues have a financial advantage only in patients with an expected survival of less than 9 months – for patients with a life expectancy greater than this, orchidectomy is the most cost-effective treatment option.

The most cost-effective androgen-with-drawal strategy would be initial treatment with an LHRH analogue followed by deferred orchidectomy after about 1 year among good responders. This policy would obviate the need for surgery in about half of the patients without substantial increase in costs compared with that of a policy of primary orchidectomy in all patients.

In conclusion, surgical orchidectomy remains the gold standard and also the cheapest. This alternative should be presented to the patient when discussing treatment modalities.

REFERENCES

1. Huggins C, Stevens RE, Hodges CV, Studies on prostatic cancer. II. The effects of castration on advanced carcinoma of the prostate gland. *Arch Surg* 1941; **43:** 209–23.
2. Huggins C, Scott WW, Hodges CV, Studies on prostatic cancer. III. The effects of fever of des-oxycorticosterone and of oestrogen on clinical patients with metastatic carcinoma of the prostate. *J Urol* 1941; 1946: 997–1006.
3. Glenn JF, Subepididymal orchiectomy: the acceptable alternative. *J Urol* 1990; **144:** 942–4.
4. Albert DD, Current status of subcapsular orchiectomy. *J Urol* 1982; **128:** 155.
5. Kaye DW, Infrapubic operations: vasovasostomy and bilateral orchiectomy. In: *Outpatient Urologic Surgery*. Lea and Febiger: Philadelphia, 1985: 217
6. Casper RF, Yen SC, Neuroendocrinology of menopausal flushes: an hypothesis of flush mechanism. *Clin Endocrinol* 1985; **22:** 293–312.
7. Charig CR, Rundle JS, Fluhing: Long term side-effect of orchidectomy in the treatment of carci-noma of the prostate. *J Urol* 1988; **139:** 478A.
8. Clayden JR, Bell WJ, Pollard P, Menopausal flushing: double blind trial of a non hormonal medication. *Br Med J* 1974; **i:** 409–12.
9. Crawford ED, Eisenberger MA, McLeod DG et al, A controlled trial of leuprolide with and without flutamide in prostatic carcinoma: data from an EORTC 30853 trial. *Semin Urol* 1990; **viii:** 166–74.
10. Eaton AC, McGuire N, Cyproterone acetate in treat-ment of post-orchidectomy hot flushes. Double-blind cross-over trial. *Lancet* 1983; **ii:** 1336–7.
11. Feldman JM, Postlethwaite RW, Glen LF, Hot flushes and sweats in men with testicular insuffi-ciency. *Arch Intern Med* 1976; **136:** 606–8.
12. Frodin Th, Alund G, Varenhorst F, Measurement of skin blood-flow and water evaporation as a means of objectively assessing hot flushes after orchidectomy in patients with prostate cancer. *Prostate* 1985; **7:** 203–308.
13. Ginsberg J, O'Reilly B, Climacteric flushing in a man. *Br Med J* 1983; **287:** 262.
14. Huggins C, Stevens RE, Hodges CV, Studies on prostatic cancer. II. The effects of castration on advanced carcinoma of the prostate gland. *Arch Surg* 1941; **43:** 209–23.
15. Jansen JE, Hendriksen ON, CPA in behanding of postorkiectomi-flushing. *Ugeskr laeger* 1989; **151:** 560–1.
16. Veterans Administration Co-operative Urological Research Group, Treatment and survival of patients with cancer of the prostate. *Surg Gynecol Obstet* 1967: **124:** 1011–17.
17. Ballar JC, Byar DP, The Veterans Administration Co-operative Urological Research Group. Estrogen treatment for cancer of the prostate: early results with 3 doses of diethylstilbestrol and placebo. *Cancer* 1970; **26:** 257–61.
18. Byar DP, VACURG, Studies on prostatic cancer and its treatment. In: *Urological Pathology: The prostate* (Tannenbaum M, ed.). Lea and Febiger: New York, 1977: 241–67.
19. Nesbit RM, Baum WC, Endocrine control of pro-static carcinoma: Clinical and statistical survey of 1818 cases. *J Am Med Assoc* 1950; **143:** 1317–20.
20. Schally AV, Arimurea A, Baba Y et al, Isolation of properties of the FSH and LH-releasing hormone. *Biochem Biophys Res Commun* 1971; **43:** 393–9.

21. Leuprolide Study Group, Leuprolide versus diethylstilbestrol. *N Engl J Med* 1986; **311:** 1251–6.

22. Turkes AO, Puelling WB, Griffith H, Treatment of patients with advanced cancer of the prostate: phase III trial. Zoladex against castration: a study of the British Prostate Group. *J Steroid Biochem* 1987; **27:** 543–9.

23. Bonzani RA, Stricker HJ, Peabody JO, Menon M, Cost comparison of orchiectomy and leuprolide in metastatic prostate cancer. *J Urol* 1998; **160:** 2446–9

15.3

Combined androgen blockade

Juan Stenner, E David Crawford

CONTENTS • **Physiologic background** • **Combination therapies** • **Side-effects of combined androgen blockade** • **Costs** • **Antiandrogen withdrawal syndrome** • **Summary** • **Future directions**

More than half a century ago, hormone manipulation was instituted as the cornerstone treatment for advanced prostate cancer,[1] and it continues to be the mainstay of therapy for this disease.[2–4] Although the concepts of advanced disease and androgen ablation have changed over this time, the knowledge of tumor biology and the availability of newer methods of hormonal ablation places the treating physician in a challenging decision-making process. Issues such as patient preference, quality of life, and survival benefit have taken center stage.[5,6]

Currently, over 50% of patients diagnosed with prostate cancer are found to have advanced disease.[7–9] All of them may be amenable to hormone manipulation. It is important to define advanced prostate cancer not only in those patients with infiltrated lymph nodes (D1) and soft tissue or bony metastasis (D2), but also in those whose prostate-specific antigen (PSA) levels rise after radical therapy (e.g. surgery, brachytherapy, radiotherapy) (D1.5), and in those with high serum PSA levels or persistently elevated serum acid phosphatase levels without objective evidence of metastasis (D0) (Table 15.3.1; see also Appendix, page 357). Since patients

with prostate cancer are now being detected early in the course of their disease,[4] an intrastage migration is observed.[10,11] With the use of diagnostic tools such as transrectal ultrasound (TRUS) and serum PSA measurement, fewer patients present initially with widespread painful osseous metastasis; more frequently, they present with minimal skeletal metastatic deposits.[2]

Table 15.3.1 Stage D prostate cancer	
D1	Pelvic lymph nodes
D1.5	Rising PSA after failed local therapy
D2	Metastatic disease in bone and/or other organs
D2.5	Rising PSA after nadir level
D3	Hormone-refractory prostate cancer
D3S	Hormonally sensitive
D3I	Hormonally insensitive

PSA, prostate-specific antigen.

Combined androgen blockade (CAB) is directed at removing all available androgens, including those produced by the testis, and other androgens produced by the adrenals. After the establishment of androgen dependence of prostate cancer by Huggins and Hodges in 1941,[1] and the observation that all patients eventually fail orchiectomy, Huggins and Scott[12] attempted total androgen ablation by performing both orchiectomy and adrenalectomy. Due to the lack of appropriate steroid replacement, this treatment had catastrophic results. Hypophysectomy was no more successful for total androgen deprivation.[13] These surgical approaches were soon abandoned. Estrogens became the medical alternative to surgical castration, and the introduction of newer drugs, such as aminoglutethimide, ketoconazole, and spironolactone, offered a pharmacologic method of adrenal androgen blockade. Knowledge that the concentration of dihydrotestosterone (DHT) remained high (up to 40%) within the prostate tissue after castration, and the fact that all the patients inevitably escaped this type of hormone manipulation and died, led to the investigation of other means of controlling the stimulus of androgens produced in other parts of the body. An initial report by Labrie et al[14] on the clinical use of CAB with a luteinizing-hormone-releasing hormone (LHRH) agonist plus flutamide created the enthusiasm for studying and, later, for the widespread use of this alternative therapy.

Although somewhat controversial, many papers have addressed the value of CAB.[15] The clinical evidence has shown that there may not only be a symptomatic benefit to combination therapy, but also a survival benefit. Others have failed to show a survival advantage, but have confirmed the symptomatic benefit.[4] Many of the trials that failed to show a therapeutic advantage were either of a small sample size and thus had only a low power to detect any differences of clinical or statistical significance,[16] or involved a follow-up period that was too short to observe any differences. Meta-analysis has not been useful to confirm or refute the therapeutic benefit of CAB[15] because of the different characteristics of the clinical trials included. Current analysis of the data supports the use of CAB, particularly as antiandrogen monotherapy has been shown to be neither equivalent nor superior to CAB, and as surgical or medical castration alone is equal or inferior to the combination therapies.

This chapter discusses the physiologic background that sets the foundation and rationale for the use of CAB, the different alternative therapies, the side-effects (including the flare phenomenon), the antiandrogen withdrawal syndrome, and the optimal timing for the initiation of treatment. Finally, the conclusions provide some insight into possible future directions for this treatment modality.

PHYSIOLOGIC BACKGROUND

Three major endocrinologic axes are known to affect the growth of normal, benign, and neoplastic prostate tissue:[13] the hypothalamic–pituitary-testis axis, the hypothalamic–pituitary–adrenal axis, and the secondary hypothalamic-pituitary–testis/adrenal axis. Each axis acts independently of and in concert with the others to create the hormonal milieu needed within prostate tissue for its normal function. Aside from this most important hormonal control of the prostate, the paracrine, autocrine, and intracrine effects of locally produced factors also regulate the rate of cell reproduction and death.[17,18] Some, if not all, of the factors involved in the hormonal escape during androgen blockade in the treatment of this neoplasia are thought to involve these latter systems.

LHRH, also known as gonadotropin-releasing hormone (GnRH), is produced in the hypothalamic parts of the brain and, following release into the pituitary portal blood vessels, acts on the pituitary gland to stimulate the secretion of luteinizing hormone (LH) and follicle-stimulating hormone (FSH). LHRH thereby regulates, indirectly at least, the functions of both the ovaries and the testes and their steroid secretions.[19] LH is secreted in a pulse-like fashion, and these pulses are stimulated by a corresponding episode of LHRH secretion from the hypothalamus. The secretion of LHRH and LH are driven by a free-running LHRH pulse generator, which is controlled by the negative feedback of gonadal hormones.[20,21] Neither LHRH nor LH has any role in the regulation of LHRH pulsatility, thereby excluding both short- and ultrashort-loop feedback. The effect of LHRH and LHRH agonists is through binding to a specific receptor on the cell membrane of the target organ.[22] When the hormone (or agonist) binds to the receptor, it initiates a cascade of events that includes microaggregation of the hormone–receptor complex, internalization, release of second messengers, mobilization of calcium, and exocytosis.[23] LHRH also stimulates the synthesis of its own receptors, second messengers, and gonadotropin subunits.[24] Gonadectomy results in an increase in LHRH receptors at the pituitary level. Continuous exposure of the pituitary gland to LHRH or its agonists results, after an initial stimulation, in a loss of responsiveness and virtual abolition of LH secretion (downregulation or desensitization).[25]

Testosterone, mainly produced by the Leydig cells in the testis, is controlled by a direct action of LH. This gonadotropin interacts directly with its own specific high-affinity receptors, which are located only on the Leydig cells. Testosterone regulates the secretion of LH and its own rate of synthesis by a negative-feedback mechanism.

Androgens function on target cells by binding to an intracellular component: the androgen receptor. This moiety binds to specific sequences of DNA on those genes regulated by androgens and modulates the rate of specific gene transcription.[26] The ultimate effect is seen in the regulation of the development, growth, and function of prostate tissue. Although testosterone is the most abundant steroid circulating in the bloodstream, DHT is the most potent androgen. DHT has the highest affinity for the androgen receptor and the majority of the androgen-mediated activity is due to this hormone. Testosterone binds to the androgen receptor with a much lower affinity.[27]

Adrenal androgens comprise a significant fraction of the steroid output of the human adrenal glands. Dehydroepiandrosterone (DHEA), dehydroepiandrosterone sulfate (DHEA-S) and androstenedione (4-dione) are weak or inactive androgen precursors that in peripheral tissue (including the prostate) are converted into testosterone and DHT.[28] Adrenocorticotropic hormone (ACTH), produced by the pituitary gland, is generally accepted as a regulating or permissive factor for adrenal androgen secretion.[29] Many other factors influence the secretion of these adrenal steroids.[13] Although there is a wide variation in the normal circulating concentration of adrenal androgens, the adult plasma levels of DHEA-S are 100–500 times higher than those of testosterone,[30] thus providing high levels of substrate required for its conversion into androgens in the peripheral tissue.

Data for the role of adrenal androgens in the growth of prostate tissue come from two sources. First, levels of DHT in prostate tissue after castration remain high (25–40% of baseline levels).[30–32] Secondly, serum levels of androgen metabolites drop by only 50–70% after removal of all testicular androgens,[33] suggesting an active transformation of adrenal androgens in peripheral tissue. Using the adrenal precursors, the prostate synthesizes its own active androgen (DHT).

There are other secondary factors with variable degrees of action on the physiology of androgen secretion; for example, growth hormone and prolactin are secreted as a result of stimulation by somatostatin, growth hormone-releasing hormone (GHRH), thyrotropin-releasing hormone (TRH), and dopamine.[13]

DHT is synthesized from testosterone by the nuclear-membrane-bound enzyme 5α-reductase in androgen-sensitive and androgen-insensitive tissue. Growth of the normal prostate and proliferation of benign and neoplastic prostatic epithelial and stromal cells require DHT. Type 1 and type 2 isoenzymes and genes have been identified for 5α-reductase.[34] Type 1 is mainly expressed in the skin and in the liver.[35] Immunohistochemical analysis has shown that only the type 2 isoenzyme is expressed in the human prostate.[36] The expression of this enzyme is predominantly in the stromal cells. There appears to be no expression of this enzyme in the epithelial cell. Thus, DHT exerts its effect as a paracrine hormone on the epithelial cells of the prostate. Although skin synthesizes a great amount of DHT through 5α-reductase type 1, it is mainly used in situ. The contribution to prostate growth by DHT produced in the skin remains unknown.

COMBINATION THERAPIES

Since CAB blends many different alternative therapies, the combination of surgical castration and antiandrogens, and of medical castration with antiandrogens will be discussed. Some alternative combinations that aim to reduce costs or side-effects, such as estrogens and antiandrogens, and, although not fully studied, 5α-reductase inhibitors and antiandrogens, will also be addressed. Focus will be on the response rate, time to progression, survival, symptomatic benefit, and the advantages and the disadvantages for each modality of combination therapy compared to the monotherapy employed in each clinical trial.

The standard hormone therapy for advanced disease has been orchiectomy alone, to which all hormone combination therapies are compared. Orchiectomy has a 20–57% rate of disease regression, a median interval to progression of 7.7–18.5 months, and a median overall survival of 16–35.5 months.[37,38] The major drawbacks of surgical castration are, of course, the irreversibility and psychological impairment that it produces in some patients.

Surgical castration and antiandrogens

Orchiectomy and nilutamide
In response to treatment, the combination of orchiectomy and nilutamide[39] facilitates regression and stabilization of the disease for 78% of patients, including subjective and objective responses (64% with placebo). The median interval to objective progression was 20.8 months (14.9 months with placebo). A statistically significant difference in response and progression rate was achieved between this combination therapy and orchiectomy alone.

The median survival time was 27.3 months (24.2 with placebo) and the cancer-specific survival was 37 months (30 months with orchiectomy alone; $p = 0.07$, NS). Compared to monotherapy, the combination showed substantially different pain relief at 1, 3, and 6 months. Quality of life, measured only by the Karnovsky score, was the same for both types of therapy.

Orchiectomy and flutamide
The available data on the combination of orchiectomy and flutamide[40] show a chemical response rate of 81% (measured by PSA) compared with a rate of 61% for orchiectomy alone. The time to progression for patients treated with combination therapy was 21 months. When a subset of good-risk patients was analyzed (i.e. those with good performance status and minimal metastatic skeletal deposits), time to progression was 49 months. Survival for patients treated with orchiectomy plus flutamide was 31 months, while for the subset of good-risk patients it was 52 months. Overall, there was no statistically significant advantage in time to progression or survival of the combination therapy over orchiectomy alone. There were no treatment-related deaths and the incidence of severe toxicity (grade 2/3) was low.

Orchiectomy and cyproterone
No results for the overall effectiveness of the combination of orchiectomy and cyproterone acetate compared with orchiectomy alone have been published. The European Organization for Research and Treatment of Cancer (EORTC) protocol 3085 is the largest clinical trial that has reported some outcome data on the use of this combination. The initial results and a further survival analysis[41–43] have shown that progression and survival rates for the combination arm were no different from monotherapy. There are no data on response rate, median interval to progression, or duration of survival. Likewise, symptom improvement, quality of life, and advantages or disadvantages to the combination of the steroidal antiandrogen cyproterone acetate and orchiectomy are not addressed in those reports.

Orchiectomy and bicalutamide
At this time, no clinical trial has been reported for the combination of bicalutamide (Casodex) and orchiectomy versus orchiectomy as monotherapy.

Conclusions
Overall, the advantages of the combination of surgical castration and antiandrogens are: metastasis-related pain is alleviated more effectively; tumor markers are normalized; the objective response rate is increased; and the time to progression is prolonged. The disadvantages are: the side-effects of adding an antiandrogen: the long-term cost of the drug; and that the combination did not show a survival benefit in all the trials.

Medical castration (LHRH agonists) plus an antiandrogen

Leuprolide and flutamide
The overall response rate for patients treated with the LHRH agonist leuprolide in combination with the antiandrogen flutamide is 43.6% (35.3% for leuprolide and placebo; p = NS).[44] Complete response was achieved in 7.9% of the patients on CAB (7.1% leuprolide alone) and partial response was achieved in 35.7% (28.2% for orchiectomy and placebo). The median progression-free survival time was 16.5 months for the combination and 13.9 months for the patients treated with leuprolide alone (p = 0.039). The median length of survival was 35.5 months in the combination group versus 28.3 months in the leuprolide and placebo group.[44] Differences between the treatment arms in progression-free survival and overall survival were particularly evident for patients with minimal disease and better performance status (0–2). Neither the symptomatic benefit to the patients treated in this trial nor the quality of life was reported. The advantage of the combination therapy was a 26% improvement in the overall survival rate. The disadvantages are mainly the side-effects of the drugs, the cost, and the administration of the LHRH agonist

and dosage regimen for the antiandrogen, but new depot formulations permit longer intervals between LHRH analog administration.

Goserelin and flutamide
The overall, complete, and partial response rates of the combination of the LHRH agonist goserelin and flutamide are 60%.[45] The chemical response rate, as measured by acid phosphatase, is 70%. Orchiectomy alone has a chemical response rate of 57%. A statistically significant difference was seen in the median time to subjective and objective progression. The median time to subjective progression was 21.75 months in patients on combination therapy and 13 months for patients treated with orchiectomy alone. The average time to objective progression was 33.25 months for those patients treated with the LHRH analog and flutamide, while it was only 21.25 months for those treated with orchiectomy alone. The time to first objective or subjective progression was 17.75 months versus 11.5 months (p = 0.002) in favor of the combination treatment. The median duration of survival is 27.1 months on orchiectomy and 34.4 months on CAB. Disease-specific survival for orchiectomy is 28.8 months and for CAB treatment it is 43.9 months (p = 0.007). Patients with less severe disease tend to benefit the most from this combination therapy. Symptomatic control and quality of life was better for this combination therapy, when analyzed by the following subjective parameters: World Health Organization (WHO) performance status, pain score, weight loss, and urologic symptoms. Progression-free intervals (free of symptoms and better quality of life) was also better for the combination therapy: 13 months for the orchiectomy group versus 21 months for CAB. Clearly, the combination of goserelin acetate and flutamide have a response rate, overall median time to progression, symptomatic control, and survival advantage over orchiectomy alone. The disadvantages of this CAB protocol are a higher incidence of side-effects and withdrawal of 7% of the population from treatment because of liver or gastrointestinal toxicity.

LHRH agonist and bicalutamide

At the present time, there are no data related to response rate, time to progression, symptomatic benefit, or survival for the combination of an LHRH agonist plus bicalutamide (Casodex) versus an LHRH agonist alone. A trial comparing this regimen to an LHRH agonist and flutamide[46] showed that the bicalutamide combination is as effective as the flutamide combination, with the advantages of fewer side-effects (diarrhea) and a convenient once-daily dosing.

Buserelin acetate and cyproterone acetate

The combination of buserelin acetate and cyproterone acetate has not been shown to be more efficacious, compared with orchiectomy alone or buserelin plus only 2 weeks of cyproterone acetate, in blocking the flare phenomenon. Although the published results are from a study with a very small sample size and immature data, the use of the steroidal antiandrogen to the LHRH agonist buserelin does not appear to confer any benefit. This form of CAB did not show any difference compared to monotherapy (either buserelin alone or orchiectomy) with respect to response rate, degree of pain relief, time to progression, or duration of survival.[47] The addition of cyproterone acetate has been shown to eliminate the biologic and biochemical signs of exacerbation (the flare phenomenon, discussed later in this chapter) that occur with the use of LHRH analogs.[48]

Estrogens and antiandrogens

Reducing the dose of estrogens and adding an antiandrogen has the theoretical advantages of (1) decreasing the well-known complications of estrogens, (2) blocking the effect of residual circulating androgens, and (3) lowering the cost of combined androgen blockade.[49] No large randomized clinical trial has been conducted to evaluate this alternative. In 1981, Geller[50] proposed this possibility. An analysis of 23 stage D2 patients, treated with the steroidal antiandrogen megestrol acetate and diethylstilbestrol, showed no advantage over either surgical castration or estrogen alone in the median time to progression of disease.[51] The combination of steroidal antiandrogens and low-dose estrogens has proved to be effective in reducing serum testosterone to castration levels.[52] The efficacy and clinical benefit of this combination compared to monotherapy remain to be seen.

Other combinations

LHRH antagonists

The clinical usefulness of LHRH antagonists in the treatment of advanced prostate cancer is beginning to be reported.[53] These new agents seems to be useful as a primary single drug treatment for metastatic prostate cancer. The use of the LHRH antagonists avoids the initial transient stimulation that occurs with the use of LHRH agonists in monotherapy. The use of these novel substances in combination with antiandrogens warrants controlled clinical trials.

Finasteride and flutamide

Finasteride, a 5α-reductase type 2 inhibitor, has been shown to have a direct inhibitory effect on prostate cancer cell lines.[54] In addition, the combination of finasteride and flutamide has been shown to decrease the size of rat ventral prostate.[55] Clinical response in the treatment of advanced prostate cancer with finasteride as monotherapy has not been dramatic.[56] Since the drug only blocks the conversion of testosterone to DHT and does not lower serum levels of testosterone, an escape is seen through the low binding capacity of testosterone to the androgen receptor that continues to stimulate the growth of the tumor. Theoretically, the combination of flutamide and finasteride could have an effective tumor control, while maintaining serum levels of testosterone and decreasing the side-effects of hormone manipulation. A very small, non-randomized, clinical trial of flutamide and finasteride in stage C and D1 sexually active patients showed a chemical response (measured by PSA) and durable response (up to 24 months) rate in 22 of 23 treated patients. Eighty-six percent of the men maintained their sexual function.[57] In an uncontrolled clinical trial with finasteride (5 mg orally, twice daily) and flutamide (125 mg orally, twice daily), we have treated 61 patients who failed to respond to therapy for apparent clinically localized disease, radical prostatectomy, radiation therapy, or cryosurgery as evidenced by rising PSA levels. The chemical response rate was 60%, with undetectable serum PSA levels. With an average of 12 months of follow-up, four patients have failed this treatment method as indicated by continued increase in PSA levels. All five patients who were sexually potent at the start of therapy remained potent (unpublished data). A randomized, controlled, clinical trial with adequate follow-up will show the effectiveness of this combination therapy, which seems to give good tumor control together with preservation of sexual function in patients with low tumor burden (i.e. stage D1.5).

SIDE-EFFECTS OF COMBINED ANDROGEN BLOCKADE

The major side-effects of androgen-deprivation therapy are a result of castration levels of serum testosterone, including loss of libido, psychologic impairment, loss of potency, anemia, malaise, and muscle wasting. The reported incidence of side-effects for each type of combination therapy and for each type of castration is given in Table 15.3.2. The majority of the studies that analyze the clinical efficacy of combined androgen blockade and report the incidence of side-effects do not address the long-term effect of combination therapy. For approximately 40% of patients treated with surgical or medical castration alone, vasomotor symptoms (hot flashes) persist for over 8 years.[58] It is not known if the incidence and degree of anemia, osteoporosis, and pathologic fractures are increased with the use of CAB compared with castration alone.

Aside from the most common side effects shown in Table 15.3.2, a few patients with surgical castration taking the antiandrogen nilutamide had to stop their medication because of

interstitial pneumonitis.[59] With the use of the intranasal administration of buserelin acetate, now rarely used, there is a very low possibility of severe nasal irritation and epistaxis.[47] Buserelin acetate and cyproterone acetate are associated with a 40–45% incidence of hot flashes and 7% of gynecomastia, as well as a very low incidence of angina pectoris, congestive heart failure, and gastrointestinal disturbances.[43,47]

The lethal complications reported with the use of estrogens include myocardial infarction, pulmonary embolism, congestive heart failure, and cerebrovascular accidents. The non-lethal complications include nausea, vomiting, edema, impotence, hot flashes, depression, and gynecomastia. The lethal complications are greatly diminished or eliminated with the use of low doses (diethylstilbestol (DES) 1 mg/day), but the non-lethal complications still occur.[49] With the combination of low-dose cyproterone acetate (50 mg twice daily) and mini-dose DES (0.1 mg daily) orally, used in only 64 patients, breast tenderness was observed in 16%, fatigue in 10%, depression in 3%, jaundice in 2%, hot flashes in 2%, and deep vein thrombosis in 2%.[52]

Although the incidence of side-effects may be high (>60% hot flashes or 13% diarrhea), the majority of the patients do not need to discontinue the medication for these reasons.[44] Only 9% of the patients treated with goserelin acetate and flutamide had their therapy modified because of side-effects, these being mainly gastrointestinal and liver toxicity.[45] Some of the gastrointestinal side-effects resulting from the use of antiandrogens, particularly flutamide, can be overcome by decreasing the dose.

The side-effects of the combination of flutamide and finasteride in the small reported series and in our own experience are loss of libido in 14%, mild diarrhea in 33%, gynecomastia in 19%, breast tenderness and/or enlargement in 63%, and 17% mild gastrointestinal disturbances. However, no patient had to withdraw from the studies due to these side effects.[57,60]

Table 15.3.2 Incidence of side-effects of combined androgen blockade

Side-effect	Surgical castration (%)			Medical castration (%)		
	Alone[39,45,59]	+ Nilutamide[39,59]	+ Flutamide[40]	LHRH-A[44,46]	LHRH-AL + flutamide[44]	LHRH-AG + flutamide[45]
Hot flashes	22–67	28–77	–	58–60.8	63.6	68
Gynecomastia	6–8	4	–	8–12.7	13.3	19
Anemia	7	4	3.0	–	–	–
Increased liver enzymes	3–5	8	1.2	–	–	5–9
Osteoporotic fractures	13.6	–	–	–	–	–
Diarrhea	–	–	3.3	4.9	13.6	–
Visual disturbances	3–14	27–40	–	–	–	–
Nausea/vomiting	6	10–13	–	14.2	11.8	–
Dyspnea	7	6	–	–	–	–
Peripheral edema	–	–	–	4.9	4.9	–

LHRH-A, luteinizing hormone-releasing hormone agonist; LHRH-AL, LHRH combined with leuprolide acetate; LHRH-AG, LHRH combined with goserelin acetate.

The flare phenomenon

The use of LHRH agonists induces an initial LH or gonadotropin hormone release. A subsequent increase in the LH-dependent production of androgens from the testis is observed.[61–63] The rise in serum androgen levels is coupled with an increase in serum levels of alkaline phosphatase and PSA.[63,64] These biochemical manifestations of tumor activity are thought to be due to a temporary rise in testosterone.[65] This can become serious and life-threatening[63,65] in those symptomatic patients who show high tumor burden, neurologic manifestations of spinal cord compression by bony metastases, or uremia from urinary flow obstruction. This entity was recognized early in the use of these agents,[66] and then several reports confirmed the phenomenon.[61–66] Both chemical and clinical disease flare appear in 4–33% of patients treated with LHRH agonists as monotherapy,[65] while less than 10% of the patients have only a clinical disease flare.[65] It became clear that this biologic effect does not generate an acceleration of tumor growth that would impair the beneficial effect of these compounds. Qayum et al[67] showed that another possible explanation for this phenomenon is a direct stimulus by LHRH analogs on cancer cells. Prostate cancer cell lines, as well as benign and malignant tumors, contain high-affinity LHRH receptors.[67–69] Animal studies have shown that the cellular activity of cancer induced by LHRH analogs occurs before the increased production of testosterone, and can continue even in the absence of this and other androgens. An initial, simultaneous administration of either ketoconazole, estrogens, steroidal antiandrogens (cyproterone acetate), or pure antiandrones (flutamide, nilutamide, bicalutamide) prevents the initial and temporary detrimental effect occasionally observed with the use of a LHRH agonist as monotherapy.[65] Early reports using the LHRH antagonists seem to avoid this flare phenomenon.[53]

COSTS

Since all forms of hormone therapy for advanced or metastatic prostate cancer are mostly palliative, not only efficacy but also costs are extremely important. Expenditure for LHRH alone in the treatment of prostate cancer in the USA was calculated to be US$328 million in 1993.[3] Relative charges for a patient on the combination of leuprolide and flutamide are in the order of US$9000 per year, compared to the one-off expenditure of US$3000 for orchiectomy alone.[70] Based on the timing of hormone manipulation, if the clinical trials prove that early is superior to delayed hormone therapy, this issue may become substantial and impose economic burdens for CAB as therapy for prostate cancer. The addition of other drugs to conventional castration, mainly antiandrogens, could have a cost benefit favorable to society, viewed as the cost per life-year gained.[71] The issue of quality-of-life benefit will need to be included in cost–benefit analysis.

ANTIANDROGEN WITHDRAWAL SYNDROME

The antiandrogen withdrawal syndrome (AAWS) is the characteristic biochemical and clinical response observed when the drug is removed from therapy after evidence of disease progression in those patients treated with CAB. It was initially described with the use of flutamide,[72] and has now been observed with other steroidal antiandrogens, pure antiandrogens, progestational agents, and estrogens also.[73] Patients on monotherapy with antiandrogens do not seem to manifest this response. Whether this is a therapeutic advantage of CAB with antiandrogens or a major drawback of these drugs is not known. Some authors have postulated that the AAWS is the factor that causes the difference in survival for the combination groups in CAB trials.[73] However, other interim endpoint results, such as time to progression, are also different. The AAWS does not seem to be the reason for the survival difference, as these other interim results, a reflection of the therapeutic intervention, are usually measured before any maneuver is performed (i.e. antiandrogen withdrawal). Focus on the molecular basis of this response was directed by the findings on the paradoxically stimulatory effect of flutamide on the LNCaP prostate cancer cell line.[74] It has been shown that LNCaP expresses a mutated androgen receptor that is stimulated by the antiandrogen in a dose-dependent fashion. This and other mutations on the androgen receptor have been documented on metastatic and hormonally independent prostate cancer tissue.[74] Castration induces the synthesis of androgen receptors.[27] Amplification of these receptors has been observed in 30% of prostate cancer specimens.[75] An amplified mutated androgen receptor that is stimulated by antiandrogens could explain the response observed from stopping the paradoxically stimulatory effect of these drugs. A greater than 50% decline in PSA from baseline is observed in 28–80% of patients treated with 'antiandrogen withdrawal' after evidence of disease progression. A symptomatic improvement is seen in 25–56% of patients. The median exposure to CAB is 16–96 months, the median time to response is less than 6 weeks, and the median duration of response is 4–14.5 months (range 2–30 months).[73] The patients most likely to respond are those with longer exposure time to the antiandrogen and those with higher serum PSA values.[73,74]

Timing

A great degree of controversy still exists with respect to the issue of when androgen ablation should be initiated, despite the known efficacy of CAB. Symptomatic patients should be treated immediately. The controversy remains for those diagnosed with asymptomatic, advanced disease. Due to the known side-effects of the alternative options and the cost of CAB, the decision is not trivial for many of those men with a good performance status and an active sexual life. With the assumption that tumor-doubling time ranges from days to several months, around 75% of the tumor's life has

elapsed by the time of diagnosis. Thus, the concept of 'early' therapy is really a misnomer, and many of these patients may have a near-lethal tumor burden at the time of presentation.[76] Approximately 10% of patients treated with hormone therapy live for 10 years and may be cured. Theoretically, waiting until the tumor burden is uncontrollable may exclude those patients from this option. Until now, there have been no randomized controlled trials that address this issue, although some inferences could be made from the existing data. Animal studies have demonstrated an inherent survival advantage for those animals receiving early androgen ablation or extirpation of the primary tumor coupled with the prompt initiation of systemic therapy.[77]

The re-evaluation of the survival data in the Veterans Administration Cooperative Urological Research Group (VACURG) study[78] provided new evidence on the issue. From this study, it was concluded that younger patients with high-grade tumors (Gleason score 7–10) and stage D disease appeared to derive a survival benefit from the initiation of hormone therapy at the time of diagnosis. Other retrospective analyses[79,80] have shown that in surgically proven stage D1 patients the progression-free interval is prolonged by early hormone manipulation, and there is also a trend for longer survival. Finally, the NCI trial INT-0036 with LHRH agonist plus flutamide[44] showed a substantial benefit for those patients with good performance status and lower tumor burden treated with CAB at the time of diagnosis, suggesting that the best results are seen in those patients treated early in the course of their disease. On the other hand, patients with advanced prostate cancer may have a long asymptomatic disease period. However, there is no definitive evidence that early hormone therapy prolongs life in all patients. Men die from the androgen-insensitive cell population that is unaffected by hormone manipulation. Aside from the potential side-effects of CAB and its cost, the risk of this early therapy could, theoretically, select the androgen-independent clones of prostate cancer cells and lead the disease into a phase for which there is currently no efficient alternative therapy. More scientific investigation is needed regarding the dynamics of androgen-resistant phenotypic tumors. Nevertheless, physicians and patients must play an active role in the decision-making process, weighing up the risks and benefits of the alternative therapeutic options. Early CAB is the form of treatment that will delay the interval of disease progression, prolong the symptom-free interval, preserve the quality of life, and, eventually, permit the simultaneous use of other systemic therapies at a time at which the tumor burden is more likely to respond.

The concept of intermittent therapy involves the initiation of androgen deprivation and then, following a predefined response, halting the treatment to allow the tumor to repopulate with androgen-sensitive cells. Due to a continuous block of the androgen-dependent growth, some of these tumor cells become hormonally independent. Due to the reversible nature of medical castration, the use of intermittent therapy would allow the tumor cells to escape from this hormone-independent growth. In vitro and animal models of prostate cancer suggest that intermittent androgen suppression delays progression to the androgen-independent state, but does not prevent it.[81] With a highly heterogeneous group of prostate cancer patients, treated with various forms of intermittent combinations of androgen blockade, Goldenberg et al[82] reported that patients, during an off-treatment period, had an improved sense of well-being and near-normal sexual function. For those patients with D2 disease, the mean overall survival was 52 months. Intermittent androgen suppression therapy has the theoretical advantage of reduced toxicity and cost, but the survival advantage remains to be proven in randomized, controlled trials.

SUMMARY

In summary, the changing concept of advanced prostate cancer and the intrastage migration observed has shifted the use of hormone manipulation towards patients with lower tumor burdens. Blocking the production of testicular androgens and the effect of adrenal androgens have been shown to be more effective in controlling symptoms and prolonging the time to progression than castration alone. The treatment of 'purely asymptomatic' patients with CAB remains controversial. The differences between the different trials may be due to the fact that not all combination alternatives are equally effective. From the survival point of view, the addition of flutamide to orchiectomy does not result in a substantial survival advantage. The combination therapy with leuprolide (LHRH agonist) plus flutamide is better than LHRH agonist alone, and the combination therapy with goserelin acetate (LHRH agonist) plus flutamide is better than orchiectomy alone. Survival rates in combined androgen blockade trials with a LHRH agonist plus an antiandrogen (flutamide) is slightly better than orchiectomy plus an antiandrogen. We believe that the difference may be due to a synergistic (additive) effect of an LHRH agonist plus an antiandrogen that is not observed with steroidal antiandrogen (cyproterone acetate) due to a progestation-like activity of this compound. The greatest survival advantage seen with CAB is in those patients with a better prognostic profile, i.e. those with minimal disease or a lower tumor burden and a good performance status. For those patients on CAB with evidence of progressive disease, the antiandrogen should be withdrawn.

From the data presented here, the new gold standard for the treatment of advanced prostate cancer is not total androgen blockade by any means, but rather combined androgen blockade with an LHRH agonist plus an antiandrogen. However, this needs to be substantiated in a large clinical trial. Such a trial would compare orchiectomy with and without an antiandrogen to an LHRH agonist with or without an antiandrogen. The stated treatment confers the best survival advantage with the least side-effects. The clinical and economic consequences of starting patients in either one of these alternative combination therapies should be weighed-up by the physician and discussed with the patient.

FUTURE DIRECTIONS

As the trend in advanced disease shifts toward an earlier diagnosis (as seen with the large screening trials), more patients will be diagnosed with a lower tumor burden and better performance status. Since this population is the most likely to benefit from early CAB, a significant impact on the mortality rate from advanced prostate cancer will be observed in the near future. Research into the biological behavior of this tumor, the molecular causes of the hormonal independence of cancer cells, the interaction of different compounds currently in use, and the novel approaches to hormone manipulation with less secondary effects, linked to a quality-of-life oriented therapy, will open up new avenues in the treatment of patients with advanced prostate cancer.

REFERENCES

1. Huggins C, Hodges CV, Studies on prostatic cancer. The effect of castration, of estrogen and of androgen injection on serum phosphatases in metastatic carcinoma of the prostate. *Cancer Res* 1941; **1:** 293–7.
2. Crawford ED, Changing concepts in the management of advanced prostate cancer. *Urology* 1994; **44:** 67–74.
3. Gee WF, Holtgrewe HL, Albertsen PC et al, Practice trends in the diagnosis and management of prostate cancer in the United States. *J Urol* 1995; **154:** 207–8.
4. Schellhammer PF, Combined androgen blockade for the treatment of metastatic cancer of the prostate. *Urology* 1996; **47:** 622–8.
5. Kornblith AB, Herr HW, Ofman US, Scher HI, Holland JC, Quality of life of patients with prostate cancer and their spouses. The value of a data base in clinical care. *Cancer* 1994; **73:** 2791–800.
6. Cassileth BR, Soloway MS, Vogelzang NJ et al, Patients' choice of treatment in stage D prostate cancer. *Urology* 1989; **33:** 57–62.
7. Catalona WJ, Smith DS, Ratliff TL, Basler JW, Detection of organ-confined prostate cancer is increased through prostate-specific antigen-based screening. *J Am Med Assoc* 1993; **270:** 948–54.
8. Epstein JI, Incidence and significance of positive margins in radical prostatectomy specimens. *Urol Clin North Am* 1996; **23:** 651–63.
9. Kupelian P, Katcher J, Levin H, Zippe C, Klein E, Correlation of clinical and pathologic factors with rising prostate-specific antigen profiles after radical prostatectomy alone for clinically localized prostate cancer. *Urology* 1996; **48:** 249–60.
10. Mettlin CJ, Murphy GP, Ho R, Menck HR, The National Cancer Data Base report on longitudinal observations on prostate cancer. *Cancer* 1996; **77:** 2162–6.
11. Schwartz KL, Severson RK, Gurney JG, Montie JE, Trends in the stage specific incidence of prostate carcinoma in the Detroit metropolitan area, 1973–1994. *Cancer* 1996; **78:** 1260–6.
12. Huggins C, Scott WW, Bilateral adrenalectomy in prostatic cancer; clinical features and urinary excretion of 17-ketosteroids and estrogen. *Ann Surg* 1945; **122:** 1031–41.
13. Daneshgari F, Crawford ED, Endocrine therapy of advanced carcinoma of the prostate. *Cancer* 1993; **71:** 1089–97.
14. Labrie F, Dupont A, Belanger A et al, Combination therapy with flutamide and castration (LHRH agonist or orchiectomy) in advanced prostate cancer: a marked improvement in response and survival. *J Steroid Biochem* 1985; **23:** 833–42.
15. Prostate Cancer Trialists' Collaborative Group, Maximum androgen blockade in advanced prostate cancer: an overview of 22 randomized trials with 3283 deaths in 5710 patients. *Lancet* 1995; **346:** 265–9.
16. Blumenstein BA, Some statistical considerations for the interpretation of trials of combined androgen therapy. *Cancer* 1993; **72**(suppl 12): 3834–46.
17. Donna M, Peehl DM, Cellular biology of prostatic growth factors. *Prostate* 1996; **6**(suppl): 74–8.
18. Culig Z, Hobisch A, Cronauer MV et al, Regulation of prostatic growth and function by peptide growth factors. *Prostate* 1996; **6**(suppl): 392–405.

19. Lincoln DW, Gonadotropin-releasing hormone (GnRH): basic physiology. In: *Endocrinology*, 3rd edn (DeGroot LJ, ed). WB Saunders: Philadelphia, 1995: 218–29.

20. Lincoln DW, Fraser HM, Lincoln GA et al, Hypothalamic pulse generators. *Recent Prog Horm Res* 1985; **41:** 369–419.

21. Wetzel WC, Valenca MM, Merchenthaler I et al, Intrinsic pulsatile secretory activity of immortalized luteinizing-hormone-releasing-hormone-secreting neurons. *Proc Natl Acad Sci USA* 1992; **89:** 4149–53.

22. Moyle WR, Campbell RK, Gonadotropins. In: *Endocrinology*, 3rd edn (DeGroot LJ, ed). WB Saunders: Philadelphia, 1995: 230–41.

23. Crowley WF Jr, Filicori M, Spratt DI, Santoro NF, The physiology of gonadotropin-releasing hormone (GnRH) secretion in men and women. *Recent Prog Horm Res* 1985; **41:** 473–526.

24. Katt JA, Duncan JA, Herbon L et al, The frequency of gonadotropin-releasing hormone stimulation determines the number of pituitary gonadotropin-releasing hormone receptors. *Endocrinology* 1985; **116:** 2113–15.

25. de Koning JA, van Dieten MJ, van Rees GP, Refractoriness of the pituitary gland after continuous exposure to luteinizing hormone releasing hormone. *J Endocrinol* 1978; **790:** 311–18.

26. Kallio PJ, Palvimo JJ, Janne OA, Genetic regulation of androgen action. *Prostate* 1996; **6**(suppl): 45–51.

27. Hiipakka RA, Liao S, Androgen physiology. In: *Endocrinology*, 3rd edn (DeGroot LJ, ed). WB Saunders: Philadelphia, 1995: 2336–47.

28. Lawrence N, Parker DN, Adrenal androgens. In: *Endocrinology*, 3rd edn (DeGroot LJ, ed). WB Saunders: Philadelphia, 1995: 1836–47.

29. Bélanger B, Caron S, Bélanger A, Dupont A, Steroid fatty acid esters in adrenals and plasma: effects of ACTH. *J Endocrinol* 1990; **127:** 505–11.

30. Labrie F, Dupont A, Bélanger A, Complete androgen blockade for the treatment of prostate cancer. In: *Important Advances in Oncology* (de Vita VT, Hellman S, Rosenberg SA, eds). JB Lippincot: Philadelphia, 1985: 193–217.

31. Geller J, Rationale for blockade of adrenal as well as testicular androgens in the treatment of advanced prostate cancer. *Semin Oncol* 1985; **12**(suppl 1): 28–35.

32. Crawford ED, De Antoni EP, Labrie F, Schoder FH, Geller J, Endocrine therapy of prostate cancer: optimal form and appropriate timing. *J Clin Endocrinol Metab* 1995; **80:** 1062–78.

33. Moghissi E, Ablan F, Horton R, Origin of plasma androstanediol glucuronide in men. *J Clin Endocrinol Metab* 1984; **59:** 417–21.

34. Russell DW, Wilson JD, Steroid 5α-reductase: two genes/two enzymes. *Annu Rev Biochem* 1994; **63:** 25–61.

35. Thigpen AE, Silver RI, Guileyardo JM, Casey ML, McConnell JD, Russell DW, Tissue distribution and ontogeny of steroid 5α-reductase isozyme expression. *J Clin Invest* 1993; **92:** 903–10.

36. Silver RI, Wiley EL, Thigpen AE, Guileyardo JM, McConnell JD, Russell DW, Cell type specific expression of steroid 5α-reductase 2. *J Urol* 1994; **152:** 438–42.

37. Beland G, Elhilali M, Fradet Y et al, Total androgen blockade for metastatic cancer of the prostate. *Am J Clin Oncol* 1988; **11**(suppl 2): S187–90.

38. Brisset JM, Nilutamide (Anandron) in prostatic cancer: review article. In: *Urology. Prostate Cancer* (Khoury S, Chatelain C, Murphy G, Denis L, eds). FIIS/RGP: Paris, 1990: 381–9.

39. Jankegt RA, Abbou CC, Bartoletti R et al, Orchiectomy and nilutamide or placebo as treatment of metastatic prostatic cancer in a multinational double-blind randomized trial. *J Urol* 1993; **149:** 77–83.

40. Crawford ED, Eisenberg MA, McLeod DG, Wilding G, Blumenstein BA, Comparison of bilateral orchiectomy with or without flutamide for the treatment of patients with stage D2 adenocarcinoma of the prostate: results of NCI intergroup study 0105 (SWOG and ECOG). *J Urol* 1997; **157:** 336.

41. Robinson MRG, Hetherington J, The EORTC studies: is there an optimal endocrine management for M1 prostatic cancer? *World J Urol* 1986; **4:** 171–5.

42. Robinson MRG, A further analysis of European Organization for Research and Treatment of Cancer protocol 30805. Orchidectomy versus orchidectomy plus cyproterone acetate versus low-dose diethylstilbestrol. *Cancer* 1993; **72**(suppl 12): 3855–7.

43. De Voogt HJ, Klijn JGM, Studer U et al, Orchidectomy versus buserelin in combination with cyproterone acetate, for 2 weeks or continuously, in the treatment of metastatic prostatic cancer. Preliminary results of EORTC trial 30843. *J Steroid Biochem Mol Biol* 1990; **37:** 965–9.

44. Crawford ED, Eisenberg MA, McLeod DG et al, A controlled trial of leuprolide with and without

flutamide in prostatic carcinoma. *N Engl J Med* 1989; **321:** 418–24.

45. Denis JL, Carneiro de Moura JL, Bono A et al, Goserelin acetate and flutamide versus bilateral orchiectomy: a phase III EORTC trial (30853). *Urology* 1993; **42:** 119–29.

46. Schellhammer P, Sharifi R, Block N et al, Maximal androgen blockade for patients with metastatic prostate cancer: outcome of a controlled trial of bicalutamide versus flutamide, each in combination with luteinizing hormone-releasing hormone analogue therapy. *Urology* 1996; **47**(suppl IA): 54–60.

47. Klijn JGM, de Voogt HJ, Studer UE et al, Short-term versus long-term addition of cyproterone acetate to buserelin therapy in comparison with orchidectomy in the treatment of metastatic prostate cancer. *Cancer* 1993; **72**(suppl 12): 3858–62.

48. Schroder FH, Cyproterone acetate – mechanisms of action and clinical effectiveness in prostate cancer treatment. *Cancer* 1993; **72**(suppl 12): 3810–15.

49. Cox RL, Crawford ED, Estrogens in the treatment of prostate cancer. *J Urol* 1995; **154:** 1991–8.

50. Geller J, Albert J, Yen SS, Geller S, Loza D, Medical castration of males with megestrol acetate and small doses of diethylstilbestrol. *J Clin Endocrinol Metab* 1981; **52:** 576–80.

51. Geller J, Megestrol acetate plus low-dose estrogen in the management of advanced prostatic carcinoma. *Urol Clin North Am* 1991; **18:** 83–91.

52. Goldenberg SL, Bruchovsky N, Gleave ME, Sullivan LD, Low-dose cyproterone acetate plus mini-dose diethylstilbestrol – a protocol for reversible medical castration. *Urology* 1996; **47:** 882–4.

53. Gonzalez-Barcena D, Vadillo-Buenfil M, Cortez-Morales A et al, Luteinizing hormone-releasing hormone antagonist Cetrorelix as primary single therapy in patients with advanced prostatic cancer and paraplegia due to metastatic invasion of spinal cord. *Urology* 1995; **45:** 275–81.

54. Bologna M, Muzi P, Biordi L, Festuccia C, Vicentini C, Finasteride dose-dependently reduces the proliferation rate of the LnCap human prostatic cancer cell line in vitro. *Urology* 1995; **45:** 282–90.

55. Fleshner NE, Trachtenberg J, Sequential androgen blockade: a biological study in the inhibition of prostatic growth. *J Urol* 1992; **148:** 1928–9.

56. Presti JC Jr, Fair WR, Andriole G et al, Multicenter, randomized, double-blind, placebo controlled study to investigate the effect of finasteride (MK-906) on stage D prostate cancer. *J Urol* 1992; **148:** 1201–12.

57. Fleshner NE, Trachtenberg J, Combination finasteride and flutamide in advanced carcinoma of the prostate: effective therapy with minimal side effects. *J Urol* 1995; **154:** 1642–6.

58. Karling P, Hammar M, Varenhorst E, Prevalence and duration of hot flushes after surgical or medical castration in men with prostatic carcinoma. *J Urol* 1994; **152:** 1170–3.

59. Beland G, Elhilali M, Fradet Y et al, Total androgen ablation: Canadian experience. *Urol Clin North Am* 1991; **18:** 75–82.

60. Mackenzie SH, Waxman S, Walsh R, Crawford ED, Androgen deprivation therapy using finasteride and flutamide to treat PSA failure following therapy for clinically localized adenocarcinoma of the prostate. In: *Proceedings of the 75th Annual Meeting SCS of the AUA*, Vail, CO, 1996: 195.

61. Allen JM, O'Shea JP, Mashiter K, Williams G, Bloom SR, Advanced carcinoma of the prostate: treatment with a gonadotrophin releasing hormone agonist. *Br Med J* 1983; **286:** 1607–9.

62. Warner B, Worgul TJ, Drago J et al, Effect of very high dose D-Leucine⁶–gonadotropin-releasing hormone proethylamide on the hypothalamic–pituitary testicular axis in patients with prostatic cancer. *J Clin Invest* 1983; **71:** 1842–53.

63. Schroeder FH, Lock TMTW, Chadha DR et al, Metastatic cancer of the prostate managed with buserelin versus buserelin plus cyproterone acetate. *J Urol* 1987; **137:** 912–18.

64. Kuhn JM, Billebaud T, Navratil H et al, Prevention of the transient adverse effects of gonadotropin-releasing hormone analogue (buserelin) in metastatic prostatic carcinoma by administration of an antiandrogen (nilutamide). *N Engl J Med* 1989; **321:** 413–18.

65. Mahler C, Is disease flare a problem? *Cancer* 1993; **72**(suppl 12): 3799–802.

66. Faure N, Lemay A, Laroche B et al, Preliminary results on the clinical efficacy and safety of androgen inhibition by an LHRH agonist alone or combined with an antiandrogen in the treatment of prostatic carcinoma. *Prostate* 1983; **4:** 601–24.

67. Qayum A, Gullick W, Clayton RC, Sikora K, Waxman J, The effects of gonadotrophin releasing hormone analogues in prostate cancer are mediated through specific tumour receptors. *Br J Cancer* 1990; **62:** 96–9.

68. Limonta P, Dondi D, Moretti RM, Maggi R, Mota M, Antiproliferative effects of luteinizing hormone-releasing hormone agonist on the human prostatic cancer cell line LNCaP. *J Clin Endocrinol Metab* 1992; **75:** 207–12.

69. Pályi I, Vincze B, Kálnay A et al, Effect of gonadotropin-releasing hormone analogs and their conjugates on gonadotropin-releasing hormone receptor-positive human cancer cell lines. *Cancer Detect Prev* 1996; **20:** 146–52.

70. Montie JE, A glimpse at the future of some endocrine aspects of prostate cancer. *Prostate* 1996; **6**(suppl): 56–61.

71. Hillner B, McLeod DG, Crawford ED, Bennett CL, Estimating the cost effectiveness of total androgen blockade with flutamide in M1 prostate cancer. *Urology* 1995; **45:** 633–40.

72. Kelly WK, Scher HI, Prostate specific antigen decline after antiandrogen withdrawal. *J Urol* 1993; **149:** 607–9.

73. Scher HI, Zhang ZF, Nanus D, Kelly WK, Hormone and antihormone withdrawal: implications for the management of androgen-independent prostate cancer. *Urology* 1996; **47**(suppl 1A): 61–9.

74. Moul JW, Srivastava S, McLeod DG, Molecular implications of the antiandrogen withdrawal syndrome. *Semin Urol* 1995; **13:** 157–63.

75. Visakorpi T, Hytinen E, Koiviston P et al, Amplification of androgen receptor gene associated with tumor recurrence in prostate cancer patients receiving androgen withdrawal therapy. In: *Basic and Clinical Aspects of Prostate Cancer.* AACR: Philadelphia, PA, 1994: abstr A-41.

76. Fair WR, Heston WDW, Overview of cancer biology and principles of oncology. In: *Campbell's Urology,* 6th edn (Walsh PC, Retik AB, Stamey TA, Vaughan ED, eds). WB Saunders: Philadelphia, 1992: 1031–52.

77. Isaacs JT, The timing of androgen ablation therapy and/or chemotherapy in the treatment of prostatic cancer. *Prostate* 1984; **5:** 1–7.

78. Byar DP, Corle D, Hormone therapy for prostate cancer: results of the Veterans Administration Cooperative Urological Research Group's studies of cancer of the prostate. *NCI Monogr* 1988; **7:** 165–70.

79. Zincke H, Bergstralh EJ, Larson-Keller JJ et al, Stage D1 prostate cancer treated by radical prostatectomy and adjuvant hormonal treatment. Evidence for favorable survival in patients with DNA diploid tumors. *Cancer* 1992; **70** (suppl): 311–23.

80. Kramolowski EV, The value of testosterone deprivation in stage D1 carcinoma of the prostate. *J Urol* 1988; **139:** 1242–4.

81. Akakura K, Bruchovsky N, Goldenberg SL, Rennie PS, Buckley AR, Sullivan LD, Effects of intermittent androgen suppression on androgen-dependent tumors. *Cancer* 1993; **71:** 2782–9.

82. Goldenberg SL, Bruchovsky N, Gleave ME, Sullivan LD, Akakura K, Intermittent androgen suppression in the treatment of prostate cancer: a preliminary report. *Urology* 1995; **45:** 839–45.

16 Chemotherapy: Relapse

16.1

Chemotherapy in advanced prostate cancer

Cora N Sternberg, Alessandra Ianari, Don WW Newling

CONTENTS • **Classification of patients relapsing after initial hormonal therapy** • **Development of hormone-refractory endocrine-insensitive disease** • **Response criteria in clinical trials of hormone-treated patients** • **Response to second-line therapy** • **Endocrine manipulations** • **New agents** • **Non-chemotherapeutic, non-hormonal therapies** • **Conclusions**

The wide spectrum of possible hormonal manipulations in advanced prostate cancer affects how patients relapsing after first-line palliative therapy can be assessed and subsequently treated. Patients with so-called 'hormone-refractory disease' now comprise a heterogeneous group. Some of these patients will have received testicular ablative therapy, some testicular and adrenal ablation, and others only androgen receptor antagonism. Two additional groups of patients are now appearing, which further complicates the problem. These are patients who have received neoadjuvant therapy prior to hopefully curative procedures, and patients who have received intermittent therapy in an attempt to delay the development of true endocrine resistance and improve their quality of life.[1]

Recent experience suggests that responses to subsequent endocrine manoeuvres may be seen following disease progression during initial testicular androgen deprivation with or without antiandrogens. While the significance of such responses and their underlying mechanisms remain unclear, it is likely that modest therapeutic benefits may be observed and may be explained by a modified response to hormones via molecular changes in cytosolic receptors. In addition, direct effects of various pituitary and hypothalamic hormones, as well as neuropeptides and biogenic amines, have also been shown to influence prostatic cell proliferation in culture. Empirical efforts at drug development have failed to produce cytotoxic agents with established activity against prostate cancer. However, with the rapid accumulation of fundamental biological knowledge about prostate cancer growth and differentiation in the laboratory, there is likely to be an impact on our ability to identify potentially active classes of drugs. A large number of compounds and modalities of treatment are in advanced stages of preclinical development, and will soon be evaluated clinically against this disease. Once a patient is deemed incurable, a potential important end-point of treatment is to achieve an acceptable quality of life status, even if survival is not prolonged.[2]

CLASSIFICATION OF PATIENTS RELAPSING AFTER INITIAL HORMONAL THERAPY

A methodological classification of prostate cancer, based on hormone sensitivity, possible antitumor effects and host factors (particularly the level of testosterone in the blood) is given in Table 16.1.1. The table is not intended as a recommendation for sequential therapeutic manoeuvres, and is not meant to suggest that the whole range of hormonal manipulations should be carried out before alternative therapies are tried. The patients in the first category are those with cancers thought to be non-curable, and who have not yet received any hormonal therapy. The second cohort consists of patients who have not undergone complete testicular androgen ablation, and have received some form of incomplete antiandrogen therapy, for example monotherapy with low-dose antiandrogens or oestrogens, neoadjuvant therapy prior to radiotherapy or prostatectomy, or intermittent therapy. This group of patients may remain androgen-sensitive in response to secondary castration, either by medical or by surgical means in 30% of cases. The response may well last between 12 and 18 months. The addition of castration, either medical or surgical, converts this group of patients to a similar status as those patients in the third group, that is, patients who relapse after primary combined hormonal manipulation or maximal androgen blockade.

The third cohort of patients is divided into two categories. Of those who have received medical or surgical castration alone, 8–30% will respond to the addition of an antiandrogen therapy (i.e. adrenal androgen blockade). They will also respond to corticosteroids, and to other hormonal manipulations, such as luteinizing hormone-releasing hormone (LHRH) antagonist and prolactin inhibitors. The second category in this third cohort includes those who have received maximal androgen blockade. Of these patients, 5–10% will also respond to corticosteroids, and to withdrawal of the agent that is blocking the androgen receptor. In addition, they may in some cases respond to LHRH antagonist, prolactin inhibitors somatostatin. The fourth cohort consists of those patients who initially underwent some form of maximal androgen blockade, and are now refractory to additive endocrine manipulations.[3]

DEVELOPMENT OF HORMONE-REFRACTORY ENDOCRINE-INSENSITIVE DISEASE

Controversy abounds over the origin of the androgen-independent cancer stem cells. One view is that these cells evolve early in carcinogenesis. However, after studies in the Shionogyi mouse breast cancer model, it was thought that the evolution of androgen-independent stem cells may be a gradual process that occurs in a low-androgen environment (i.e. below castration levels).[4] This led to the suggestion that periodic withdrawal of androgen suppression may extend the time of hormone dependence.[5]

Studies have shown that patients primed with testosterone before the use of chemotherapy have a shorter survival than do patients who receive chemotherapy alone.[6] This may indicate a continued sensitivity of prostate cancer to androgens. The finding of a decreasing prostate-specific antigen (PSA) and objective tumour improvement after flutamide withdrawal (the flutamide withdrawal syndrome) has been interpreted as evidence that continued manipulation of androgen-dependent growth may be therapeutically feasible.[7]

An important advance is the recognition of a neuroendocrine component of cells in the prostate. Small cell carcinoma of the prostate is an extremely aggressive tumour, associated with rapid proliferation and spread, particularly to soft tissue, which occurs in younger patients, and is rapidly fatal. This small cell carcinoma of the prostate is similar to small cell carcinomas in other organs, and should be suspected when a tumour is found in a young person already metastatic, with a low PSA. This tumour is never endocrine sensitive, and should be treated as are other small cell carcinomas in other organs, with initial combined cisplatin-based chemotherapy.[8] Abrahamsson[8] has recently shown that the development of hormone-refractory prostate cancer may be associated with proliferation of elements of a variety of neuroendocrine cells – 'small cells'.

Table 16.1.1 Methodological classification of prostate cancer based on hormone sensitivity

Category		Tumour factors	Host factors
Androgen-dependent	Endocrine-naive No prior hormone therapy	Anti-tumour effect: 1. Androgens are withdrawn 2. Antiandrogens are administered	Physiological levels of androgens in the blood
Androgen-dependent	Endocrine-sensitive: 1. Relapse after neoadjuvant therapy 2. Intermittent therapy – planned discontinuation of hormones 3. Relapse on antiandrogens alone	Decrease in proliferation if: 1. Androgens are withdrawn 2. Antiandrogens are administered (except group 3)	Non-castrate levels of androgens in the blood

Androgen-independent	Endocrine-sensitive	Decrease in proliferation in response to:
		
		1. Castration alone:
		  (a) adrenal androgen blockade
		  (b) corticosteroids
		  (c) other hormonal manipulations.
		2. Maximal androgen blockade:
		  (a) corticosteroids
		  (b) withdrawal of agents that bind to steroid hormone receptors
		  (c) other hormonal manipulations
			Castrate levels of testosterone

Hormone-independent	Androgen-independent and endocrine-insensitive	Insensitive to all hormonal manipulation(s)	Castrate levels of testosterone

RESPONSE CRITERIA IN CLINICAL TRIALS OF HORMONE-TREATED PATIENTS

Before considering the response criteria to be used in trials of new agents in patients relapsing after primary therapy, one must consider that the definition of progression on first-line therapy may be variable. This category of patients is heterogeneous. For instance, a patient who is assessed as progressing because of a rising PSA will have much longer to live than a patient whose primary tumour progresses to bone metastases or soft tissue metastases.[9]

RESPONSE TO SECOND-LINE THERAPY

Patients with measurable disease including the primary tumour

Measurable soft tissue disease occurs in a minority of patients with metastatic prostate cancer after relapse on primary therapy. While measurement of the primary tumour has been used in some studies to assess second-line therapy, variations in other pathological processes in the prostate gland make a distinction between tumour and hyperplastic benign change difficult and not reproducible. The demonstration of response or progression in soft tissue masses and their effects on the ureters or bladder may usually be measured by means of computed tomography (CT) when planning further local therapy.

Bone disease

Measurement of the response in bone to first- or second-line therapy poses many problems. The unequivocal disappearance of an osteolytic lesion and its replacement by osteoblastosis or normal-appearing bone is the only indisputable evidence of response to a given therapy. However, patients with metastatic prostate cancer most often have osteoblastic rather than osteolytic metastases. Progression of disease in the bone may be manifested by an increasing number of metastatic deposits, increasing size of the pre-existing lesions or increasing pain associated with bone lesions, without evidence of fracture. The difficulty caused by the presence of other bone pathology, the development of pathological fractures, subsequent new bone formation, as well as the effects of endocrine therapy on bone metabolism itself, can often confuse the issue and make the measurement of response to second-line therapy in these metastases particularly difficult.[10]

Subjective parameters

The use of subjective parameters, such as the measurement of pain or performance status, either individually or as a part of general quality of life assessment, plays an important role in assessing response to second-line therapy. The assessment of these parameters must be clearly defined and must be part of an acceptable spectrum of subjective measurements.[11]

Tumour-specific biochemical parameters

Metastatic prostate cancer can result in changes in a number of biochemical factors that are measurable in the blood or urine. Some of these are tumour specific (e.g. PSA and acid phosphatase), some reflect tumour burden (e.g. lactate dehydrogenase) and some reflect changes in the host tissues brought about by the presence of the tumour. This last group would include the measurement of alkaline phosphatase and hydroxyproline excretion. Scher and Fosså[12] have shown that the use of PSA as an outcome measure in patients treated with second-line therapy may indicate activity against the tumour, but is not always associated with prolonging survival or preventing subsequent objective progression. However, in second- and even third-line therapy it remains a useful indication to identify an agent with an antiproliferative effect. Thus, it should be used as an indication to investigate an agent further, while not definitely assuming the agent to be effectively antiproliferative. Recently, evidence has accumulated that certain agents, particularly suramin, somatostatin, vinblastine, epirubicin and, in prostatic cell cultures can diminish production of PSA without impairment of prostatic cancer cell proliferation.[13]

Recently, Wilding[14] has summarized the difficulties, by looking at a variety of hypothetical end-points for agents that act by different mechanisms to impair tumour proliferation and considering what effects these might have on the bone scan image, PSA level, etc. His suggestions are included in Table 16.1.2.

ENDOCRINE MANIPULATIONS

Antiandrogen withdrawal

This phenomenon was first identified by Scher and Kelly.[15] During total androgen blockade the androgen receptor in the tumour cells may mutate, causing cell growth stimulation by the antiandrogen rather than inhibition of proliferation. If the antiandrogen is discontinued in these patients, serum PSA subsequently decreases. This occurs in 15–25% of patients. Further clinical evidence suggests that castration levels of testosterone may be necessary for the mutation to take place. Consequently, the antiandrogen withdrawal effect is almost exclusively seen in patients after total androgen blockade.[15]

Oestrogens and corticosteroids

A significant number of patients with progressing hormone-refractory prostate cancer after total androgen blockade will respond to oestrogens. Oestrogens appear to be particularly useful in patients who have large pelvic tumours.[16] Significant PSA reduction is achieved in 20% of the patients receiving corticosteroids as their only secondary therapy. Corticosteroids seem to work mainly by diminishing adrenal androgen production, but may in addition have a separate effect on prostate cancer cells.[17]

Antifungal agents

Ketoconazole is an oral imidazole derivative with antifungal properties that works by inhibiting adrenal androgen synthesis and by inhibiting the cytochrome P450III enzyme system. In 48 patients treated with the combination of ketoconazole and hydrocortisone, 67% had a 50% decline in PSA and 50% had a decline of more than or equivalent to 80%, with responses lasting up to 1 year.[18] In a previous study, ketoconazole was combined with doxorubicin to produce a more than 50% reduction in PSA on three separate occasions in 55% of patients, with measurable disease regression in 7/12 (58%). Cardiac and mucocutaneous toxicities were seen.[19]

Liarozole is another imidazole derivative. A

Table 16.1.2 Patterns of response and hypothetical means of response evaluation

Criteria	Endocrine	Cytotoxic	Dedifferentiation	Anti-angiogenic	Antimetastatic	Cystostatic	Radiotherapy
Measurable disease	↓	↓	↔	↔	↔	↔	↓
Bone scan	↓↔(↑)	↔	↔	↔	↔	↔	↓↑
PSA	↓	↓	↑(↔)	Any	Any	↔	Any
Symptoms	↓	↓	↓	↓	↓	↓	↓
Progression-free survival	↑	↑	↑	↑	↑	↑	Any

↓, decrease; ↔, no change; (↑), flare; ↑, increase.

significant difference in survival was reported for patients who responded with a decline in PSA of more than 50%. A dose–response relationship may have been demonstrated. Although gastrointestinal tolerance is acceptable, cutaneous symptoms analogous to those encountered with retinoids and muscle fatigue were seen. Both of these agents appear to act via induction of differentiation and accumulation of all-*trans*-retinoic acid.[20]

Estramustine and combinations

Estramustine (Estracyt), a nitrogen mustard derivative of oestradiol, has shown activity in patients refractory to prior hormonal therapy. In the USA, responses have reportedly been low (0–4%), while in Europe response rates have generally been higher (of the order of 30–50%).[21,22] Estramustine inhibits microtubule assembly in a mechanism distinct from vinblastine. When estramustine was combined with vinblastine in three separate randomized trials, cumulative data revealed a greater than 50% decrease in PSA in 35/82 (43%) of patients, with measurable disease regression in 8/19 (42%).[23–25] Phase III trials are in progress to study this prospectively. Estramustine has also been combined with navelbine (Vinorelbine) in a phase I–II study.[26–28]

The combination of estramustine and etoposide was first introduced in 1994, with updated results reported in 1996. Etoposide, a podophyllotoxin derivative, is known to inhibit topoisomerase II at the nuclear matrix level. Although estramustine is best known as an antimicrotubule agent, it appears to act synergistically with etoposide. The mechanism of action may be different from that in combination with vinblastine. Of 95 patients, the first 52 were treated with a dose of estramustine 15 mg/kg per day and oral etoposide 50 mg/m^2 per day for 21 days every 28 days. The remaining 43 patients were treated with a reduced dose of estramustine of 10 mg/kg per day and allowed prior chemotherapy. Fifty of 95 (53%) patients had a greater than 50% decline in PSA, with no difference between the two groups. The authors concluded that the 10 mg/kg per day dose was equally effective and, importantly, was associated with less nausea. These results are of interest in view of the limited activity of etoposide as a single agent.[29]

The combination of estramustine plus paclitaxel (Taxol), an agent which also binds tubulin, may also be of interest. The combination of estramustine and paclitaxel, as a 96-hour infusion, showed responses in over 50% of cases.[30]

Chemotherapy

Despite the wide disparity in reports suggesting efficacy of 40–80%, hormone-refractory prostate cancer is resistant to most chemotherapy, and no standard chemotherapy regimen has been defined. Objective tumour regression occurs in less than 10–20% of patients.[31] The median survival in most older studies was 30–40 weeks. No single agent or combination of agents has consistently been shown to improve survival in randomized trials.

As mentioned previously, clinical trials have been hampered by the preponderance of bony metastases as the major parameter by which response is measured. Conclusions of many earlier studies were elusive due to the evaluation of lesions by means that are themselves difficult to evaluate, such as bone scans, intravenous pyelogram, digital rectal examinations and peripheral oedema. When trials were limited to patients with a bidimensionally measurable parameter, only 10–20% of patients with advanced prostate cancer were eligible.[32] Evaluating decline in PSA will hopefully facilitate the identification of new active agents. No chemotherapy regimen has been defined.

Anthracyclines

Low-dose weekly doxorubicin is considered by many oncologists in the USA as first-line therapy in hormone-refractory prostate cancer. Response rates for doxorubicin range from zero to more than 50%, depending upon the response criteria utilized. In Europe, a doxorubicin analogue, epirubicin, is often used. Mitoxantrone, another anthracycline, was combined with low-dose prednisone in a randomized trial and compared with prednisone alone. Of 161 patients randomized, 30/80 (38%) had a palliative response (pain reduction or decreased analgesic use) with the combination versus 17/81 (21%) with prednisone as a single agent. Response duration was longer with the combination (43 weeks versus 18 weeks). Although no difference in survival was observed, improvement in quality of life was accomplished with mitozantrone plus prednisone.[33] This improvement in the quality of life has been used by the US Food and Drug Administration (FDA) to accept the combination of mitozantrone and prednisone for hormone-relapsed prostate cancer.

5-Fluorouracil and cisplatin

Continuous-infusion 5-fluorouracil was combined with cisplatin in a study at Duke University of 49 patients; 40% showed a greater than 50% decline in PSA. Ten of 29 (35%) patients with bi-dimensional parameters, attained an objective response. Therapy was well tolerated in this elderly population, and home infusion reduced the need for hospitalization.[34]

NEW AGENTS

A new platinum analogue, Pro-plat (Bristol Meyers), has shown promise in phase II studies against prostate cancer cells. The European Organization for Research and Treatment of Cancer (EORTC) is planning to start a randomized phase III trial of this agent plus hydrocortisone against hydrocortisone alone in the near future.

Suramin

Palliation of pain with decline in PSA has been shown with the growth factor inhibitor suramin in combination with hydrocortisone. In published studies, approximately 40–70% of patients have a greater than 50% decrease in PSA, and 20–40% show an objective response rate.[35] There is a wide variability in schedules, conflicting response rates, and a high rate of neurotoxicity. Trials are difficult to interpret due to the concomitant use of corticosteroids, and failure to recognize regression due to flutamide withdrawal. Eisenberger et al[36] have proposed three different peak plasma serum concentrations as targets for treating patients. Toxicity was most frequently seen at the highest dose. Reyno et al[37] administered suramin as a simple, intermittent bolus injection. There appears to be no advantage to continuous infusion schedules, and intermittent dosing schedules are easier. Investigators from the Memorial Sloan–Kettering Cancer Center have also shown that suramin administration could be simplified, while maintaining drug concentrations.[38] A prospective evaluation of hydrocortisone and suramin from the same institution in patients who had disease progression after flutamide withdrawal and hydrocortisone demonstrated only limited activity.[39] A large cooperative group trial of suramin plus hydrocortisone versus hydrocortisone alone is ongoing. The mechanism of suramin-mediated anti-tumour activity still needs to be clarified.

Somatostatin

Although this may be considered by some as a hormonal therapy, its principal action again appears to be on a hormone-independent growth factor pathway. Although some activity has been observed in a number of small phase II studies, somatostatin has not as yet been proven to offer any survival advantage.[40]

Radiation therapy and bone-seeking isotopes

Bone pain is often the most debilitating component of metastatic prostate cancer and should be approached systematically. Focal irradiation to palliate bone pain for solitary, painful bone metastases may be supplemented by hemibody irradiation for the palliation of widespread metastases.

Strontium-89, a pure β-emitter with a half-life of 50 days, is a bone-seeking radionuclide, with a high uptake in osteoblastic metastases, and remains in tumour sites for up to 100 days. It delivers a high dose of radiation to prostate cancer metastases, with a low dose to normal tissues. Strontium-89 has recently been found to be effective in palliation of bone pain, with subjective response in more than 75–80% of patients. It may be most useful as an adjuvant to local field radiation therapy, and may prevent the development of new painful metastases.[41,42] It is the only agent approved for general use. Other radionuclides, such as rhenium-186 and samarium-153 conjugated to ligands with affinity to bone, emit both γ energies that provide images and β energies that are therapeutic.

Recent experimental work with a hormone-independent Dunning tumour in Copenhagen rats has shown that the early administration of rhenium-186 has a dramatic influence on the survival of rats with metastatic prostate cancer. The early administration of bone-seeking isotopes in the treatment of patients with relapse after primary endocrine therapy is presently undergoing investigation in a phase I–II clinical trial.[43]

NON-CHEMOTHERAPEUTIC, NON-HORMONAL THERAPIES

Gene therapy

Gene therapy, or the transfer of genetic material into human cells for therapeutic purposes, may constitute a novel, potential treatment modality that can be used in addition to surgery, chemotherapy, radiotherapy and systemic immunotherapy. A greater frequency of p53 mutations and altered Rb gene product have been reported in hormone-refractory prostate cancer.[44] Replacement of mutant p53 or Rb with an engineered wild-type gene or its protein product and restoring normal antiproliferative

effects has not yet been attempted in patients with prostate cancer. Another approach to hormone-refractory patients may be to restore androgen receptor positivity to cells that have become independent, and then to treat these patients once again with antiandrogens. This molecular strategy could be made possible by the techniques of cell transfection using recombinant DNA complementary to the androgen receptor DNA.[45]

Immunotargeting

The approach of immunotargeting of cytotoxic drugs or bacterial cytotoxins gives an important new direction and an opening for further pre-clinical and applied research. Radioactive antibodies have the potential advantage of localizing directly to tumour cells, rather than to bone. A phase I immunolocalization trial of monoclonal antibody (mAb) Prost 30 labelled with 10 mCi radioiodine showed that Prost 30 can localize to disseminated sites of prostate cancer and may have therapeutic potential.[46] Another antibody, CYT-356, has been conjugated with yttrium-90, a β-emitter, and is under clinical investigation.[47]

Angiogenesis inhibitors

Tumour angiogenesis may represent an important process during the metastatic cascade of prostate cancer. A number of angiogenesis inhibitors working through different mechanisms are under development at this time, and some of these are currently undergoing clinical trials. Among these are TNP-470, suramin pentosine, vitamin D_3 analogues and thalidomide.[48]

Receptor antagonists

The use of a variety of growth factor receptor antagonists, for example endothelin-1 receptor antagonist or bombesine receptor antagonist, is a promising new line of therapy.[49] At the moment some agents are ready to enter phase II studies, and a clinical trial is underway with one such agent, FRABJC 225 + doxorubicin at the Memorial Sloan–Kettering Cancer Center and the University of Virginia.

Summary

What is evident from this list of possible agents is that many of them would not be appropriately tested and would be unlikely to show any effect in far advanced disease. If we accept the concept that there are endocrine-independent cells early on in the development of a clinical prostate cancer, then new methods need to be devised for testing the activity of these agents at this stage of the disease, at which they will hopefully achieve clinical usage. Clearly, to set up a phase II study of gene therapy or angiogenesis inhibition in patients with very low-volume disease or who are only deemed as being at risk of developing subsequent disease within present methodologies would be worth consideration. It has even been suggested that these agents should initially be tested in a phase I trial for toxicity in patients who are either healthy volunteers or deemed to be at risk of developing prostate cancer because of their family history. The agents should later be tested against placebo in patients with early stage disease prior to prostatectomy, but who may be cured by prostatectomy or radiotherapy, evaluating these agents on histological grounds in place of clinical grounds. With the development of new molecular markers of cancer cell activity, and in particular markers of metastatic potential, it is possible that for many of these agents new evaluation criteria must be devised.[3]

CONCLUSIONS

After failure of initial hormonal therapy, various treatment options are available that may provide objective remission and palliate the symptoms of disease. Hormone-refractory prostate cancer remains a challenge, but it is not as resistant to treatment as was previously believed. A trial of flutamide withdrawal should be considered in patients progressing on maximal androgen blockade. In patients who have not been on maximal androgen blockade, one can consider adding an antiandrogen or estramustine, either alone or in association with chemotherapy. Agents such as ketoconazole and liarozole, which inhibit retinoic acid breakdown, may then be tried. Chemotherapy and suramin may be efficacious in selected patients. Whenever possible, patients should be considered for well-controlled clinical trials. Future studies may focus on dietary modification. An increased understanding of the biology of the disease will direct future therapeutic strategies. While progress in the management of metastatic prostate cancer is urgently awaited, advances in molecular biology will offer future hope to patients.

The performance of clinical trials in patients with hormone-refractory prostate cancer represents a challenge for the working scientific clinician. First, the application and interpretation of response criteria are problematic. Second, the heterogeneity and unavoidable selection of patients entered into trials, in terms of previous treatment, clinical presentation, co-morbidity and patients' expectations, make it difficult to transfer results from single-institution studies to general daily practice. Third, most patients with progressive hormone-refractory prostate cancer will sooner or later suffer from cancer-related subjective and psychological distress, which, beyond all the aims of any clinical trials, must be met by the responsible clinician with empathy and efforts to palliate. This requires communication skills of the clinicians when seeing the patient and his family.

THE 'TAKE-HOME' MESSAGE

The doctor's challenge is to increase our understanding of and scientific approach to the management of hormone-refractory prostate cancer and, at the same time, to be the individual patient's advocate and help him in his struggle with an incurable malignancy.

REFERENCES

1. Newling DWW, McLeod D, Solowy M, Di Silverio F, Smith P, Proceedings of the International Workshop in Prostatic Cancer and BPH; Panel V: Distant Disease. *Cancer* 1992; **70:** 365–7.
2. Sternberg C, Ianari A, Hormone refractory metastatic prostate cancer. *Urology* 1996; **46:** 258–63.
3. Newling DWW, Fosså SD, Andersson L et al, Assessment of hormone refractory prostate cancer. *Urology* 1997; **49**(Suppl 4A): 46–53.
4. Logothetis CJ, Hoosein NM, Hsieh JT, The clinical and biological study of androgen independent prostate cancer (AIPCa). *Semin Oncol* 1994; **21:** 620–9.
5. Bruchovsky M, Snoek R, Rennie PS, Akakura K, Goldenberg SL, Gleave M, Control of tumor progression by maintenance of apoptosis. *Prostate* 1996; **6**(suppl): 13–21.
6. Manni A, Bartholomew N, Caplan R et al, Androgen priming and chemotherapy in advance prostate cancer: evaluation of determinants of clinical outcome. *J Clin Oncol* 1988; **6:** 1456–66.
7. Scher HI, Zhang ZF, Cohen L, Kelly WK, Hormonally relapsed prostatic cancer: lessons from the flutamide withdrawal syndrome. *Adv Urol* 1995; **8:** 61–95.
8. Abrahamsson PA, Neuroendocrine differentiation and hormone refractory prostate cancer. *Prostate* 1996; **6**(suppl): 3–8.
9. Newling DWW, Dennis L, Vermeylen K, Orchiectomy vs goserelin and flutamide in the treatment of newly metastatic diagnosed prostate cancer. Analysis of the criteria of evaluation use in the EORTC Genitourinary Group study. *Cancer* 1993; **72:** 3793–8.
10. Jones WG, Alasa H, Van Oosterom A, Kotake T, Objective response criteria in phase II and phase III studies. In: *Progress and Controversies in Urologic Oncology* (Schröder FH, Klijn JGM, Kurth KH, Pinedo HM, Splinter TAW, De Voogt HJ, eds), vol 2. AR Liss: New York, 1988: 243–61.
11. Newling DWW, Parameters of response and progression in prostate cancer. In: *Treatment of Prostate Cancer – Facts and Controversies* (Schröder FH, ed). Wiley-Liss: New York, 1990: 25–48.
12. Scher HI, Fosså SD, Prostate cancer in the era of prostate specific antigen. *Curr Opinion Oncol* 1995; **7:** 281–91.
13. Thalman GN, Sikes RA, Chang SM, Johnston DA, von Eschenbach, Chung LW, Suramin induced decrease in PSA expression with no effect on tumor growth in the LnCaP model of human prostatic cancer. *J Natl Cancer Inst* 1996; **88:** 794–801.
14. Wilding G, quoted in Eisenber MA and Nelson WG, How much can we rely on PSA as an endpoint for evaluation of clinical trials? A word of caution. *J Natl Cancer Inst* 1996; **88:** 779–81.
15. Scher H, Kelly WK, Flutamide withdrawal syndrome: its impact on clinical trials in prostate cancer. *Clin Oncol* 1993; **11:** 1566–72.
16. Ferro MA, Use of intravenous stilbestrol in patients with prostatic cancer refractory to conventional hormonal manipulations. *Urol Clin North Am* 1991; **18:** 139–43.
17. Fosså SD, Jahnsen JK, Karlsen S et al, High dose MPA vs prednisone in hormone resistant prostatic cancer. A pilot study. *Eur Urol* 1985; **11:** 11–16.
18. Small EJ, Egan B, Ralphe L, Advanced prostate cancer patients who have progressed after flutamide withdrawal retain hormonal sensitivity to ketoconazole. *J Urol* 1996; **155:** 608A [abstract].
19. Sella EJ, Kilbourn R, Amato R et al, Phase II study of ketoconazole combined with weekly doxorubicin in patients with androgen independent prostate cancer. *J Clin Oncol* 1994; **12:** 683–8.
20. Smith J, Abdriole G, Ahmann F et al, Effects of liarozole (LIA) on PSA-levels in patients with relapsed stage D prostate cancer. *Proc Am Soc Clin Oncol* 1996; **15:** 250 [abstract].
21. Halpern J, Catane R, Oral estramustine phosphate (Estracyt): a broad phase II study. *J Med* 1984; **15:** 35–43.
22. Konyves I, 1984; Estramustine phosphate (Estracyt) in the treatment of prostatic carcinoma. *Int Urol Neprol* 1989; **21:** 393–7.
23. Seidman AD, Scher HI, Petrylak D, Dershaw DD, Curley I, Estramustine and vinblastine: use of prostate specific antigen as a clinical trial endpoint for hormone refractory prostatic cancer. *J Urol* 1992; **147:** 931–4.
24. Amato RJ, Logothetis CJ, Dexeus FH, Sella A, Kilbourn RG, Fitz K, Preliminary results of a phase II trial of estramustine (EMCYT) and vinblastine (VLB) for patients with progressive hormone refractory prostate carcinoma (HRPC). *Proc Am Assoc Cancer Res* 1991; **32:** 186 [abstract].
25. Hudes GR, Greenberg R, Krigel RL et al, Phase II study of estramustine and vinblastine, two microtubule inhibitors, in hormone refractory

prostate cancer. *J Clin Oncol* 1992; **10**: 1754–61.

26. Reese D, Burris H, Belledgrun A et al, A phase I–II study of navelbine (Vinorelbine) and estramustine in the treatment of hormone refractory prostate cancer (HRPC). *Proc Am Soc Clin Oncol* **15**: 259 [abstract].

27. Pienta KJ, Redman B, Hussain M et al, Phase II evaluation of oral estramustine and oral etoposide in hormone refractory adenocarcinoma of the prostate. *J Clin Oncol* 1994; **12**: 2005–12.

28. Pienta KJ, Flaherty LE, Hussain M, Esper PS, Naik H, Redman BG, Report of an extended phase II trial of oral estramustine and oral etoposide in the treatment of hormone refractory prostate cancer patients. *Proc Am Clin Oncol* 1996; **15**: 261 [abstract].

29. Scher HI, Sternberg CN, Heston WD et al, Etoposide in prostatic cancer; experimental studies and phase II trial patients with bi-dimensionally measurable disease. *Cancer Chemother Pharmacol* 1986; 18: 24–6.

30. Hudes G, Nathan F, Chapman AE, Combined antimicrotubule therapy of metastatic prostate cancer with 96 hr paclitaxel (P) and estramustine (EM): activity in hormone refractory disease (HRPC). *Proc Am Soc Clin Oncol* 1995; **14**: 237 [abstract].

31. Yagoda A, Petrylak DP, Cytotoxic chemotherapy for advanced hormone resistant prostate cancer. *Cancer* 1992; **71**: 1098–109.

32. Sternberg C, Hormone refractory metastatic prostate cancer. *Ann Oncol* 1992; **3**: 331–5.

33. Moore MJ, Tannock I, Osoba D et al, Chemotherapy with mitoxantrone and low dose prednisone provides useful palliation for some patients with hormonal resistant prostate cancer (HRPC). *J Urol* 1996; **155**: 610A [abstract].

34. Walther PJ, Hall SC, Walker RA, Continuous infusion 5-fluorouracil combined with cisplatin in the treatment of androgen independent metastatic prostate carcinoma. *J Urol* 1996; **155**: 579A [abstr 1072].

35. Clark JW, Suramin and prostate cancer. Where do we go from here? *J Clin Oncol* 1995; **13**: 2155–7.

36. Eisenberger MA, Simibaldi VJ, Reyno LM et al, Phase I and clinical evaluation of a pharmacological guided regimen of suramin in patients with hormone refractory prostate cancer. *J Clin Oncol* 1995; **13**: 2174–86.

37. Reyno LM, Egorin MJ, Eisenberg MA, Sinibaldi VJ, Zuhowski EG, Sridhara R, Development and validation of pharmacokinetically based fixed dosing scheme for suramin. *J Clin Oncol* 1995; **13**: 2187–95.

38. Kelly WK, Scher HI, Mazumdar M et al, Suramin and hydrocortisone: determining drug efficiency in androgen independent prostate cancer. *J Clin Oncol* 1995; **13**: 2214–22.

39. Kelly WK, Curley T, Leibertz C, Dnistrian A, Schwartz M, Scher HI, Prospective evaluation of hydrocorticosone and suramin in patients with androgen independent prostate cancer. *J Clin Oncol* 1995; **13**: 2208–12.

40. Mahler C, Denis L, Treatment of hormone refractory disease. *Semin Surg Oncol* 1995; **11**: 770–83.

41. Porter AT, McEwan AJB, Powe JE et al, Results of a randomized phase III trial to evaluate the efficacy of strontium-89 adjuvant to local field external beam irradiation in the management of endocrine resistant metastastic prostate cancer. *Int J Radiother Biol Phys* 1993; **25**: 805–13.

42. Crawford ED, Kozlowski JM, Debruyne FMJ et al, Strontium-89 therapy for the palliation of pain due to osseous metastases. *J Am Med Assoc* 1995; **274**: 420–4.

43. Geldof AA, van der Tillaar PLM, Newling DWW, Teule G, Radionuclide therapy for prostate cancer lumbar metastases prolongs symptom-free in rat model. *Urology* 1997; **49**: 795–802.

44. Heidenberger HB, Sesterhenn IA, Gaddipatti JP et al, Alteration of the tumor suppressor gene p53 in a high fraction of hormone refractory prostate cancer. *J Urol* 1995; **154**: 414–21.

45. Pandha HS, Sikora K, Gene therapy for urological cancer. *Br J Urol* 1995; **75**(suppl 1): 67–74.

46. Bander NH, Dvigi C, Theodoulou M et al, Phase I immuno-localization trial of monoclonal antibody (mAb) Prost 30 in patients with prostate cancer. *J Urol* 1996; **155**: 610A [abstract].

47. Bander NH, 1996; Current status of monoclonal antibodies for imaging and therapy of prostate cancer. *Semin Oncol* 1994; **21**: 607–12.

48. Ferrer FA, Miller LJ, Andoawir RI et al, Cytokine regulation of angiogenesis factors in human prostate cancer. *J Urol* 1996; **155**(suppl 5): abstr 163.

49. Nelson JB, Chan-Tack K, Hedican SP et al, Endothelin-1 is expressed in advanced prostate cancer: Etb receptor mediated proliferation accompanies decreased Etb expression. *J Urol* 1996; **155**(suppl 5): abstr 1164.

16.2

Palliative care

Adrian Tookman, Anna Kurowska

CONTENTS • **Service delivery** • **Communication** • **Underlying principles of symptom control** • **Pain** • **Weakness and immobility** • **Anorexia** • **Nausea and vomiting** • **Constipation** • **Management of the terminal phase** • **Bereavement**

The Association of Palliative Medicine defines palliative medicine as follows:

> Palliative medicine is the appropriate medical care of patients with advanced and progressive disease for whom the focus of care is quality of life and in whom the prognosis is limited (although sometimes it may be several years). Palliative medicine includes consideration of the families' needs before and after the patient's death.

In the early stages of the illness, palliative care plays an important role as a resource in symptom management and psychological support. As the disease progresses palliative care expertise increases in importance; by the end of the illness it may well play the major role in an individual's care.

Cancer of the prostate is particularly challenging. Bone pain is very common and, in the late stages, can prove difficult to control. Disease progression is often slow, with late involvement of vital organs. Periods of disease stability leave patients with many rehabilitation problems and a long period of painful debilitation may precede death. With its focus on castration, treatment can be psychologically distressing. The management of prostate cancer, therefore, needs the skills of a variety of professionals, the relative importance of whose roles changes over the course of the illness (Figure 16.2.1).

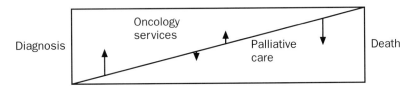

Figure 16.2.1 The interrelationship between oncology services (surgical oncology, radiotherapy and medical oncology) and palliative care services, and patient flow between services.

SERVICE DELIVERY

Palliative care must be delivered by a team with a multi-professional approach. The aim is to enable patients and their families to benefit from the significant advances that have been made recently in pain and symptom control, and thereby to maximize their quality of life. All the patient's problems should be addressed, not just their physical symptoms, but also their emotional, social, spiritual and sexual problems. Patient choice is crucial, especially regarding place of death. A variety of models of care have been adopted.

An effective palliative care service aims to deliver care in all settings (hospice, hospital and community) – a so-called 'seamless' service (Figure 16.2.2). In this way patients can be offered real choices about where they spend their illness and where they die. Most patients would choose to die in their own homes; however, the majority of cancer deaths still occur in hospital.[1]

COMMUNICATION

Patients cannot make informed choices without accurate information. Every patient should be given a clear explanation of the likely physical and functional outcome of treatment. Patients who are given this information adapt better to radical treatments.

Communication with patients with advanced illness can be difficult. Terminal illness can be seen as a failure and generate feelings of inadequacy, failure and vulnerability in the doctor. This can lead to the use of certain tactics in order to keep patients at a safe emotional distance, including:

- *Premature reassurance*: the patient is quickly reassured that symptoms can be relieved without any attempt to explore underlying emotional fears.
- *Selective attention*: the doctor concentrates on the physical symptoms to the exclusion of the patient's underlying fears.
- *Changing topics*: expression of the patient's emotional problems is ignored, and instead the doctor enquires about their physical symptoms.
- *Closed questions*: e.g. 'You're feeling much better today, aren't you?'
- *Physical avoidance*: walking past the end of the bed.

These tactics should be avoided wherever possible. Good communication will: enable patients to express their anxieties and to be

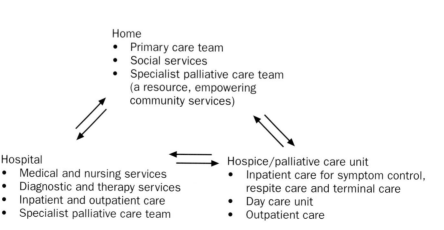

Figure 16.2.2 The tripod of care.

reassured; reduce uncertainty and inappropriate hope; and allow patients to adjust to their illness both practically and emotionally.

The principles of good communication are:

- Listen to the patient (including reflective listening, i.e. asking questions about questions).
- Deal with patient's problems before professional concerns.
- Cover each topic before proceeding to the next.
- All problems should be elicited before attempting to find a solution.
- Non-verbal clues are important.
- Clarify and summarize.
- Avoid jargon.

UNDERLYING PRINCIPLES OF SYMPTOM CONTROL

A problem-orientated individualized approach is the key to success. A positive but realistic attitude is essential, with reassurance being given that a great deal can be achieved.

The following actions should be taken *for each* symptom.

Diagnose the cause of the symptom and treat appropriately

Since the treatment of a symptom varies considerably depending on the underlying pathology, accurate diagnosis is vital. A careful history and examination are often more revealing than extensive investigations, which can be impractical and distressing. Such investigations should be ordered only if they will alter management.

If the underlying pathology remains uncertain and, because of the frailty of the patient, it is not appropriate to investigate further, symptomatic relief should be given. A therapeutic trial may elucidate the cause. For example, in a confused patient with suspected cerebral metastases who is too unwell for a computed tomography (CT) scan, response to a trial of steroids would support the diagnosis.

Explain the symptom to the patient

Fear will colour the patient's interpretation of any symptom. Explanation reassures the patient that the symptom is understood and can be treated.

Discuss treatment options

Informed choice is dependent on adequate and accurate information. A patient's sense of control is enhanced by discussion of options.

Set realistic objectives

It is frustrating to both patients and staff if expectations are set that will never be achieved.

Anticipate

In patients with advanced illness, symptoms may change rapidly. If such changes can be anticipated much distress may be avoided. For example, a patient may become unable to take oral medication as their condition deteriorates. This should be anticipated and parenteral preparations be made available. This applies particularly in the home, where a crisis, possibly leading to admission, could be avoided.

Ensure relatives remain informed and supported

It is important to acknowledge and treat the whole 'family'.

Treat all symptoms

Minor symptoms can cause considerable distress. Such symptoms seem trivial in the context of advanced carcinoma of the prostate, but may have major significance to the individual concerned. A patient's social and emotional problems are as important as their physical problems.

PAIN

Pain is probably the most feared symptom of cancer.[2] Given that, eventually, 70–80% of patients with prostate cancer develop skeletal metastases, it is not surprising that bone pain is an extremely common symptom. Prostate cancer generally metastasizes to the pelvis, spine and proximal long bones. Considerable

Table 16.2.1 The 'pain experience'

Type of pain	Examples
Physical	Due to carcinoma of the prostate (e.g. bone pain)
	Due to treatment (e.g. constipation due to opioids)
	Due to debility (e.g. pressure sores)
	Due to concurrent disease (e.g. shingles)
Emotional	Depression
	Despair
	Anxiety
	Fear (virtually universal)
	Anger
Social	Isolation
	Financial problems
	Personal/family relationships
	Making a will/funeral arrangements
Spiritual	Spirituality – spiritual issues including the search for meaning, the unanswerable questions related to a diagnosis of a fatal illness
	Religious belief – although formal religious belief can give comfort, it can also create problems related to the guilt and possible retribution for past misdemeanours. Patients may feel let down by their god
Sexual	Loss of sexual role within a relationship can be particularly important in cancer of the prostate, with its treatments often leading to impotence and loss of sexual drive

morbidity from bone metastases is seen because of the long clinical course of this disease. Pathological fractures tend not to occur because of the osteoblastic reaction.

Pain is a 'total experience'. To enable an individual patient to have total pain control, all aspects of their pain experience must be considered (Table 16.2.1). The management of physical pain is pivotal in achieving good control, but all the factors listed in Table 16.2.1 must be considered. Many of the non-physical causes of pain have no definitive solution. Usually some help can be given, even if only to encourage the expression of such worries. By listening to the patient, value is given to their problems.

Evaluation

Pain can be alleviated or modified in all patients. Proper pain assessment leads to effective management. The majority of patients have pain at more than one site.[3] Each pain should be evaluated individually. In order to establish the cause of the pain it is essential to take a careful history noting:

- the site of pain and any radiation
- the type and severity of pain
- when the pain started and any subsequent changes
- exacerbating and alleviating factors.

Physical examination often confirms diagnosis. Occasionally it may be necessary to investigate using radiographs, isotope bone scans, CT scans, etc.

Treatment

Treatment of pain depends on the underlying pathology. Pain can be managed:

- by modifying the pathological process (by hormone therapy, radiotherapy or chemotherapy, as discussed elsewhere in this book)
- by elevating the pain threshold by pharmacological means
- by interrupting pain transmission.

Table 16.2.2 outlines the common causes of pain in patients with carcinoma of the prostate. In-depth discussion of pain management will focus mainly on bone pain, as this is the most common cause of pain in this group of patients.

Modifying the pathological process

Relatively simple treatments can modify the disease. The physician who is palliating the patient with cancer of the prostate must be familiar with systemic management. A close professional relationship with the clinical oncology team is crucial in order to avail the patient of all therapeutic options that could help control their symptoms. Of particular interest is the role of steroids in palliation. These have always had a clear role in the management of certain well-defined problems (e.g. acute management of cord compression or of pelvic pain from a mass lesion). However, steroids also have a role in *direct* disease management in prostate cancer. Replacement doses of steroids (e.g. hydrocortisone 20 mg twice daily) suppress the adrenal axis, which in turn can modify the disease process, palliate symptoms and, on occasion, produce a useful remission.[4,5]

Local radiotherapy

This is discussed elsewhere. A single fraction of treatment may be more suitable for certain patients than a fractionated course. Such decisions are dependent on the proposed site of radiotherapy and the condition of the patient. A physician who is aware of the various treatment schedules available is best placed to refer his or her patient appropriately and negotiate optimal treatment.[6,7]

Strontium-89

Radioactive strontium is a radiopharmaceutical that provides a single dose systemic treatment. It targets metastatic bone lesions, causing transient side-effects and minimal toxicity, while bringing the possibility of long-lasting pain relief.

Strontium mimics the bone-seeking activity of calcium. Strontium-89, its radioactive isotope, is an almost pure β-emitter (maximum energy 1.46 MeV). Its long half-life (50.6 days) enables prolonged radiation to be delivered to bone, while its short range of penetration (3.2–3.5 mm in bone; 6–7 mm in soft tissue) ensures minimal radiation to surrounding healthy tissue.[8] After intravenous injection strontium-89 is taken up in areas of osteogenesis (such as bone metastases). It is retained in these sites and 'washed out' of normal bone. Its biological half-life in normal bone is 14 days, which is considerably shorter than its biological half-life in bony metastases. The dose to bone marrow is approximately one-tenth the dose to diseased bone.[9]

The efficacy of strontium in relieving metastatic bone pain in multiple myeloma and cancer of the prostate was investigated by Firusian et al,[10] with favourable results and minimal myelosuppression. American trials subsequently reported 80% response rates in prostate cancer, 89% response rates in breast cancer and total relief of pain in 22%.[11] Studies in Canada with strontium-89 have looked at its role as adjuvant therapy with local field radiotherapy. The group of patients who received adjuvant strontium-89 showed improved pain control at 3 and 6 months, and a significant delay in disease progression.[12] A UK study compared strontium-89 with local field radiotherapy and strontium-89 with hemibody radiation. No overall effects on survival were found; however, strontium-89 was at least as effective in

Table 16.2.2 Common causes of pain in patients with advanced carcinoma of the prostate and an indication of their relative morphine sensitivity

Cause of pain	Morphine sensitivity	Reason for pain	Some suggested treatments
Bone pain	Partially morphine sensitive	Mechanical disruption of bone Fracture of bone Stimulation of chemical mediators that activate osteoclasts	NSAIDs Opioids *Second line* Radiotherapy (local to deposit, generalized, e.g. hemibody or 'systemic' strontium-89). Prophylactic surgery and fixation of fractures. Chemotherapy/hormones. Bisphosphonate therapy
Nerve pain	Classically morphine insensitive	Nerve compression/irritation/infiltration	Amitriptyline. Antiepileptics. Membrane stabilizers (e.g. flecainide, mexiletine) *Second line* Nerve blocks. Steroids, hormones. Radiotherapy/chemotherapy
Musculoskeletal pain	Morphine insensitive	Common with bony involvement Can occur secondary to weakness and debility Arthritis	NSAIDs Benzodiazepines Physiotherapy Massage *Second line* Trigger point injection. Joint injections. Acupuncture
Colic	Morphine insensitive (may be due to opioid)	Stretching of hollow viscus secondary to an obstructive lesion (usually constipation in patients with prostatic cancer; malignant obstruction uncommon)	Treat constipation (laxatives) Stop/reduce drugs causing hyperperistalsis
Capsular stretching	Partially morphine sensitive	Usually due to liver metastases	Opioids NSAIDs Steroids *Second line* Hormones/chemotherapy
Pain of cerebral metastases	Partially sensitive	Pain caused by tumour expansion in an enclosed space and raised intracranial pressure Relatively uncommon in prostate cancer	Steroids Benzodiazepines Weak opioids *Second line* Radiotherapy
Pain due to large tumour mass	Partially morphine sensitive	Mass lesion compressing viscera and infiltrating coexistent adjacent structures (e.g. nerve plexus)	Opioids Treatment of nerve pain and/or bone pain Steroids *Second line* Treat 'tumour bulk' by radiotherapy, hormones chemotherapy, surgery or embolization

NSAIDs, non-steroidal anti-inflammatory drugs.
*The second-line treatments listed should be considered when appropriate.

producing pain relief, cheaper than local field radiotherapy, and it was suggested that it might prevent the development of new sites of pain.[13]

Strontium-89 is available in 60 centres in the UK. It must be administered by authorized personnel. Patient selection is important when considering its use. Criteria for deciding patient suitability include:

- Multiple bony metastases with multiple sites of pain.
- A 'superscan' or isotope bone scan is a relative contraindication. The high overall uptake will spread the strontium throughout the skeleton, giving a low total dose to metastatic lesions and higher haemopoietic toxicity.
- Patients should have a good marrow reserve and a 'normal' blood count (a drop of platelets of 30% should be expected).
- Severe renal impairment is a contraindication (strontium is excreted by the kidney).
- Previous radiotherapy is not a contraindication.
- Calcium medication should be stopped because of competition with strontium.
- If chemotherapy is a future treatment option, strontium-89 treatment should be considered with caution as it will affect marrow reserve.

Strontium is given by intravenous injection. The standard recommended dose is 150 MBq. Warmth and slight dizziness may occur during injection. Within 24–72 hours patients may experience a 'flare' of their pain (25% in our series), which can be treated with an increased dose of analgesic or, if severe, with a single dose of dexamethasone. Patients can experience a mild non-specific malaise for several weeks. The blood count must be closely monitored, since the platelet count and the white blood count will fall by approximately 30%. The nadir of this fall is at 5 weeks.

Improvement in pain typically occurs 3 weeks after treatment, and some response would be expected in over 80% of patients. This response should be maintained in approximately 50% of responders for many months (differing response rates in different series).

Bisphosphonates

Bisphosphonates inhibit osteoclast activity and hence bone resorption. In malignant disease bisphosphonates are the drug of choice for hypercalcaemia, providing the most consistent, rapid and effective treatment. A clinical response is seen in 48 hours (e.g. improvement in mental state) and normal calcium levels are achieved in 1 week.

Biphosphonates also have an established role in the management of metastatic bone pain. Destruction of bone, an integral part of the formation of lytic metastases, is substantially mediated by osteoclasts. Tumours that metastasize to the skeleton often release substances that cause osteoclast stimulation, which results in increased bone resorption. Inhibiting osteoclast activity is a possible way of modifying the progressive osteolytic process. There are tightly regulated physiological processes governing bone turnover where the resorption (osteoclast mediated) and formation (osteoblast mediated) of bone are closely linked. Although osteosclerotic metastases are characteristic of prostate cancer, bone resorption is also accelerated. Following the relative success of bisphosphonates in breast cancer, significant palliation of bone pain in patients with hormone-resistant prostate cancer have been reported.[14–16]

Generally, intravenous bisphosphonates are used in the management of bone pain. Oral bisphosphonates are not as reliable; they are poorly absorbed from the gastrointestinal tract (1–10% of dose is absorbed). Absorption is reduced further by food ingestion, especially products containing calcium. Side-effects with oral bisphosphonates include nausea and diarrhoea.

Clearly, bisphosphonates have a role in the management of painful bony deposits in prostate cancer. However, the precise place of these drugs in treatment and, in particular, the optimal dose and regimen are still to be elucidated.

Elevating the pain threshold

Opioids

The World Health Organization describes a three-step ladder for the prescribing of analgesics:

1. Non-opioid ± adjuvant
2. Weak opioid ± non-opioid ± adjuvant
3. Strong opioid ± non-opioid ± adjuvant

It should be noted that co-analgesics and adjuvants can be used at each step for treating that element of the pain that is opioid insensitive. Analgesics should be prescribed regularly, and inadequate pain control at one step requires a move to the next step rather than to an alternative drug of similar efficacy. Non-opioids include aspirin, paracetamol and non-steroidal anti-inflammatory drugs (NSAIDs). Weak opioids include codeine, dihydrocodeine and dextropropoxyphene (as in co-proxamol). Tramadol might also be included in this class. Tramadol is approximately double the strength of codeine. It has a dual mechanism of action, part opioid and part by blocking reuptake of monoamines, leading to fewer adverse opioid side-effects.

Oral morphine is the strong opioid of choice and is the mainstay of the treatment of pain in advanced disease. It is safe, predictable and reliable when prescribed appropriately and correctly. The correct use of strong opioids has made a major impact on the management of pain in patients with advanced cancer. But unfounded fears about the use of strong opioids, ignorance of the way in which opioids should be prescribed and an inability to recognize pain that is morphine resistant all continue to hamper optimum management.

The misconceptions about strong opioids are as follows:

- *Addiction*, that is, psychological dependence and craving, does not occur.[17] Chemical dependence does occur with opioids, hence withdrawal should be gradual when the patient no longer needs the opioid, such as when the pain is controlled by some other means (e.g. the pain of a bony metastasis may settle when the bone is irradiated).

- *Tolerance* is the progressive increase of dose to achieve the same effect in chronic treatment. There is little evidence of tolerance to morphine's analgesic effect. In chronic pain management, when patients are treated over long periods with oral opioids, the rate of rise in dose is slow and there are long periods without any dose increase.[18] Increasing doses of morphine in cancer patients are invariably due to disease progression. Tolerance does develop to some of the side-effects (notably nausea and sedation), this being of benefit to the patient.

- In cancer patients where the opioid dose is titrated against the patient's pain, clinically significant *respiratory depression* does not occur.[19] Indeed, a double dose at bedtime can be given safely. The explanation lies in the fact that pain is the physiological antagonist of the depressant effects of opioids on respiration. Respiratory depression can and does occur if the underlying cause of the pain is removed and the morphine dose not adjusted.[20]

- Morphine is often not started until the patient is virtually moribund, hence the erroneous assumption that morphine *hastens death* because of the close conjunction of the two events. Early prescribing of morphine may in fact prolong life, because control of pain enables the patient to sleep, eat better and increase physical activity.

- In the past morphine was often prescribed in the form of a cocktail (usually with chlorpromazine as antiemetic and/or cocaine for an enhanced sense of well-being). Unfortunately, as the dose of morphine was titrated upwards, the toxic effects of the other drugs (sedation and hallucinations) emerged. Hence the common misconception that morphine has significant *sedative and hallucinogenic properties*.

Morphine can be safely and reliably used by adhering to the following guidelines:

- Morphine should be given orally unless the patient cannot tolerate oral medication.

- It must be prescribed regularly to pre-empt pain. (Use on an as-required basis will result in poor pain control, increased incidence of side-effects and the use of higher doses overall.)
- Extra doses must be co-prescribed to be used as necessary:
  - (a) breakthrough analgesia – for pain that breaks through the regular dose, to be taken as and when the pain arises;
  - (b) incident analgesia – for incident pain (pain that occurs with movement, weight bearing, dressing change or some other incident), to be taken 30 minutes before the incident, if predictable.
- It must be given an adequate trial at an adequate dose.
- Side-effects should be anticipated so that they can be prevented (Table 16.2.3).

The development of a slow-release morphine preparation (MST) has revolutionized the management of cancer pain by enabling patients stabilized on 4-hourly morphine to be converted to a twice daily regimen (see Table 16.2.4 for dose equivalents).

Table 16.2.4 Equivalent doses of opioids

Dose of oral morphine/Dose of injected diamorphine = 2 : 1 or 3 : 1

10 mg morphine sulphate orally 4 hourly
(60 mg oral morphine in 24 hours)
is equivalent to
30 mg slow release morphine twice daily
(60 mg oral morphine in 24 hours)
is equivalent to
5 mg subcutaneous diamorphine hydrochloride
4 hourly
(30 mg subcutaneous diamorphine in 24 hours)
is equivalent to
30 mg diamorphine in a 24-hour subcutaneous
infusion (syringe driver)

Table 16.2.3 Side-effects of morphine

- **Constipation** is virtually universal. A laxative should always be co-prescribed with regular opioids unless there is a specific contraindication, such as bowel obstruction

- **Nausea and vomiting** are less common (35% of patients). If the patient has a predisposition to vomiting, then regular antiemetics should be started. Opioid-induced nausea is self-limiting, and antiemetics can often be stopped after 14 days

- **Drowsiness** occurs in about 50% of patients. It wears off after a week on a stable dose. Explanation and reassurance are usually all that is necessary

- **Other side-effects** include confusion, sweating, dry mouth, itch, hallucinations and myoclonus. If severe, they may be an indication to use an alternative strong opioid

---

Table 16.2.5 Subcutaneous infusion of opioid

Consider a continuous subcutaneous infusion when:

Patient is unable to take oral medication

- Problems swallowing:
  - dysphagia (due to tumour obstruction or neuromuscular incoordination)
  - aspiration
- Nausea or vomiting
- Drowsiness or unconscious:
  - in the terminal phase of the illness
- Patient is unable to take large numbers of tablets

Parenteral route is preferred

- Absorption problems
- Pain responds better to injections of opioid rather than oral opioid (*rare*)

For patients who are unable to take oral morphine, injectable diamorphine is the drug of choice. It is highly soluble, and therefore smaller volumes are needed. Because of the 'first-pass effect', the dose of parenteral morphine is one-half to one-third the dose of oral morphine (see Table 16.2.4). The preferred route of administration is subcutaneous injection (it is less painful). For patients on a regular opioid who need parenteral administration, a subcutaneous infusion pump should be used (Table 16.2.5).

In the last few years there has been interest in using alternative opioids and/or rotating opioids. A recent paper suggests that accumulation of toxic metabolites of certain opioids might explain cases of opioids toxicity and that these symptoms can often be relieved by opioid rotation.[21] A trial with an alternative opioid should be considered when dose escalation with morphine, or any other opioid, is ineffective in controlling pain or leads to intolerable and unmanageable side-effects.

Alternative opioids

Like morphine, **hydromorphone**[22] is a μ-selective full opioid agonist. The major pharmacological actions of the two drugs are the same. Hydromorphone is available in both normal and slow-release formulations. It is thought to be 5–10 times more potent than morphine. Generally, a ratio of 7.5 : 1 is used when converting from morphine to hydromorphone. For example, 10 mg morphine is equivalent to a 1.3 mg hydromorphone capsule.

Fentanyl is a short-acting step-3 analgesic. A transdermal preparation is available. The patches are designed to last for 72 hours. Peak plasma concentrations are achieved after 12–24 hours, and after removal a deposit remains in the skin for 24 hours. The major use of the fentanyl patch is when the oral route is not ideal (e.g. in patients with nausea, vomiting, dysphagia). Non-compliant patients can often be better managed with transdermal preparations. Fentanyl is not intended for the opioid naive and is not suitable for patients who need rapid dose titration. It is for patients with a stable demand of opioid.[23]

Methadone has effects generally similar to those of morphine. It probably has a role in patients who appear to develop insensitivity to morphine and those whose pain responds poorly to morphine and suffer major adverse side-effects.[24] It is particularly useful in patients with renal failure who have become very drowsy on morphine. The effects of methadone, unlike those of morphine, are not altered in renal failure. It is a difficult drug to use because of its long half-life and slow terminal elimination phase. Accumulation, leading to sedation, is a potential problem for most patients. Close supervision is needed (a steady state is not reached for 2–3 weeks). Once pain control is achieved, the frequency of dosing can be dropped to either two or three times daily.

Phenazocine has also been used in morphine-intolerant patients, especially when drowsiness is the main problem. It is five times as potent as morphine (i.e. 5 mg phenazocine is equivalent to 25 mg morphine). It is said to cause less central effects than morphine. Although there is much anecdotal evidence supporting this finding, there have been no convincing formal studies.

Oxycodone is an effective and well-tolerated opioid, which has been extensively used in the USA. Its high bioavailability leads to a more predictable pharmacokinetic profile compared to morphine. Oral and controlled-release preparations will shortly be available in the UK. Oxycodone is slightly more potent than morphine (1.3 : 1).

Non-steroidal anti-inflammatory drugs

NSAIDs inhibit prostaglandin synthesis and have a key role in the management of bone pain. The choice of drug depends on several factors, such as availability, cost, toxicity and fashion. Diclofenac (± misoprostol), naproxen and flurbiprofen are generally used by the authors. Occasionally, patients require subcutaneous infusion, in which case ketorolac or diclofenac can be used. The main adverse effects are gastrointestinal, including gastric erosions, peptic ulcers and haemorrhage. Further risks include precipitation of bronchospasm and renal failure.

Interrupting pain transmission

Nerve blocks are highly effective when used in a selected group of patients (approximately 4% of patients with pain will benefit). Various 'injection techniques' can be used. Although some of these techniques need expertise and specialized equipment to perform, simple techniques can be performed at the bedside.

A nerve block should not be offered as a 'last resort' without consideration of the likelihood of success. Nerve blocks can be considered when there is:

- unilateral pain
- localized pain
- pain due to involvement of one or two nerve roots
- abdominal pain arising from the 'upper' gut
- rib pain.

The patient needs careful assessment as to the cause of the pain before a block is carried out. This assessment will determine the exact site at which the pain pathways should be interrupted. Many procedures can be performed using local anaesthetics and steroids. These blocks are safe procedures that can give good pain relief outlasting the effect of the anaesthetic. The pain relief from a nerve block may be transient, and repeated blocks may be necessary.

Major neurolytic procedures carry the risk of serious side-effects. For example, intraspinal neurolysis for nerve root pain can produce urinary and faecal incontinence, coeliac plexus block for upper abdominal pain can cause postural hypotension, and cordotomy for unilateral pain is a major procedure, with side-effects that can be permanent.

WEAKNESS AND IMMOBILITY

Weakness is a common and distressing symptom in patients with advanced carcinoma of the prostate. When due to general debility it is very difficult to treat. Reversible causes such as anaemia, cord compression and cerebral metastases must be excluded. A patient who is immobile and confined to bed will lose muscle strength.[25] A normal person loses 10–15% of his or her muscle strength when completely rested for 1 week, and it takes 60 days to restore that strength. It is therefore not surprising that muscle weakness quickly develops in the immobile cancer patient.

It is important to acknowledge the problem and explain to the patient that it is a result of the illness. This allows realistic goals to be set, which in itself can reduce the patient's distress. Even very sick patients need to feel a sense of control over their lives, and often simple measures such as a wheelchair can help them achieve this.

Steroids improve weakness in up to 60% of patients.[26,27] The response, however, is often short lived (a few weeks), and side-effects such as proximal myopathy and poor wound healing must be set against the benefits. Therefore patients must be carefully selected and the time at which steroids are introduced has to be judged carefully.

ANOREXIA

This symptom occurs in about 70% of patients with advanced cancer. It is important to decide whose problem it is – the patient's or the carers'. The family needs to understand that, as death approaches, it is normal to lose interest in

---

Table 16.2.6 Causes of anorexia

- Tumour bulk and associated biochemical abnormalities (hypercalcaemia, uraemia)
- Oral problems (e.g. thrush)
- Constipation
- Drugs, radiotherapy
- Depression or anxiety
- Fear of vomiting may lead to avoidance of food (as opposed to true anorexia)
- Psychological factors such as anxiety and depression can manifest as lack of appetite

Table 16.2.7 Common causes of nausea and vomiting in advanced cancer

Cause	Symptomatic treatment
Drugs	If possible withdraw the drug
Metabolic (hypercalcaemia, uraemia, etc.)	Treatment with centrally acting antiemetics (e.g. cyclizine/haloperidol)
Bowel obstruction	
Gastric stasis	Treat with prokinetic antiemetics (e.g. domperidone) and/or H_2-receptor antagonist
Squashed stomach syndrome*	
Gastric irritation (e.g. NSAIDs, gastric ulceration)	H_2-receptor antagonist
Constipation	Laxatives
Raised intracranial pressure	Steroids

*Squashed/small stomach syndrome is a constellation of alimentary symptoms seen in patients with large epigastric mass/gross hepatomegaly. It is manifested as early satiation, epigastric fullness, flatulence, hiccoughs, nausea, vomiting and heartburn.

food. At this stage the goal of eating is enjoyment, not optimal nutrition.

Presentation of food is important – it should be in small portions and attractively arranged. If the factors outlined in Table 16.2.6 have been attended to and it is still felt to be a problem for the patient, steroids can be tried as an appetite stimulant. Up to 75% of patients will respond with increased appetite, but the effect usually lasts for only 3–4 weeks.[26–29]

NAUSEA AND VOMITING

Nausea and/or vomiting occur in approximately 40% of patients with far-advanced cancer. Rational treatment depends on establishing the underlying cause (Table 16.2.7). If an antiemetic is appropriate, most nausea and vomiting can be controlled using just three antiemetic drugs (Table 16.2.8).

Table 16.2.8 Drugs for controlling nausea and vomiting

- Neuroleptic (e.g. haloperidol)
- Antihistamine (e.g. cyclizine)
- Prokinetic (e.g. domperidone)

CONSTIPATION

The need to treat constipation is usually a consequence of failing to use prophylactic laxatives (virtually all patients on opioids should have a regular laxative). A rectal examination, to assess for impaction, is essential in any patient complaining of constipation. Use a laxative that combines a softener and stimulant (e.g. co-danthramer).

MANAGEMENT OF TERMINAL PHASE

When a patient who has advanced cancer of the prostate enters into the terminal phase (normally a day or so prior to death) all medication should be reviewed. All drugs should be stopped apart from those aimed at symptom control. Communication is vital, and explanation should be given to patients and their carers about anticipated changes in the patients' condition. Reassurance should be given that symptoms will remain controlled and the patient kept comfortable. Often it is appropriate to use a syringe driver to administer medications.

The rules of symptom control should always be followed, even at this stage of the illness. Symptoms should be evaluated and treatment instituted. It is important to anticipate problems and to communicate well with all concerned. It has been shown that 'peaceful' death leads to far fewer bereavement problems in the family.

Analgesia

Analgesia should be continued even if a patient becomes unconscious. The patient may still perceive pain, and abrupt withdrawal of opioids can result in an unpleasant physical withdrawal reaction. If a patient is on regular opioids they will need to be continued at an equivalent dose subcutaneously. If the patient will require more than a few injections, a 24-hour subcutaneous infusion should be started.

Agitation

Causes of agitation must be looked for and treated (e.g. retention of urine requires catheterization). However, it is not uncommon for patients to become agitated and confused shortly before death. If a tranquillizer is indicated, use subcutaneous midazolam 5–10 mg 4–6 hourly. Midazolam up to 60 mg per 24 hours can be combined with diamorphine in a syringe driver.

Bronchial secretions

Changing the patient's position may be helpful. Subcutaneous hyoscine hydrobromide 600 µg 4 hourly, as required, is useful and can be added to the syringe driver together with the diamorphine and midazolam. If there is no response to repeated doses of hysocine, intramuscular bumetanide 2 mg should be tried.

Crises

In some circumstances drugs should be prescribed for a potential crisis. For example, if it is likely that the patient may have a major bleed (haemoptysis, haematemesis) prescribe diamorphine and midazolam as a 'crisis pack' to be given in such an event. Such crises can be of great distress to the patient and family and need to be handled with speed and sensitivity.

BEREAVEMENT

Support offered to the family both during the patient's illness and at the time of the patient's death not only helps them to cope better but reduces the likelihood of future complications.[30] Evidence suggests that there is higher physical and psychiatric morbidity and possibly increased mortality in those recently bereaved.[31] People avoid grieving individuals because they feel helpless, awkward and embarrassed. They do not wish to feel sad themselves and they fear releasing strong emotions.

Bereavement counseling

It is important to interpret normal reactions to loss (denial, developing awareness, resolution). Many people who are undergoing a normal grief reaction interpret their symptoms as evidence of psychiatric illness. Reassurance can be given that such reactions are expected and will resolve with time.

It is important to identify those who are likely to have a difficult bereavement, since they are at risk of developing psychiatric illness (e.g. psychosis, clinical depression, extreme anxiety states) in the bereavement period. Some individuals may resort to alcohol, drugs, denial, idealization, etc., as a way of coping with loss. They should be referred early to the appropriate agency (psychiatrist, bereavement counsellor, etc.).

Important risk factors for abnormal bereavement reaction

Those at increased risk of difficult bereavement[32] include those:

- with a close dependent or ambivalent relationship
- undergoing concurrent stress at the time of bereavement
- with memories of a 'bad' death (e.g. uncontrolled symptoms)
- who have a perceived low level of support (the carer's perception is more important than the actual support in determining outcome)
- experiencing strong feelings of guilt/reproach
- unable to say goodbye, who feel there are things left unsaid (e.g. sudden or traumatic deaths or absence at the time of death).

REFERENCES

1. Thorpe G, Enabling more dying people to remain at home. *Br Med J* 1993; **307:** 915–18.
2. Levin DN, Cleland CS, Dar R, Public attitudes toward cancer pain. *Cancer* 1985; **56:** 2337–9.
3. Grond S, Zech D, Dienfenbach C et al, Assessment of cancer pain: a prospective evaluation in 2266 cancer patients referred to a pain service. *Pain* 1996, **64:** 107–14.
4. Plowman PN, Perry LA, Chard T, Androgen suppression by hydrocortisone without aminoglutethimide in orchiectomised men with prostatic cancer. *Br J Urol* 1987; **59:** 225–31.
5. Harland SJ, Duchesne GM, Suramin and prostate cancer: the role of hydrocortisone. *Eur J Cancer* 1992; **67:** 1295.
6. Price P, Hoskin P, Easton D et al, Prospective randomized trial of single and multifraction radiotherapy schedules in the treatment of painful bony metastases. *Radiother Oncol* 1986; **6:** 247–55.
7. Needham PR, Hoskin PJ, Radiotherapy for painful bone metastases. *Palliative Med* 1994; **8:** 95–104.
8. Blake GM, Zivanovic MA, McEwan AJ, Ackery DM, Sr-89 therapy: strontium kinetics in disseminated carcinoma of the prostate. *Eur J Nucl Med* 1986; **12:** 447–54.
9. Blake GM, Aivanovic MA, Blaquiere RM, Fine DR, McEwan AJ, Ackery DM, Strontium-89 therapy: measurement of absorbed dose to skeletal metastases. *J Nucl Med* 1988; **29:** 549–57.
10. Firusian N, Mellin P, Schmidt CG, Results of strontium-89 therapy in patients with carcinoma of the prostate and incurable pain from bone metastases: a preliminary report. *J Urol* 1976; **116:** 764–8.
11. Robinson RG, Spicer JA, Preston DF, Wegst AV, Martin NL, Treatment of metastatic bone pain with strontium-89. *Nucl Med Biol* 1987; **14:** 219–22.
12. Porter AT, McEwan AJ, Strontium-89 as an adjuvant to external beam radiation improves pain relief and delays disease progression in advanced prostate cancer: results of a randomised control trial. *Semin Oncol* 1993; **20**(3 suppl 2): 38–43.
13. Bolger JJ, Dearnaley DP, Kirk D et al, Strontium-89 (Metastron) versus external beam radiotherapy in patients with painful bone metastases secondary to prostatic cancer: preliminary report of a multicentre trial. *Semin Oncol* 1993; **20**(3 suppl 2): 32–3.
14. Vorreuther R, Biphosphonates as an adjunct to palliative therapy of bone metastases from prostatic carcinoma. A pilot study on clodronate. *Br J Urol* 1993; **72:** 792–5.
15. Cresswell SM, English PJ, Hall RR, Roberts JT, Marsh MM, Pain relief and quality of life assessment following intravenous and oral clodronate in hormone escaped metastatic prostate cancer. *Br J Urol* 1995; **76:** 360–5.
16. Collins MK, Senkus E, Gadd J, Horwich A, Dearnaley DP, High dose outpatient clodronate infusion for pain control in hormone refractory metastatic prostate carcinoma: a phase I/II

study. *British Prostate Group Autumn Meeting*, Leicester November 1995 [abstract].

17. Porter J, Jick J, Addiction rare in patients treated with narcotic. *N Engl J Med* 1980; **302**: 123.

18. Portenoy RK, Foley KM, Chronic use of opioid analgesics in non-malignant pain: report of 38 cases. *Pain* 1986; **25**: 171–86.

19. Walsh TD, Opiates and respiratory function in advanced cancer. Recent results. *Cancer Res* 1984; **89**: 115–17.

20. Hanks GW, Twycross R, Lloyd JW, Unexpected complication of a successful nerve block. *Anaesthesia* 1981; **8**: 1–2.

21. de Stoutz ND, Bruera E, Suarez-Almazor M, Opioid rotation for toxicity reduction in terminal cancer patients. *J Pain Symptom Management* 1995; **10**: 378–84.

22. Hays H, Hagen N, Thriwell M et al, Comparative clinical efficacy and safety of immediate release and controlled release hydromorphone for chronic severe cancer pain. *Cancer* 1994; **74**: 1808–16.

23. TTS–Fentanyl Multicentre Study Group, Transdermal fentanyl in cancer pain. *J Drug Dev* 1994; **6**: 93–7.

24. Fainsinger R, Schoeller T, Bruera E, Methadone in the management of cancer pain: a review. *Pain* 1993; **52**: 137–47.

25. Kottke FJ, The effects of limitation of activity upon the human body. *J Am Med Assoc* 1966; **196**: 825–30.

26. Bruera E, Roca E, Cedaro L, Carraro S, Chacon R, Action of oral methylprednisolone in terminal cancer patients: a prospective randomized double-blind study. *Cancer Treatment Rep* 1985; **69**: 751–4.

27. Hanks GW, Trueman T, Twycross RG, Corticosteroids in terminal cancer – a prospective analysis of current practice. *Postgrad Med J* 1983; **59**: 702–6.

28. Willox JC, Corr J, Shaw J, Richardson M, Calman KC, Drennan MI, Prednisolone as an appetite stimulant in patients with cancer. *Br Med J* 1984; **288**: 27.

29. Farr WC, The use of corticosteroids for symptom management in terminally ill patients. *Am J Hospice Care* 1990; **7**: 41–6.

30. Parkes CM, *Bereavement: Studies of Grief in Adult Life*. Penguin Books: London, 1986.

31. Parkes CM, Effects of bereavement on physical and mental health – a study of the medical records of widows. *Br Med J* 1964; **2**: 274–9.

32. Parkes CM, Risk factors in bereavement: implications for the prevention and treatment of pathologic grief. *Psychiatr Ann* 1990; **20**: 308–13.

FURTHER READING

Buckman R, *How to Break Bad News. A Guide for Health Care Professionals.* Papermac: London, 1992.

Doyle D, Hanks GW, MacDonald N (eds), *Oxford Textbook of Palliative Medicine.* Oxford University Press: Oxford, 1994.

Kaye P, *Breaking Bad News. A Ten Step Approach.* EPL: Northampton, 1996.

Stedeford A, *Facing Death: Patients, Families and Professionals.* Sobell: Oxford, 1994.

Twycross RG, *Pain Relief in Advanced Cancer.* Churchill Livingstone: Edinburgh, 1994.

17

The future

Louis Denis

CONTENTS • Introduction • Epidemiology and natural history • Pathology • Prostate growth • Diagnosis and staging • Treatment • Treatment of endocrine-escaped or endocrine-resistant disease • Innovative treatment of hormone-resistant or hormone-insensitive disease • Conclusions

INTRODUCTION

Predicting the future is always a risky business, especially for a subject as complex as prostate cancer. Indeed, there are great controversies regarding almost any aspect of this disease, ranging from natural history to endocrine treatment. We happen to believe that there is really no substantial reason for controversy if experts express their views with moderation and keep their focus on a couple of simple facts that are of prime importance in the growth of the prostate and for the outcome of treatment of prostate cancer. These simple facts are that:

- we are dealing with a disease of the middle-aged man, with a slowly growing tumour that takes about 20 years to develop from a focal lesion to a full-blown metastatic cancer, with prognostic factors that determine the course of the disease and the outcome of treatment;
- most importantly, with the present state of therapeutic knowledge, cancer of the prostate outside the prostate capsule is an incurable disease.

In 1994, a Consensus Workshop on Screening and Global Strategy for Prostate Cancer was organized in Antwerp, involving a number of research and clinical organizations, to address this complex situation from a variety of angles in order to come to a balanced view on the assessment of and answers to four basic questions. These questions are presented in Table 17.1, and were answered as accurately as possible by a number of ad hoc working parties.[1]

EPIDEMIOLOGY AND NATURAL HISTORY

Before elaborating on future trends in the basic scientific knowledge and clinical management of prostate cancer, we should like to emphasize that looking into the past helps to understand the future and that advances in basic research as well as results from randomized clinical trials must fit into a pattern of progress. This progress is on a broad front, and does not take place in quantum leaps but rather in a slow but steady fashion, as is typical of the slow growth of the disease itself.

Table 17.1 Questions on prostate cancer
1. Is there an acceptable method for the early detection of prostate cancer available on a population basis?
2. Do the current results provide encouragement for proceeding to develop widespread, randomized trials?
3. What is the proper way to conduct such efforts and what other important issues should be considered?
4. What are the bases for the treatment of patients with prostate cancer when discovered?

Some good minds, good laboratories, organized clinics, and collaboration between institutions, researchers, clinicians and patients mixed with patience always form the basis for future success. The introduction of prostate-specific antigen (PSA) as a marker for prostate diseases, and almost simultaneously the introduction of the spring-loaded biopty gun that allows for painless transrectal biopsies performed under visual guidance by transrectal ultrasound (TRUS), doubled the diagnosis of prostate cancer and quadrupled the diagnosis of localized disease.[2] This avalanche of new cases of prostate cancer per year has been enhanced further by the increased life expectancy of human populations, the coming of age of the post-war baby boom and the increased awareness of prostate disease in the elderly population. It took a few years for epidemiologists to take into account and analyse the obvious shift in the pattern of prostate cancer incidence. When this was done, it led in 1998 to a downward revision in the incidence of prostate cancer, which was accompanied by a small but persistent decrease for two years in the number of deaths from prostate cancer.[3,4] The net result was a considerable shift in cancer staging at the time of diagnosis of non-metastatic disease – first in the USA and later in some European countries.[5]

This led initially to a huge discrepancy between incidence and mortality rates, and attracted considerable attention from epidemiologists, health economists, biostatisticians,

family practitioners, and health authority analysts trying to forecast the repercussions of prostate cancer on general health policies and cost to society. This situation was enhanced by a surge in radical prostatectomies and radiotherapy for early localized disease, as urologists and radiotherapists were alike given a unique opportunity to cure the greatest number of patients. This huge number of curative treatments for early prostate cancer – somewhat overshadowed by overtreatment in up to 10% of all cases – led to a backlash from therapeutic nihilists.

Even in 1998, there were still editorials in oncological journals claiming that early prostate cancer diagnosed by biopsy is identical to the latent microscopic cases found at autopsy, that even successful treatment causes more harm than good, and that prostate cancer is a non-entity for public health since the cumulative loss of life years is minimal.[6] We know, of course, that at least 85% of the cancers detected are clinically important cancers, that, on the basis of life years lost, prostate cancer ranks third among male cancers, and that prostate cancer is a major health problem in a number of countries with an aging population and a lifestyle with a high-fat, high-calorie diet and lack of exercise.[7] This kind of basic ignorance fuels the controversy around population screening for prostate cancer. On the one hand, it is reported that, on the basis of an analysis of 280 234 cases diagnosed between 1973 and 1993

Table 17.2 Advantages and disadvantages of screening for prostate cancer

Advantages

I. Possible cure for cases detected by screening

II. Less-radical treatment with identical cure rate

III. Reassurance for those with negative test results

IV. Cost saving by treating upfront

Disadvantages

I. Longer morbidity for cases whose prognosis is unaltered (length and lead bias)

II. Overtreatment of clinically unimportant cancers

III. False reassurance for those with false-negative results

IV. Diversion of scarce resources to screening programme

V. Hazards of screening test (biopsy, anxiety)

in the population-based Surveillance, Epidemiology and End Results (SEER) Program, indirect evidence suggests that screening in men over 50 years of age decreased the incidence of distant disease, which may influence the mortality rate.[8] Indeed, the WHO criteria to justify population screening for cancer are almost completely fulfilled for prostate cancer, with the exception that we still lack detailed knowledge of its natural history in its early stages and that there is no evidence that screening with the available modalities and treatments can lead to a reduction in mortality.[9] Despite the tremendous advances made in clinical sciences and the positive results of large demonstration series, one has to face up to the advantages and disadvantages of population screening for prostate cancer. These are listed in Table 17.2. The future lies with the completion of randomized, prospective screening trials for prostate cancer, which should bring us an answer, not only on mortality but also on the quality of life and on cost/efficacy to society.[10]

PATHOLOGY

The gap in our understanding of the natural history of early prostate cancer is caused by the differing growth potential of prostate cancer cells. Undifferentiated tumours carry a poor prognosis while well-differentiated tumours carry in general a good prognosis, unless the biopsy specimen is not representative of the tumour. The volume and stage of the tumour are also independent prognostic factors – but these point more to a particular instance of time in the life of the tumour than to its actual potential for growth. To help resolve this problem, it is of the utmost importance that surgical pathology reports on prostate specimens, and specifically on biopsy specimens, be meticulous regarding the presence or absence of carcinoma and associated lesions such as prostate intraepithelial neoplasia (PIN) and atypical adenomatous hyperplasia (AAH), as well as in their use of agreed definitions of terms.[1] The histological grading according to Gleason[11] is widely accepted, but is influenced by a number of factors, including intra- and interobserver variations. The introduction of a standardized methodology and syntactic structural analysis of materials may be of help here, but confirmation of prognostic factors is the first priority. Next to the development of syntactic structural analysis with a minimal spanning tree (MST), histological markers remain the best bet for future improvements.

Out of over 30 additional prognostic markers reported in the literature so far, research has confirmed that the proportion of neuroendocrine cells, microvessel density, tumour suppressor genes (*p53* and *p27*) and angiogenesis inhibitors (TSP, E-cadherin expression, Ki-67 and apoptic index (AI)) are helpful in the better prediction of tumour progression, and can aid decision making regarding the need for aggressive treatment, as well as furthering our understanding of the neoplastic potential of a particular malignancy.[11-17]

Most laboratories already use some of these markers, but a concerted effort is needed to develop a routine pattern based on validated results. So far, we believe that microvessel density, the presence of neuroendocrine cells, p53, Ki-67 and E-cadherin could add in the prediction of a perfect Gleason grading. It should be pointed out here that, although prostate biopsies have become routine, they do have limitations, and efforts must be made to decrease the large number of false-negative results.[18]

PROSTATE GROWTH

The development of a set of validated prognostic markers on histological tissue should allow the identification of approximately two-thirds of the patients who require aggressive treatment in the early stages of the disease.[19] These markers, of course, are products of the endocrine, biochemical and molecular processes involved in the pathogenesis of prostate cancer. The classic 5α-dihydrotestosterone (DHT) dependence results in the DHT androgen receptor (AR) complex associating with hormone-responsive elements (HRE) in the genome to modulate, together with other transcription factors, the expression of androgen-responsive genes. The extrinsic factor interacts with a host of intrinsic factors known as growth factors that promote or inhibit cell proliferation. The interrelationship of stimulatory and inhibitory actions is pivotal to the growth of the prostate. The fibroblast growth factor family (FGF 1–10) plays a major role in this process. The complexity of the system is enhanced by the presence of α and β oestrogen receptors that predominate in the stroma cells. As already mentioned, the neuroendocrine cells are subject to a number of growth processes. The production of vascular endothelial growth factor (VEGF) and the specific morbidity caused by exocrine gene products produced by metastatic prostate cancer cells give us a glimpse of the complete picture,

and should allow the development of a number of specific drugs to counteract these processes.[20,21]

Understanding of the molecular biology offers a reasonable interpretation of the possible primary preventive effect of nutritional intervention by eliminating the fat effect and supporting the inhibitory or protective effects of phyto-oestrogens primarily found in flavonoids and lignans.[22,23]

DIAGNOSIS AND STAGING

Primary prevention will play a role in the future in preventing the clinical development of the disease, but current efforts to decrease mortality are based on diagnosis of the disease at a localized stage and on providing curative treatment.

It is important to examine the prostate by touch via a digital rectal examination (DRE) or by imaging with TRUS in order to diagnose some cancers that are in a curable stage but are completely passed over by the PSA serum determination. It is ironic that a non-cancer-specific test would be recognized as the most important biological marker for prostate cancer. The simple PSA > 4 ng/ml test is not perfect, and a number of variations have been developed, taking account of density, age, free versus bound PSA, etc., but they have not demonstrated effective superiority over the simple test. More time and research will determine if total bound PSA, human glandular kallikrein 2 (hK2) or prostate-specific membrane antigen (PSMA) will outperform the ubiquitous PSA test.[24]

The disappointing results on diagnosis of curable prostate cancer by TRUS have been offset by its excellent performance as a guided biopsy instrument in the now-classic six-core biopsy set. By adding colour Doppler flow (to identify neovascularity) and a blood vessel image enhancer, it is hoped to improve the yield of accurate diagnoses. However, so far the methodology has not provoked any wave of general enthusiasm.[25,26]

Accurate histological diagnosis, and particularly according a Gleason score to the tissue material, requires collaboration between expert pathologists and urologists. Incomplete material or negative biopsies undergo a second biopsy, if indicated. However, staging prostate cancer is a different matter, and over- and under-staging (but mostly the latter) in the tumour classification of the UICC TNM system remains a clinical problem.[27]

Most clinical staging relies on the presence of abnormalities in the diagnostic tools such as DRE, TRUS and PSA, and this works in the extreme values of very good or very bad. It is claimed that use of a transrectal coil with magnetic resonance (MRI) imaging can detect extracapsular disease, but once again the lack of enthusiasm on the part of clinicians points to problems in introducing this test as a clinical routine. The recently introduced polymerase chain reaction (PCR) technique offers hope of identifying tumour cells in the plasma. Research is ongoing, and the value of the test is ambiguous. Even when they are identified, we do not know if the detected cells are representative of invasive disease.

Clinicians usually work by elimination of metastatic disease, relying on a bone scan or a PSA < 10 ng/ml. The bone scan is rarely positive in men with PSA < 10 ng/ml, but the image forms a baseline for any future comparisons in the course of the disease. The only sure way to diagnose N-node-negative patients is to perform a pelvic node dissection. Radioimmunoscintography and spectroscopic evaluation of the prostate may become important in the lymph node evaluation, and the results of ongoing studies are awaited.[28,29] The net result is that we have to take account of the inaccuracy of our clinical diagnosis and staging when planning the management of locally advanced disease.

TREATMENT

There is a world of difference between the choice between attempting curative treatment of localized disease and attempting control of locally advanced or metastatic disease.

Treatment of localized disease

Sufficient progress has been made in the perfection of local treatment by surgery and radiotherapy to allow us to state that contemporary series on treatment outcomes should not be mixed with earlier reports dealing with patients in later stages of the same TNM category. In most cases with modern management, extracapsular disease is minimal and quite different from seminal vesicle invasion or node-positive patients in the initial evaluation from the treatment. This length time bias for minimally advanced disease offers an extra time frame of treatment, which allows for follow-up evaluation of signs of clinical aggression, but unfortunately also carries the drawback of new types of complications arising during the long time of treatment.

The treatment options are presented in Table 17.3. It is clear that a policy of watchful waiting in older patients with low-volume and well-differentiated tumours is appropriate, particularly when other significant diseases (comorbidity) are present. The chronological age for this indication hovers around 70 years (but this figure might go up, with a 77-year-old astronaut in space!). These patients are counselled, and reassured with their choice, and their PSA is measured at regular intervals.

Table 17.3 Treatment options for localized prostate cancer

1. Watchful waiting or deferred treatment
2. Radiotherapy:
    External-beam
    Brachytherapy
3. Surgery:
    Retropubic
    Perineal
4. Investigational:
    Cryotherapy
    Laser therapy
    High-intensity focused ultrasound

It should again be emphasized that untreated cancers from a previous era were generally more advanced than localized cancers detected by DRE and PSA examination. The 10-year follow-up is crucial, since a pooled analysis showed 19% for well-differentiated versus 42% for moderately differentiated versus 74% for poorly differentiated cancers at risk for metastasis, but the metastatic rate risk was higher than estimated in previous reports.[30] Since the studied cohorts are not comparable, we must wait for the results of a number of controlled clinical trials of screening, such as the ERSPC and PLCO trials, or trials of treatment for localized disease, such as the PIVOT and Finasteride Prostate Cancer Prevention Trial studies.[31–34]

Both forms of curative treatment have considerably improved, and, once again, future publications will show the contemporary complication rates to be far more acceptable than those reported previously.[35]

The understaged cases, the early pT3 after radical prostatectomy and the clinical T3 receiving curative radiotherapy (approximately one-third of all treated cases), will receive considerable attention in the near future. The surgically treated patients with PSA > 0.5 ng/ml will be subjected either to additional radiotherapy or to medical treatment in randomized trials. The radiotherapy-treated patients are already subjected to simultaneous or neoadjuvant endocrine treatment based on the first favourable results of randomized trials.[36] It will be a matter of time to transfer these studies to patients with localized disease submitted to curative radiotherapy.

The advantage of neoadjuvant therapy in radiation treatment is the decrease in tumour volume, which may result in a reduction of normal tissue complications.

Treatment of metastatic disease

Endocrine therapy of advanced prostate cancer was, is and will remain a palliative treatment where quality of life should be a major endpoint of any study. This point has been overlooked a number of times in the five decades of

---

Table 17.4 First-line endocrine treatments in clinical use

Androgen withdrawal
Surgical castration:
  Bilateral orchiectomy
  (subcapsular, subepididymal)
Medical castration:
  Oestrogens, progesterones,
  LHRH analogues, antagonists

Androgen blockade
Steroidal antiandrogens:
  Cyproterone
  Chlormadinone
  Megestrol
Non-steroidal antiandrogens:
  Flutamide
  Nilutamide
  Bicalutamide

---

clinical investigations on the benefit and complications of endocrine treatment in all stages of prostate cancer. Not only do we have a wide choice of treatments, such as the monotherapies presented in Table 17.4, but, in addition, combinations, especially the LHRH analogues and non-steroidal antiandrogens known as maximal androgen blockade (MAB) or combined androgen blockade (CAB), have been tested over and over again in controlled trials seeking superior treatments.[37]

The percentage of patients first diagnosed with metastatic disease has been steadily decreasing over the last decade, and this represents a new challenge to the clinician dealing with advanced disease in its earliest stages. This automatically means that we shall be giving endocrine treatment for longer periods of time with new complications, such as long-term depression, anaemia and osteoporosis, to name but a few. The duration of endocrine treatment in the future is presented in Table 17.5.

Table 17.5 Endocrine therapy over time	
Indication at stage	**Duration**
Metastatic pain	2 years
Metastatic	3–5 years
Locally advanced at recurrence	5–7 years
Rising PSA in prevention	5–15 years
Neoadjuvant	3–8 months
Adjuvant	3–? years
Primary prevention	5–20 years

We believe that the search for the best 'classic' endocrine treatment is now over. A meta-analysis of MAB versus monotherapy showed a small advantage for MAB in survival, but this was not statistically significant.[38]

The bottom line is simple. Only patients with minimal disease may profit – but this profit is at the expense of their serum testosterone, the toxicity of the added antiandrogen and the possibility that the antiandrogen may turn agonist in the course of the treatment.[39] Two trends emerge from the confusion. First there is active interest in monotherapy with antiandrogens in the earliest stages of the disease. The 'old' progestative antiandrogens such as cyproterone acetate are being re-evaluated as monotherapy, and bicalutamide 150 mg a day has been shown to be equivalent to castration in a large randomized trial with a follow-up of four years.[40] Secondly, there is the trend to use endocrine therapy for selected purposes such as reducing tumour volume to improve or facilitate radio- and brachytherapy in neoadjuvant fashion or to control tumour growth by intermittent treatment. Randomized trials of the latter indication are in progress.

New developments in endocrine treatment will mainly focus on drugs adding to the concept of preserving serum testosterone by combining finasteride with antiandrogens. The first results look promising.[41]

The result of this situation in endocrine therapy is a renewed focus on the fact that 20–30% of all treated cancers are either resistant to endocrine therapy or show a relative decrease in serum PSA values. These are the patients, diagnosed after 3–6 months of endocrine treatment, who will progress and die of the disease. This is an important group of patients who will join the group of relapsed, hormone-resistant disease – but in much earlier stages with smaller tumour volume. We hope that in the near future these patients will receive most of the attention in future clinical trials with chemotherapy, immunotherapy and gene therapy.

TREATMENT OF ENDOCRINE-ESCAPED OR ENDOCRINE-RESISTANT DISEASE

Endocrine treatment of metastatic prostate cancer usually results in a temporary remission of 3–18 months, after which we are confronted with debilitated patients for whom most treatment successes are anecdotal and for whom chemotherapy is an extra burden. We have found consensus that patients in this condition should receive palliative treatment, since any cytotoxic or alternative treatment seems unfair to patients and treatment evaluation alike.

The results of chemotherapy at this late stage of the disease are so poor that efficacy is now judged on quality of life and pain relief rather than mere survival. Palliative treatment, including pain control, has to be perfected, and radiotherapy and strontium-89, as well as hydrocortisone, should be considered in the treatment schedules.

There is hope that new drugs or combinations will be tested in the earlier stages of endocrine resistance and insensitivity as a pathway to innovative treatment.

INNOVATIVE TREATMENT OF HORMONE-RESISTANT OR HORMONE-INSENSITIVE DISEASE

The metastatic pathway of prostate cancer cells is presented in Figure 17.1, from which it is

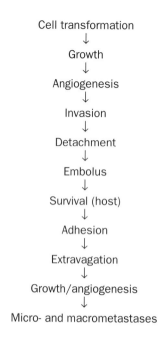

Cell transformation
↓
Growth
↓
Angiogenesis
↓
Invasion
↓
Detachment
↓
Embolus
↓
Survival (host)
↓
Adhesion
↓
Extravagation
↓
Growth/angiogenesis
↓
Micro- and macrometastases

Figure 17.1 Metastatic pathway. Innovative treatment strategies are being developed against a number of steps in this process.

possible to see different steps where opportunities for treatment exist. This field is complex, with at least a dozen gene technology companies involved, and there are many potential applications in prostate cancer, ranging from the detection of the *HPC1* familial gene for prostate cancer to several gene therapy strategies to control the disease.

Gene therapy

Gene therapy involves the transfer of genetic probes to the patient in order to:

- repair defects in tumour suppressor genes or block oncogenes;
- enhance natural cytotoxic and immunostimulatory defence mechanisms in the host;
- deliver toxic substances or induce sensitivity to toxic substances.

Corrective therapy using an adenovirus vector carrying *p53* and *p21*, cytoreductive therapy with a herpes simplex virus carrying a thymidine kinase gene, and the projected use of a suicide gene are already in phase I trials.[42] So far, tumour regression has been observed and there is real promise for the future.

Immunotherapy

Cytokines have exhibited both direct and indirect cytotoxic and immunomodulatory effects on prostate cancer cells. Tumour cells can be modified to express interleukin-2 (IL-2), granulocyte–macrophage colony-stimulating factor (GM-CSF) or interferon-γ (IFN-γ) by retrovirally mediated gene transfer. Direct immunotherapy depends on the presence of cancer-specific antigens, which, when bound to major histocompatibility complex (MHC) proteins, can be recognized by T cells. Prostate-specific membrane antigen (PSMA) is one such specific antigen. The key process here depends on the presentation of this antigen by the host's antigen-presenting cells (dendritic cells) to circulating T cells. The technical problems involved with this approach have been solved, and phase I/II trials are in progress.[43]

Small molecules and other therapy

A number of unconventional new drugs are being developed and tested for more selective treatment of prostate cancer. FGN-1, an apoptosis-inducing compound, is being evaluated in preclinical models as a preventive drug. Several angiogenesis inhibitors (suramin, somatuline, thalidomide) are in phase I/II studies. The study of receptors is a rapidly growing field, and growth factor receptor tyrosine kinases are another target for clinical trials.

These innovative treatments may seem futuristic, but there is promise in this field to identify future patients, predict prognosis and cure prostate cancer very early on, or even to alter the path of the disease in established cases.

CONCLUSIONS

The management of prostate cancer has finally received the first injection of significant research funds to tackle its many problems on a broad front.

Collaboration at consensus meetings has provided a clinical forum where evidence-based data on all aspects of the disease have been scrutinized and transformed into reliable guidelines.

Research funding is now being spent on fundamental questions in several fields that will attract further investment from the pharmaceutical industry. Until these questions have been answered, we shall have to treat our patients with our minds on the science and our hearts on the patients. This practice of medicine is still more or less an art, and we hope that urologists, general practitioners, oncologists and scientists will collaborate to the benefit of our patients with both targets in focus way into the next century.

REFERENCES

1. Denis LJ, Murphy GP, Schröder FH, Report of the Consensus Workshop on Screening and Global Strategy for Prostate Cancer. *Cancer* 1995; **75:** 1187–207.

2. Smart C, Prostate cancer facts and fiction. *J Surg Oncol* 1997; **66:** 223–9.

3. Wingo PA, Landis S, Ries LAG, An adjustment to the 1997 estimate for new prostate cancer cases. *CA* 1997; **47:** 239–42.

4. Landis SH, Murray T, Bolden S, Wingo PA, Cancer Statistics, 1998. *CA* 1998; **48:** 6–49.

5. Mettlin C, Public health impact of prostate cancer early detection. *Prostate* 1997; **31:** 71–3.

6. Weyler J, Prostate cancer: screening or watchful waiting? *Ann Oncol* 1998; **9:** 9–11.

7. Report from the UICC Council Group on Prostate Cancer, UICC General Assembly, 1998, or the occasion of the 17th World Congress against Cancer.

8. Smart CR, The results of prostate carcinoma screening in the US as reflected in the Surveillance, Epidemiology and End Results Program. *Cancer* 1997; **80:** 1835–44.

9. Wilson JMG, Jungner G, *Principles and Practice of Screening for Disease*. Public Health Paper, No. 34. WHO: Geneva.

10. Denis L, Screening for prostate cancer: the good, the bad and the ugly. In: *Progress in Oncology* (Khayat D, Hortobagyi GN, eds). Springer-Verlag: Paris, 1999.

11. Gleason DF, Histologic grading in clinical staging of prostatic carcinoma. In: *Urologic Pathology: The Prostate* (Tannenbaum M, ed.). Lea & Febiger: Philadelphia, 1997: 171–98.

12. Mydlo JH, Kral JG, Volpe M et al, An analysis of microvessel density, androgen receptor, p35 and HER-2/neu expression and Gleason score in prostate cancer. *Eur Urol* 1998; **34:** 426–32.

13. Stapleton AMF, Zbell P, Kattan MW et al, Assessment of the biologic markers p53, Ki-67, and apoptotic index as predictive indicators of prostate carcinoma recurrence after surgery. *Cancer* 1998; **82:** 168–75.

14. O'Reilly MS, Holmgren L, Shing Y et al, Angiostatin: a circulating endothelial cell inhibitor that suppresses angiogenesis and tumor growth. In: *Proceedings of Cold Spring Harbor Symposium*, 1994: 471 (abst).

15. Schlechte H, Lenk SV, Löning T et al, p53 tumour suppressor gene mutations in benign prostatic hyperplasia and prostate cancer. *Eur Urol* 1998; **34:** 433–40.

16. di Sant'Agnese AP, Neuroendocrine differentiation in prostatic carcinoma: an update. *Prostate* 1998; **8:** 74–9.

17. Giroldi LA, Schalken JA, Decreased expression of the intercellular adhesion molecule E-cadherin in prostate cancer: biological significance and clinical implications. *Cancer Metastasis Rev* 1993; **12:** 29–37.

18. Beerlage HP, de la Rosette JJMCH, de Reijke TM, Considerations regarding prostate biopsies. *Eur Urol* 1998; **35:** 303–12.

19. Borre M, Nerstrom B, Overgaard J, The natural history of prostate carcinoma based on a Danish population treated with no intent to cure. *Cancer* 1997; **80:** 917–28.

20. Aaronson S, Growth factors and cancer. *Science* 1998; **254:** 1146–53.

21. Chou E, Simons JW, The molecular biology of prostate cancer morbidity and mortality: accelerated death from ejaculate poisoning? *Urol Oncol* 1997; **3:** 79–84.

22. Wynder EL, Fair WR, Editorial: Prostate cancer – nutrition adjunct therapy. *J Urol* 1996; **156:** 1364–5.

23. Griffiths K, Adlerkrentz H, Boyle P et al, *Nutrition and Cancer*. Isis Medical Media: Oxford, 1996.

24. Murphy GP, Partin A, Workshop on Prostate Markers. *Cancer* 1998; **83:** 2233–8.

25. Louvar E, Littrup PJ, Goldstein A et al, Correlation of color Doppler flow in the prostate with tissue microvascularity. *Cancer* 1998; **83:** 135–40.

26. Ragde H, Kenny GM, Murphy GP, Landin K, Transrectal ultrasound microbubble contrast angiography of the prostate. *Prostate* 1997; **32:** 279–83.

27. Sobin LH, Wittekind Ch, *UICC TNM Classification of Malignant Tumours. SH Edition*. Wiley-Liss: New York, 1997.

28. Podoloff DA, Neal CE, Babaiau RJE, Detection of lymph node metastasis in prostatic carcinoma with In-111 labeled CYT356. *Radiology* 1993; **189:** 334–40.

29. Kurhaewwicz J, Vignerou DB, Hricak H et al, 3D H-1 MR spectroscopic imaging of the in situ prostate with high spatial resolution. *Radiology* 1996; **198:** 795–805.

30. Chodak GW, Thisted RA, Gerber GA et al, Results of conservative management of clinically localized prostate cancer. *N Engl J Med* 1994; **330:** 242–8.

31. Standaert B, Denis L, The European Randomized Study of Screening for Prostate Cancer: an update. *Cancer* 1997; **80:** 1830–4.

32. Gohaghan JK, Prorok PC, Kramer BS, Cornett JE, Prostate cancer screening in the Prostate, Lung, Colorectal and Ovarian Cancer Screening Trial of the National Cancer Institute. *J Urol* 1994; **152:** 1905–9.

33. Wilt TJ, Brawer MK, The Prostate Cancer Intervention versus Observation Trial: a randomized trial comparing radical prostatectomy versus expectant management for the treatment of clinically localized prostate cancer. *J Urol* 1994; **152:** 1910–14.

34. Thompson IM, Coltman CA, Crowley J, Chemoprevention of prostate cancer: the Prostate Cancer Prevention Trial. *Prostate* 1997; **33:** 217–21.

35. Murphy GP, Griffiths K, Denis L et al (eds), *First International Consultation on Prostate Cancer*. SCI: Paris, 1997.

36. Bolla M, Bartelink H, Gibbors R et al, Treatment of regional disease. In: *First International Consultation on Prostate Cancer* (Murphy GR, Griffiths K, Denis L et al, eds). SCI: Paris, 1997: 259–67.

37. Denis LJ, Maximal androgen blockade: facts and fallacies. *Endocrine-Related Cancer* 1998; **5:** 1–4.

38. Peto R, Communication at the Fifth Paciou Meeting, Rotterdam, 17 October 1998.

39. Scher HI, Kolvenberg GJCM, The anti-androgen withdrawal syndrome in relapsed prostate cancer. *Eur Urol* 1997; **31:** 3–7.

40. Iversen P, Anti-androgen monotherapy. In: *Progress and Controversies in Urological Oncology* (Schröder F, ed). London: Parthenon, 1999.

41. Griffiths K, Some comments on maximal androgen blockade for prostate cancer in relation to 5AR-inhibitor and anti-androgen combination therapy. *Prospectives* 1998; **8**(3): 6–8.

42. Herman JR, Lerner SP, Current status of gene therapy for prostate and bladder cancer. *Int J Urol* 1997; **4:** 435–40.

43. Tjoa BA, Simmons SJ, Bowes VA et al, Evaluation of phase I/II clinical trials in prostate cancer with dendritic cells and PSMA peptides. *Prostate* 1998; **36:** 39–44.

Appendix

Clinical classification for prostate cancer		
Stage	**TNM**	
Not palpable on rectal examination	T0	No evidence of primary tumour
A1 Focal cancer (< 3 chips)	T1	Clinically inapparent tumour, not palpable and not visible by imaging
A2 Diffuse (> 3 chips)	T1a	Tumour an incidental histological finding in < 5% of tissue resected
	T1b	Tumour an incidental histological finding in > 5% of tissue resected
	T1c	Tumour identified by needle biopsy (e.g. because of elevated serum PSA)
B1 Unilobar, < 2 cm	T2	Tumour confined within the prostate
	T2a	Tumour involves half of a lobe or less
B2 Unilobar, > 2 cm	T2b	Tumour involves more than half a lobe, but not both lobes
B3 All other, intracapsular	T2c	Tumour involves both lobes
Extending through capsule	T3	Tumour extends through the prostatic capsule
C1 Sulcus or sulci not free	T3a	Unilateral extracapsular extension
C2 > Base of seminal vesicles ± sulci	T3b	Bilateral extracapsular extension
	T3c	Tumour invades seminal vesicles
C3 > Base of seminal vesicles ± other adjacent organs	T4	Tumour fixed or invades adjacent structures other than seminal vesicles
	T4a	Tumour invades bladder neck and/or external sphincter and/or rectum
	T4b	Tumour invades levator muscles and/or is fixed to pelvic wall
Any local extension	Disseminated	
D1 Lymph node involvement	N+	
	N1 Solitary, < 2 cm	
	N2 Solitary, > 2 cm; < 5 cm or multiple < 5 cm	
	N3 > 5 cm	
D2 Other metastases	M+	
D3	Resistant to hormone therapy	

Index